Renegotiating Health Care

· ·

Leonard J. Marcus with
Barry C. Dorn, Phyllis B. Kritek,
Velvet G. Miller, and Janice B. Wyatt

Renegotiating Health Care

Resolving Conflict to Build Collaboration

Jossey-Bass Publishers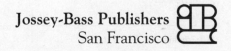
San Francisco

Substantial discounts on bulk quantities of Jossey-Bass books are available to corporations, professional associations, and other organizations. For details and discount information, contact the special sales department at Jossey-Bass Inc., Publishers. (415) 433–1740; Fax (800) 605–2665.

For sales outside the United States, please contact your local Simon & Schuster International Office.

Jossey-Bass Web address: http://www.josseybass.com

 Manufactured in the United States of America on Lyons Falls Pathfinder Tradebook. This paper is acid free and 100 percent totally chlorine free.

Library of Congress Cataloging-in-Publication Data

Marcus, Leonard J., 1952–
 Renegotiating health care : resolving conflict to build
collaboration / Leonard J. Marcus ; with Barry C. Dorn ... [et al.].
  p. cm—(Jossey-Bass health series)
 Includes bibliographical references and index.
 ISBN 0-7879-0151-2 (alk. paper)
 1. Health planning—Decision making. 2. Conflict management.
3. Negotiation. 4. Medical policy—Decision making. 5. Medical
care—Decision making. 6. Health planning—Decision making—Case
studies. 7. Conflict management—Decision making—Case studies.
8. Negotiation—Case studies. 9. Medical policy—Decision making—
Case studies. 10. Medical care—Decision making—Case studies.
I. Dorn, Barry C. II. Title. III. Series.
RA394.9.M365 1995
362.1—dc20   95–23022
                       CIP

HB Printing 10 9 8 7 6 5 4 3 2   FIRST EDITION

Contents

• •

Preface

This book is motivated by three basic premises. First, conflicts and differences are an inevitable part of our work and relationships in health care. Second, how we handle those differences affects what we can and cannot accomplish as people and as professionals. Third, to benefit from those differences, we must not only be prepared to change what we do, we must also be ready to examine and perhaps shift the very assumptions that impel why we do it.

Health care work is a constant negotiation. You are continuously engaged in making decisions, taking actions, and selecting options—sometimes on your own, and many times under the direction of others. You transact intangibles such as information, expertise, opinion, knowledge, skill, as well as tangibles such as money, equipment, space, supplies, personnel. Because your responsibilities are so closely intertwined with those of others, orchestrating mutual involvement is largely a matter of negotiation. The effectiveness of your work is dependent upon the proficiency of those exchanges.

In your hands is a set of tools in the shape of a book. Its purpose is to provide you, as a health professional, with a range of choices for what you negotiate and how you go about negotiating it. These tools are designed to fit the specific circumstances of your work: what it is you strive to accomplish set in parallel with that of others. The necessary balance of expectation among people working together is presented within a framework for constructing pragmatic collaboration. And for those instances when differences explode into disruptive conflict, there are methods to guide you toward resolution or, when necessary, toward a dignified exit affording you minimum pain.

This book is entitled *Renegotiating Health Care*. Why "re"negotiating? Because the changes emerging in health care today require us not only to improve our day-to-day negotiations. More importantly, the changes affect the very premises, expectations, relationships, and motivations that have influenced the way health care has been conducted for so many years. The ground rules that guided associations between clinicians and managers, managers and insurers, as well as patients and clinicians, to name but a few, are all changing. Old ways, manners, and rewards are no longer operative. New behaviors and incentives are being negotiated to satisfy the mutual expectations of those who have a stake in the process. These new ground rules then become the basis for continued negotiation. The intention here is to speak to the change, the "renegotiation," mindful of the ways in which this transformation affects ongoing "negotiation."

The subtitle, *Resolving Conflict to Build Collaboration*, points to our fundamental purpose as health professionals.

Conflict resolution, as a process, is considered here not only as a method for cooling a boiling dispute. Rather, it is viewed as a regular function of your work. We negotiate our differences every day. Some of these differences are resolved routinely, without much notice. In other cases, even the very same issue can explode into a major confrontation: that confrontation had its beginning usually in a simple negotiation that could have been better handled. Conflict resolution, therefore, is viewed as an integrated aspect of what you continually do to balance the array of expertise, values, and aspirations that attend even the simplest of decisions.

Collaboration refers to the combined activity of the host of people and organizations necessary for the work of health care. In the emerging health care reality, those groups and enterprises most likely to succeed are those who are best able to achieve efficient and effective collaboration. Whether it be two organizations forming a partnership, two physicians devising a primary specialty care alliance or a floor of nurses creating a better-coordinated work environment, those people who do collaborate—and do it well—are those who are most likely to survive and thrive. These successful collaborations are able to foster quality, enhance productivity, and cultivate satisfaction both for those who provide health care services and for those who receive them. The emerging system will not tolerate loners outside the flows of patient care, the networks for referral, and the systems for reimbursement.

"Build" collaboration because negotiation is an ongoing process that you formulate and reformulate every day. To aid your building process, this book offers a set of negotiation tools.

The purpose here is to highlight aspects of negotiation and conflict resolution particularly germane to health care, and to present a model that fits its unique demands and dimensions. The book is written primarily for those who work in the field. Nonetheless, those who are consumers of health services likely will also find the insights useful, just as those who are interested in general aspects of negotiation and conflict resolution may find the elements of health care to inform general theoretical and methodological understanding.

How is the book written? There are really three books in one. The first is a guidebook on the concepts, methods, and techniques of negotiation and conflict resolution. This discussion ranges from the theoretical to the practical, with an emphasis on how you can build interest-based negotiation into your everyday professional repertoire.

The second book is written by four colleagues who apply these general concepts and topics to the work and responsibilities of their arena of practice: public health and policy, management, nursing, and medicine. These chapters are intended in part for professionals in these specific fields, to offer them a way to interpret and integrate these concepts into practice. These chapters are also intended as a way for those outside these disciplines to gain a new appreciation for the perspectives, problems, and challenges of people in other professions.

The third book is a set of parables placed within the context of the typical dilemmas, conflicts, and negotiations that face people working in health care settings. These stories are interwoven throughout the text and are the most unique aspect of this book.

I am often impressed with our compulsion to create neat lists, categories, cases, and concepts to describe and understand matters of negotiation, mediation, and organization. In the process we seem to forget that each of these activities is essentially about people: what they say and do, how they feel and react, and the complex and sometimes fluky interactions that occur in the course of elaborate and highly consequential decision making. By turning people into precisely defined objects, we risk creating further confusion and misunderstanding. The "novel" is here to instruct, to illustrate, and to remind us of the inherently human aspects of negotiation.

A word of caution as you read the "novel." It is not intended to illustrate or represent the typical nurse, doctor, manager, patient, or policy maker. That would be impossible, if not ingenuous. It is also not intended to idolize, impugn, or trivialize any particular profession or type of person. Rather, it is intended to place the considerations, problems, and consequences of people living and working in health care environments into a plausible human dimension. These sections are written as metaphors as much as reflections. Read them as such. Do not take them too literally. Ponder, contemplate, and perhaps discuss with others what you find in these stories. And to keep you mindful of this note, the characters' names are all given as alliterations. Remember, look for the meaning and allow yourself to engage with these characters for who they are and for what they represent.

Finally, why did I write this book? I view life as a journey. I regard the human condition as a continuous process of evolution, shaped by our many intersecting journeys. We each can contribute or detract from that evolution in the journeys we pursue and in the manner we conduct ourselves in travel. This voyage through life is one of exploration, discovery, learning, convergences, and departures. We make our contributions; we impose our costs. We cast our goals, set our destinations, and fulfill our aspirations. The trip sees its accomplishments and its disappointments.

The journey is marked by its many meetings: intersections with others defined by our negotiations. Our origins are varied just as our destinations are different. The question is whether we can constructively conduct those meetings so that they enhance and not detract from the virtues we each hope to accomplish.

What we do in our work as health care professionals is unique. We deal with life and the quality of that life. Our society and the people who come for service depend upon us to do well, to extend and enhance the value of their own journeys.

This book hopes to nourish you for your journeys and to help our many intersecting pathways enhance the ongoing process of health care change and evolution.

Happy travels.

Boston, Massachusetts   LEONARD J. MARCUS, PH.D.
July 1995

Acknowledgments

Writing a book is a quirky task. On the one hand, one feels the loneliness of the writing duty itself. On the other hand, there is a real sense of bonding with those who have been part of the enterprise. That bonding is tangible when I think of direct collaborators. The feeling is more distant, though very present, when I think of people or events that helped to shape this book and the work that led to it.

I tend to be an organizer, just as I am an educator. I have learned over the years that the best human qualities and ideas rise when placed amid those of other fine people. I love nothing more than introducing two people to one another, a person to an idea, or an idea to a person. I have seen good things flow from the process often enough to believe in its value.

Similarly, I have met wonderful people who themselves have introduced me to new people, ideas, and settings that have enlarged my own vistas. To the extent that I have been able to share some of these vistas here, I am indebted and grateful.

Barry Dorn has been my soul mate throughout the preparation of this book: my coach, guide, and inspiration. We have traveled many momentous paths together, and he has been a good-humored and enlightening partner and friend. Phyllis Kritek was on this train when it first left the station. She often inspirited the value of the journey and encouraged the many grand destinations to which it aspires. Velvet Miller has always kept the big picture in focus. She has reminded us of the purpose of our work and the many people who can benefit by our pushing on. And Janice Wyatt has been there to keep us on track. She has grounded me in what I am doing and where I am going. As collaborators, the beauty of our mix lies in our differences and our willingness to continue struggling with them. And the specialness has been not only in the work we have each shared: there has also been an abundance of warm friendship and good laughs.

Others deserve appreciation for expanding my own understandings and horizons. Tim Dutton, director of the Hospital of Albert Schweitzer in Deschappelles, Haiti, has taught me the courage of conviction. Jim Laue, Frank Sanders, and David Matz inspired my learning and pursuit of conflict resolution and encouraged me to explore its uses for health care. Nancy Neveloff Dubler, Edward Dauer, Alexander Fleming, and Lisa Fenichel were instrumental in fostering my applications of this field to practical problems facing health care. My colleague Susan Payne was an important source of support and encouragement. Deborah Prothrow-Stith and Paul Campbell were responsible for opening doors at the Harvard School of Public Health.

My entree to conflict resolution was through the Kellogg National Fellowship Program, sponsored by the W.K. Kellogg Foundation. Its director at the time, Larraine Matusak, opened new doors and encouraged me to find, explore, and create doors that I never knew existed. That beginning with Kellogg was continued with support from the community-oriented health care initiative, directed by Ronald Richards. The National Institute for Dispute Resolution was instrumental in allowing me to launch this work, and Tom Fee, the director of the innovations program at the time, has remained a friend throughout. Vital assistance has been provided by the William and Flora Hewlett Foundation, and program officer Stephen Toben has been a steadfast source of much appreciated encouragement.

This book was first read in draft form by students in my classes and training programs, who offered crucial insights into what worked and what did not. I, and the readers who now can make use of the final version of this text, owe them a great deal of gratitude.

I am fortunate to have a number of dear friends who prodded and pulled me along through this process and who sometimes had to put up with the short end of the stick to maintain the progress of our work. There are too many people to mention individually. Deborah Leschinsky and Janine Zuromski, though, deserve special recognition for their persistence through rocky roads.

I have benefitted from a bounty of patience, encouragement, and good advice from my friends at Jossey-Bass Publishers. Trisha O'Hare assured me that this book was a worthwhile endeavor. Barbara Hill was like the trainer, keeping the runner moving along with words of reassurance. Becky McGovern offered wisdom and counsel and helped me put this project into perspective.

This book was written in the fishing village of Gloucester, Massachusetts, at the beach home of Barry and Deanne Dorn. The front porch looks out onto the Atlantic Ocean with its endless vistas, its energy and timelessness. The back of the house overlooks Gloucester harbor. I wrote facing the harbor, my Macintosh computer on the dining room table, watching the parade of boats expectantly going out to sea and wearily returning from the ocean with their bounty of fish. I composed to the harbor and pondered to the sea. The setting inspired the thoughts and encouraged the words that you find here. I am forever grateful to Barry and Deanne for their generosity.

Perhaps those who paid the dearest cost for this book are my son, Jeremy, and wife, Barbara. Their perseverance and love through this long process have allowed me the time and energy to bring this project to fruition. Jeremy's insights into baseball card trading were handy as I dissected aspects of the negotiation process. Barb has helped me to understand my dreams and has encouraged me to pursue them. Her faith and common sense has allowed me to keep life, and what I do, in perspective.

And to you, dear reader, who allows me to do what I most value: to share these ideas so that they might find new homes, new uses, and new journeys.

To Barb and Jeremy
My partners in love and in life

The Authors

Leonard J. Marcus, Ph.D., is founder and director of the Program for Health Care Negotiation and Conflict Resolution at the Harvard School of Public Health. He earned his doctoral degree at the Heller School of Brandeis University. In 1986 he was selected for the Kellogg National Fellowship Program, through which he began his concentration in negotiation and conflict resolution. He is active on the state and national levels in advancing models and uses of mediation to resolve health care disputes. He conducts mediation through the Center for Health Care Negotiation, Inc., a nonprofit mediation service he launched in 1991.

Barry C. Dorn, M.D., is clinical professor of orthopedic surgery and director of the adult orthopedic clinic at Tufts New England Medical Center. He maintains a private orthopedic practice in Winchester, Massachusetts. Dr. Dorn is a frequent speaker to medical and other health care groups across the country on the topic of negotiation and conflict resolution. He is cochair of the Society of Professionals in Dispute Resolution Health Sector and a mediator with the Center for Health Care Negotiation.

Phyllis Beck Kritek, R.N., Ph.D., is author of the recently published *Negotiating at an Uneven Table: Developing Moral Courage in Resolving Our Conflicts* (Jossey-Bass, 1994). She is professor of nursing and director of doctoral program development at the University of Texas Medical Branch at the Galveston School of Nursing. Her previous position was as dean of the School of Nursing at Marquette University. Dr. Kritek has extensively published, presented, and consulted on gender issues, conflict resolution, nursing diagnosis, nursing research, and health professional issues.

Velvet G. Miller, B.S.N., M.P.A., is director of the Division of Medical Assistance and Health Services, New Jersey Department of Human Services, and former assistant commissioner of the Bureau of Public Health Hospitals for the Massachusetts Department of Public Health. Throughout her career in public health administration, nursing, and education, she has been committed to improving health services for the poor and for people of color. Ms. Miller is a senior associate with Health Care Negotiation Associates, Inc., and a frequent speaker on issues of community-based health care collaboration.

Janice B. Wyatt, M.S., is a partner with Korn Ferry International, Boston, and the former president and chief executive officer of the MetroWest Medical Center. She has served as vice chancellor and hospital director at the University of Massachusetts Medical Center. Ms. Wyatt was honored as Massachusetts Health Care Leader of the Year by the American College of Health Care Executives. She is a senior associate with Health Care Negotiation Associates, Inc., through which she conducts organizational consultation and training.

Renegotiating Health Care

Part I

....

Conflict

1

· ·

Why Conflict?

If your work is health care, your daily routine requires constant negotiation and involves some measure of conflict. Decisions affecting a number of people have to be made. Competing priorities have to be balanced. There is the pressure of time and a constant vigilance that the job is done correctly.

Health care work is accomplished via an intricately structured set of relationships. Formal and informal rules determine who speaks to whom, who makes what decisions, and who has what information. People are organized and decisions are aligned in a cautiously defined order. The most important or momentous information, person, or decision gets the uppermost attention first, and the rest trails behind. This sequence is intended to yield systematic decision making.

And the work is done by people and for people. There is perhaps no endeavor more intimately tied to who we are, our identity, than the duties we perform or the care we receive in the health care system. Health care is at the cusp of life and death and the quality of life. Whether we are in the role of patient, provider, or manager, our values, beliefs, and personality are exposed and interlocked amid the close interpersonal proximity of health care decision making, negotiation, and conflict.

What if this complex puzzle does not smoothly fit together? What if there are differences about what or who is more important? What if a mistake occurs? What if there is a clash of personalities

among people who must closely interrelate? What if there is dissonance between the policies and procedures defining these relationships? What if people are working under different incentives? How
will this affect what we do and how we do it?

Consider the following:

* * * * * * *

It is another hectic night in the emergency department of Oppidania Medical Center. A frenzy of activity centers at the desk,
where nurses, residents, attending physicians, and emergency
medical technicians gather to exchange information, tell stories,
and take a break.

Nearby, Artie Ashwood, twenty-four, moans in one of the
beds. The monitors and machines surrounding him are beeping,
breathing, and filling him with lifesaving fluids. He has an enlarged heart, arrythmia, and shortness of breath. It has been
three hours since he came in, and it is time to decide where he
should go next. In the visitor's room, his family nervously awaits
news of his condition.

The attending physician, Dr. Beatrice Benson, oversees the
work of the medical residents. She explains, "The emergency
department is not meant for treatment. It is meant for triage.
It is our job to assess the patient and decide the next step. If the
problem is life-threatening, we admit to the intensive care unit.
If the patient does not need to be in the hospital, we discharge
with a treatment plan and instructions. If it's someplace in between, we admit for observation and treatment. So if it's an
admission, the question is, to which service?"

Ashwood's condition defies a conclusive diagnosis. His
young age concerns the staff. His symptoms could be signaling
a dangerous situation. Hoping for more information, they hold
him in the emergency room waiting for stabilization. Nurses and
residents are constantly monitoring his condition, and nothing
changes.

Suddenly, Charlotte Channing, the triage nurse at the desk,
signals the impending arrival of a multiple gunshot wound. The

door to the specially equipped trauma room is opened, and the staff moves to their places around the gurney that will hold the dying man.

Benson talks by telephone with the paramedics in the ambulance to assess the incoming patient's condition and to prepare for briefing the staff. As she turns toward the trauma room, Channing suggests that the young man with the enlarged heart be admitted to one of the floors in the hospital, since it was looking like a busy night.

Benson says, "Good idea," and walks off, preoccupied. Channing is frustrated.

◆ ◆ ◆ ◆ ◆ ◆ ◆

There are so far three people in our story. Artie Ashwood's fate is in the hands of the people who surround him. He is in great pain. He is frightened. He doesn't know what is happening to him and what it might mean for the rest of his life. People are asking questions, many of them repetitive. Some of those who speak to him seem genuinely concerned about how he is doing. Others seem to be asking questions as if they are part of a prescribed list. He is afraid of being lost in this loud mass of people. He overhears that a gunshot wound is on its way. Might the hospital explode in shots if the attackers come here to finish the job? Even more frightening, might the nurses and doctors who have been at his side forget him once someone sicker arrives? He has been waiting for a long time. Can't they just fix him up and move him along already? He is dependent upon people who seem preoccupied.

Dr. Beatrice Benson is the attending physician in the emergency department (ED). She oversees and has responsibility for the work of the ED medical residents and physicians. She simultaneously tends to many constituencies and concerns, and is interdependent with many parts of the system. She is vigilant of the patients, watchful over the residents, and in touch with other parts of the system. "Is the intensive care unit backed up?" "Yes, we can accept a patient severely cut in an accident at work." "No, we are not taking a nine-month pregnant, cocaine-addicted woman being dumped by a suburban hospital." By its very nature, her work is in the short term: her responsibility is to keep the flow of patients moving. She sees patients for a matter of hours before they disappear into the labyrinth of the hospital or out to discharge. She rarely sees them again. The long term is an abstraction. She has some power and influence, though others in the hospital understate the authority she believes is hers. There is, however, no understatement when it comes to responsibility. For a miscalculation, the lawyers will come to Dr. Benson with their suit, the administrators will challenge her about wastefulness, and the patients will complain about their delayed or inadequate care. She is constantly negotiating and continually trying to keep the system in balance.

Charlotte Channing is the triage nurse in the ED. Ostensibly her role is to screen patients and determine the severity and urgency of their conditions. In fact her function is to create order among the unpredictable flow of patients arriving at the ER. That order must align with the contingent of nurses, physicians, and other personnel staffing the shift. It is a matter of creating a fluid balance. Patients arrive at the hospital in pain or discomfort and are anxious to be seen at once. Family or friends who accompany them advocate, question, and worry. It is up to her to decide who will be seen when, by whom, and where: she holds the criteria and judges each case accordingly. Physicians, nurses, technicians, and housekeeping personnel scurry to keep the pace caring for one patient and preparing for the next. They depend on Channing to make the right calls, to hold off patients who can't yet be seen, and when the staff is overloaded, to send in only the most severely ill. Her desk is like a lightening rod for conflict. She mediates between the needs of patients, the capacity of the staff, and the personalities who may explode under the pressure and stress of the decisions she is required to make. Her greatest source of irritation are the obstacles erected by those, especially physicians, who hold greater authority and who carry far less perspective and understanding than does she.

Each of these people is part of the same reality, yet their perspectives are very different. The question is whether their distinct responsibilities, concerns, and decisions can combine in a congruent manner, allowing each to satisfactorily achieve their very reason for being in the ED this night. If they can, their interaction will be productive and mutually beneficial. If they cannot, conflict is likely. Disputing often has its roots in common experiences seen from very different perspectives and with seemingly incongruent expectations.

Different Purposes

We often begin training in health care negotiation and conflict resolution with a classic game theory simulation exercise called the "Prisoners' Dilemma." (For a discussion of the Prisoners' Dilemma and game theory, see Luce and Raiffa, 1957; Goldberg, Green, and Sander, 1957; and Rahim, 1992.) The exercise demonstrates the problem of negotiating when people have little opportunity for direct or prolonged interaction, like prisoners in different cells endeavoring to communicate. Each participant in the exercise is part of a foursome: one pair faces in one direction and another pair faces in another direction. The two pairs sit with their backs to each other, and a trainer moves messages on paper between them. In a series of transactions, they exchange X's and Y's, which when combined equate according to a formula into positive or negative points for the two sides.

To simulate conditions in real organizations, the directions for the exercise are purposefully written in an ambiguous manner. One line in the directions encourages the participants to "do the best you can to achieve a high level of benefit from the transactions." The unspoken quandary is that "high level of benefit" is intentionally left open to interpretation. Because they must begin negotiating immediately, the players often do not have a common definition for what they are trying to achieve. As a result, one of the four players may assume that "winning" means his twosome receives more points than the other pair. Another player may conclude that winning requires collecting more points while also reducing the other side's points. A third may assume that winning means each team receives an equal score. And finally, the fourth may surmise that winning means both teams get a score close to zero.

The problem is readily apparent. If each player assumes a different interpretation of "high level of benefit," there is certain to be conflict. In essence, one person is playing one game, "defeat the opponent," while his or her partner is playing another game, "let's all win."

Even among the most subdued of players, the interchange becomes passionate. At face value they are only exchanging X's and Y's—objects with no inherent value. The yelling, screaming, and pathos emerge from the underlying belief systems and perspectives that influence the players' actions during the game. Each person is playing, in part, to advance and validate his or her own belief system. It is common for someone to say during the after-exercise debriefing, "It wasn't that I was going for points. I was trying to show that we can play to win together." It is also common to hear, "I love to win, no matter what I am doing." Each party strives to justify the principles that frame his or her behavior.

The Prisoners' Dilemma parallels the situation in the ED.

◆ ◆ ◆ ◆ ◆ ◆ ◆

Artie Ashwood stares up at the tiles of the hospital ceiling. He is in a great deal of pain. He is frightened. He hopes that the people around him will care for him well.

Ashwood's condition continues to defy a conclusive diagnosis. His symptoms could be signaling a dangerous situation. Hoping for more information, Dr. Dave Donley, the resident who has been following Ashwood, holds him in the emergency room, waiting for the stabilization. Nothing changes.

Charlotte Channing signals Benson over to the triage desk and asks if anyone might be ready to move along. The waiting room is full, and the gunshot wound is stretching everyone thin. Perhaps if Benson decides on her own, things will start happening. This is a game Channing learned a long time ago. She hates having to play it, and smiles to herself every time it works.

Benson nods and calls over Dr. Donley. "We're too busy to hold this fellow any longer. Call the cardiac intensive care unit and tell them we've got an admission. Tell them to get down here right away because we're overloaded tonight."

It has been a busy shift on the CICU as well. Seven of the CICU's eight beds are filled. Six of the patients require heavy-duty care. The seventh patient was sent up by emergency three hours ago.

By the time the CICU nurses and physicians had completed the workup and admission, it became clear that emergency had misjudged this one. The patient didn't need to be in intensive care.

Three hours left in the shift, and the staff were hoping the night would calm down.

The chief resident of the CICU, Eli Ewing, knows that he is running an expensive unit. That misjudged patient not only consumed a great deal of unnecessary time and work, it also cost the hospital and some insurer a lot of money. Ewing believes he has a responsibility to screen out patients who do not require this most technical level of care.

Ewing also has a responsibility to the staff. He knows the lingo well. In the parlance of the teaching hospital, a "wall" is a resident who succeeds in keeping out admissions to the unit. A "sieve" is someone who doesn't know how to say no. Walls are liked far better than sieves.

Ewing takes the call from Donley. Still smarting from the last case, Ewing sardonically listens to the report on Ashwood's enlarged heart. Donley admits he is not certain that the patient is in a medical crisis. Ewing's reaction is abrupt: the patient doesn't need to be admitted to the CICU, and the unit is not going to take him. He suggests calling one of the general medical floors, which can do a far better and far less expensive job of baby-sitting. Ending the call abruptly, Ewing turns to the CICU staff and smiles.

Donley is perplexed. Is there something he is missing? He walks into the trauma room where Benson is now overseeing work on the patient with the gunshot wound. He explains the situation. "Tell the CICU they are taking the patient. End of story."

The back and forth goes nowhere. Forty-five minutes later, Benson emerges from the trauma room to find Ashwood still in the bed. "They just won't take him," the frustrated resident explains in defeat.

Enraged, Benson calls the CICU and demands that the chief resident get on the line. "I want you down here right now."

"Look, this guy doesn't need to be admitted to the CICU. If you want him in for observation, send him to one of the medical floors. We've already had to sweat out one misread from you guys tonight."

"Fine, then let's see what Fisher thinks about this case."

The CICU resident pauses. "Fisher? You're going to call Fisher on this? I didn't know you guys considered this so serious. OK, I'll be right down."

◆ ◆ ◆ ◆ ◆ ◆ ◆

The parties in this emergency room admission scenario are in much the same prisoners' dilemma. They have little opportunity to meet. Yet they must engage in a series of transactions and reach a set of common decisions that are utterly interdependent.

While the parties share many common objectives, their definition of "high level of benefit" is heavily influenced by their immediate context, be it a crowded emergency room or an overworked CICU staff. The emergency room weighs the care required by one patient against that needed by others flowing into the hospital. The condition and care given one patient is then measured relative to others. The CICU criteria are based on far more standard criteria. An insurer will not reimburse the hospital for this expensive level of care if the patient's condition does not warrant admission. Thus while the emergency room staff have one set of criteria for admitting a patient to the CICU, the CICU staff have a very different set.

When the emergency attending physician ordered the CICU admission, it still wasn't clear what was the problem with the patient. It could have ranged from minor to life-threatening. With limited information and a great deal of ambiguity, a decision was reached. Once the parties adopt a line of thinking, they become allegiant to it. Each believes there is much at stake, be it the patient's life, the work of the staff, money, time, or professional prestige. The interchange then becomes passionate as the parties defend principles. "The emergency department decides who is admitted and to which department they are going," maintains Benson. "Without that authority, I can't make this place work."

Ewing counters, "Only the CICU can determine who needs its care. Without that authority, this hospital would turn into expensive chaos. No physician wants to take the risk of undertreating a patient. Before you know it, every patient will be sent through the CICU as a precaution."

From their own perspective, each of the parties was trying to achieve a high level of benefit. Nonetheless, given the different definitions of benefit that they brought to the task, it was likely that they would experience a great deal of conflict in the process. The CICU resident was trying to protect the system as well as his staff. The attending physician was trying to maintain a reasonable balance in the emergency room while doing what she felt was best for the patient. The emergency room resident was mediating between the two. And the patient was hoping that the people who determined his fate could assure him the best possible level of care.

There are two common elements in the emergency room—CICU and the prisoners' dilemma scenarios. The first is interaction and the conflict inherent therein. These are different people, with different considerations, authority, and information. They reach different conclusions and advance different solutions to care for the patient. They are each trying to do their best, and since they define this criterion so differently, their interdependent work is destined to generate conflict.

The second link to the prisoners' dilemma metaphor is purpose as it affects patient care. The patient is the common thread that binds the people, institutions, and activities that we call *health care*. While the patient focus is a constant, it has so many different meanings and interpretations that it often becomes a passionate fulcrum of conflict.

The Complexity of Conflict

The first step in negotiating and resolving conflict is beginning to understand it. I emphasize *beginning* because conflict is so complex a phenomenon. Many times, even in retrospect, it is difficult to fully comprehend its origins and manifestations. (For a discussion of conflict analysis, see Likert and Likert, 1976; Potapchuk and Carlson, 1987; and Kolb and Bartunek, 1992.)

Consider yourself. You are a bundle of different desires, values, and fears. Your life experiences clash within you, expressing themselves in your dreams, apprehensions, and vulnerabilities. While you exhibit decisiveness to others, privately those different ideas, anxieties, and aspirations collide. You experience inner conflict while you appear outwardly unequivocal.

Consider that others are experiencing the same inner conflict. And their life experiences and beliefs are different from yours, making it all the more difficult for you to fathom their point of view.

Place another person in the same room with yourself. That person also is not fully aware of his or her internal dynamics. Try playing a game together. Use different rules and different interpretations of what you are trying to accomplish. One person holds a football while the other carries a baseball and bat. Both want to play ball. However, each is equipped for a different game, with very different rules and objectives. It will be difficult to organize a coherent game.

A prescription for conflict.

Now imagine adding hundreds of other people together into the same room. They all have different experiences, rule books, and objectives for the game they wish to play. They have different personalities and temperaments. To further complicate the scenario, imagine people in far-off places like Washington or Chicago mandating how they should play. Now add the drama of life and death and the passion of illness.

What a mess! Welcome to health care.

We want to understand conflict so we can modify the ingredients that vary its presence and impact. Conflict itself is inevitable. Nevertheless, it does present us with choices. As we begin to observe and understand conflict, we can modify its potential destructiveness. We can also learn from conflict. It is a vehicle to help us better perceive ourselves, the people we work with, and what we are trying to achieve together. If we truly comprehend it and learn to work with it, conflict can uncover opportunities for institutional as well as personal improvement.

What are the components of conflict? If you wanted to create it, what ingredients would you blend together?

First, formulate ambiguity. Take information that could be interpreted in different ways by different people, depending on their knowledge, values, and life experiences. Exclude some important information, and distribute what is known to different people. Bring in events that could be viewed and interpreted in disparate and contradictory ways. Create uncertainty about options and outcomes. Sprinkle a dash of vagueness over the mix.

The ambiguity itself would be inconsequential if it wasn't baked in the heat of requisite decisions and actions. Artie Ashwood presented to the emergency room without a medical chart. There was no information about his baseline medical condition. He was unclear about his medical history. It was impossible to unequivocally predict what was going to happen next. And who knows how his insurer would assess the appropriateness and necessity of care when the case is reviewed in retrospect? If the wrong decision is made, it could be unnecessarily fatal for Ashwood or unnecessarily expensive for the hospital. Yet a decision must be made.

Next add complexity. The more people involved in or affected by a decision, the greater the potential for conflict. Some people are physically present in the scenario: physicians, nurses, and patients. Others are not actually on the scene, though their presence is felt nonetheless. These are people who write the rules of reimbursement, professional conduct, and hospital policy. While one person holds the responsibility for making the decision, that decision is colored by hundreds of people who grant or who restrict the choices.

This complexity would not be so problematic if it weren't attached to stakes. While there may be only one decision on the table, such as whether or not to admit, the stakes for the many people involved differ considerably. Those stakes may be measured in terms of professional responsibility, legal or financial liability, personal pride, or a tough night on the job. They may also be measured in terms of quality of life, time, and pain.

For the person who holds the responsibility, the experience is something akin to white-water rafting. You are pushed through a torrent of decisions. There are obstacles and restrictions on all sides. You must navigate a narrow path through the water. If you veer too far in either direction, you are doomed. Some failures can be corrected. Others are fatal. Your map is ambiguous and incomplete. You find many uncharted twists and turns in the river.

Mix into the pie competition and evaluation. There are competing departments, professions, and institutions at play. Each of these wield different power, prestige, and status. Within the intricately hierarchical edifice of health care, people are arrayed on rungs of a ladder, ascending and descending on their own successes and the failures of others. The CICU resident hopes to boast to his subordinates and his superiors that he has protected the unit from another unnecessary admission, and to rise another rung on the ladder in the process. His conquest becomes someone else's conundrum. However, if his superior is admonished for wrongful refusal of a patient, the penalty is a slide down that ladder. Likewise, the attending physician in the emergency department wonders what influence she has on the floors above her. Can she keep patients flowing smoothly through the emergency room to appropriate destinations? She is dependent on the efficiency of the lab, the timeliness of the medical records department, and the cooperation of the medical services throughout the institution. What if her work and decisions are not respected? It could spell disaster for her, for her department, and for the patients dependent on her work. That consternation is amplified for the triage nurse in the emergency department. She views and experiences the logjam first and most immediately, yet she has limited capacity to dislodge it, short of her capacity to wield some persuasive influence with those in charge.

The competition and hierarchical predicaments would not be so portentous if they were not cast in the light of obligatory cooperation. Information must be exchanged. Care for ill patients must be uninterrupted in the course of movement from one department to another. A heavy work load in one area of the hospital must be alleviated by help from others. And the work must be in conformity with the rules of reimbursement, the standards of quality, and the needs of the patients.

Combine the above with stress and pressure. Time is not an abstraction in health care. It is measured in moments when a life can be saved. It is measured in colossal dollars when there is a delay in discharge for a patient who need not be in the hospital. There is little room for error or delay. With time so critical, it is imperative to synchronize actions and decisions. Given the extraordinary interdependence of health care service, procrastination on the part of one individual, department, or institution strains the entire system.

The stress and pressure is amplified by consequences. Whether measured in terms of the patient's quality of life or the institution's financial balance sheet, the implications of even routine decisions can be overwhelming. Artie Ashwood prays that he will be able to return to a normal life after this horrible night. He hopes the people caring for him have the competence and compassion to make sure that happens. Charlotte Channing and Beatrice Benson both know they are juggling an acute set of choices: a misjudgment could cost them loss of professional prestige, a liability suit, or even their license to practice. Dave Donley knows that he is building the foundation for the rest of his medical career, and he hopes it to be a beginning that will do him well for years to come. And Eli Ewing wants to show that he can handle the tough decisions required of physicians. That reputation will win him a prestigious position once his residency is over.

Put these factors in the context of change: reimbursement formulas, professional responsibilities, technology, social expectations, organizational arrangements, knowledge, information. Some people welcome these changes in the pursuit of the opportunities they present. Others recoil from them because the shifts threaten their status, comfort, or influence. The clash between comfortable security and precarious, unknown opportunity magnifies the conflict. The health care system is akin to a colossal jigsaw puzzle in which the parts—financing, organization, service, training, and people— are aligning themselves into a new order and a new fit.

Is Conflict Bad?

Thomas Schelling (1960) distinguishes two fundamental approaches to the study and understanding of conflict. One approach views it as a problem, the other as an opportunity.

Those who view conflict as pathological believe it is best silenced or eliminated. From this outlook, conflict reflects negatively upon an organization and therefore must be removed. It is an annoyance in and of itself, as are those people who raise it. The people who instigate conflict are labeled "troublemakers," and the problem is associated with them personally. When this perspective pervades a group, discussion usually descends to finger-pointing, polarization, and personalization of the issues.

This perspective by its very nature is conservative, since the true danger of conflict lies in its disruption of the status quo. The concerns of those who ignite an issue are delegitimized, as they endanger the authority and influence of those who are threatened by dissatisfaction with the current state of affairs. The actual problem is lost in the struggle to determine who has the legitimate authority to raise concerns and make decisions. One might hear some version of, "There is nothing wrong with what we are doing or how we go about doing it. The problem is with the individual who is raising the problem."

From this point of view, conflict and contest are intertwined in their meaning. The only response to conflict can be to bring it to defeat. Conflict is viewed as a threat and a source of vulnerability. Going for a win is akin to fighting for survival. It is an instinctual, self-protective response that allows for an inherently limited set of options.

If conflict is regarded as intrinsically bad and the people who raise it are treated as troublemakers, then little can be learned or gained from the problems an organization or group of people naturally encounter. Rather than considering what may be wrong or what might be fixed, attention is directed to silencing the dissenters and invalidating their concerns. The problem is that the problem itself is then compounded. Not only does the source of the original dissatisfaction remain. For those who raised the issues, the silence imposed upon their concerns adds yet another layer of frustration.

The second approach to conflict views it as a naturally occurring social phenomenon. Just as a stream meanders irregularly if not harnessed by concrete walls, so too do people and organizations vacillate in their interests, priorities, concerns, and relationships. From this perspective, conflict is acknowledged and handled as one measure of the problems or concerns that merit some measure of attention. To harness and silence differing points of view into concrete barriers would counter the values of a democratic society.

Those who foster this model encourage constructive expression of differences so they can be acknowledged, addressed, and hopefully remedied. Rather than discounting expression of dissatisfaction, they solicit it as a way to move toward resolution. This perspective recognizes that the most successful organizations are those that can efficiently and accurately respond to internal as well as external contingencies. Effective solutions are devised by accumulating a wide source of credible information and then working resourcefully to invent mutually acceptable solutions.

This approach does not imply that all expressions of conflict are inherently valid. Absolutely not. Not every issue and concern is meritorious. If someone raises a matter that is irrelevant to the purposes of an organization, is beyond reasonable expectation, or is without validity, then certainly it does not deserve action. One might question why the misinformed expectations arose in the first place, and one may want to improve information and communication as a result. That is to say, even if an issue is without merit, it may reveal something important about the conditions, people, or circumstances that spawned it.

Those who approach conflict in this way encourage its expression, endeavor to find its roots, learn from it, and, when appropriate, change conditions that merit modification. Express, learn, engage, exchange, and change form a recurring cycle of organizational practice. Often, finding the resolution is a matter of negotiation. The responsibility for enhancing the process by framing the issues constructively lies with all parties to the disagreement. If conflict is to be a value-added opportunity, its initial framing, response, and subsequent bargaining must be conducted in a manner that respects the legitimate concerns of all sides.

The approach of this book is to view constructively expressed conflict as an opportunity. We regard conflict as part and parcel of human endeavor—and part and parcel of health care. It is to be expected. If we accept that differences of opinion, and sometimes even heated differences, are predictable occurrences in health care, then we can prepare for it. We then reframe conflict as opportunity. Conflict is a plus if used as one test for determining what is and what is not working about health care. It can serve as a barometer for what needs to be changed.

◆ ◆ ◆ ◆ ◆ ◆ ◆

Channing wonders aloud what can be done to change this
nightly standoff between the emergency department and other
floors of the hospital. Sure, part of it goes with the territory.
There will always be some creative tension between the unpre-
dictability of what happens here and the order of the rest of
the hospital. Nonetheless, there has to be a better way to play
out these decisions so that people, herself included, don't get
caught in the cross fire.

Artie Ashwood's mother and girlfriend have been pacing
impatiently in the emergency department waiting room. During
those long stretches of time with no information and no decision,
each had convinced herself that Artie was going to die. Their
old animosities rose to the fore, as each was certain that Artie's
death would be a greater tragedy for her than for the other. Together they approached the triage desk, pleading to be allowed
to see Artie. Charlotte Channing explains that only one person
at a time is allowed back to see the patients. They both explode
about who Artie really wants to see. Channing patiently asks
them to sit down while she goes back to see what's happening.
She stands up and heads right for Benson.

◆ ◆ ◆ ◆ ◆ ◆ ◆

We prepare ourselves for conflict by better understanding it and
better negotiating our differences. We prepare our organizations for
it by anticipating it and by building mechanisms to resolve it early
in the process. And we incorporate a concern for it when we craft
public policies that regulate work and interactions in health care
settings.

This country is now readjusting its health system. New policies,
procedures, expectations, and pressures are putting their mark on
the everyday negotiations and interactions in all parts of the system
throughout the country. These new policies are reframing professional, fiduciary, and organizational relationships between doctors
and patients, patients and insurers, nurses and patients, doctors and

businesses, and the many others who are part of the health care system. If those relationships are framed correctly, then the system will work when a patient arrives at a hospital for care. However, if the system is not carefully designed, and appropriate incentives, restrictions, and protections are not in place, people will face great disappointment when they need care for themselves or for a member of their family. Our work as health care professionals will be a story of bitter disappointment (Thorne, 1993).

This book is a map to help you better understand conflict, negotiate choices, and build systems to improve the processes of decision making. It is not intended as a blueprint for a better health care system, a more satisfying health care career, or improved health care experiences. Rather, it is a guide to the process for getting there.

2

Moving Beyond Conflict

Picture yourself in the midst of a conflict. Let's say one other person is involved, one of your colleagues. Your discussions have become cold and tense. For both of you, the problem absorbs a great deal of time. It begins to feel like an obsession, filling your thoughts and distracting your attention.

Moving beyond conflict requires at least one of you to make a shift (see Fisher and Brown, 1988; Ury, 1991). Resolving the conflict demands both of you to make the shift. You are both caught in the momentum of conflict. To override its escalation, you elicit a motive to settle, that genuine desire to close the issue. That motivation could arise from the anticipated benefits of resolution. It could emerge from the feared consequences of escalation. Most likely it will be fostered by some combination of both. Crafting your resolution requires the ingenuity to balance the giving and the getting among you. In the process, you build a climate of mutual satisfaction, an outcome unimaginable at the outset.

Among the simulation exercises I use in conflict resolution training is the "Arms Race." In this exercise, I auction off a one-dollar bill. The bidding starts at 10 cents and goes up in increments of at least 5 cents. Before the auction begins, I inform the participants that all proceeds will be donated to my son's favorite charity (a small compensation to Jeremy for losing his dad to frequent travel). Jeremy has been raising money for multiple sclerosis, shelters for the homeless, and a hospital in Haiti. I also explain the unique rule of the game: you must pay whatever you last bid, whether or not you make the final bid. If you bid 10 cents, someone else bids 15 cents, you raise your bid to 20 cents, and then they get the dollar for a quarter, you still have to pay your last bid of 20 cents. (For a discussion of games and negotiation, see Brams, 1990).

The game has a robust beginning. People are eager to participate in the action, and the bidding climbs rapidly in small increments toward a dollar. As we approach the dollar point, the pace slows. Often bidding grinds to a halt at 95 cents. Usually ten or so people have been actively bidding, and they are now faced with a choice. Up to this point, there was a relatively small risk for a potentially profitable outcome. After all, they reason, "This guy is selling a dollar, and I can get it for 25 cents."

I walk over to the person with the 90-cent bid. I suggest, "You might as well bid the dollar. This way, at least you come out even. Otherwise, you'll pay 90 cents and have nothing to show for it." (Yes, I recognize that this is manipulation. It is purposely done to demonstrate a common phenomenon in conflict escalation. The game effectively portrays the dynamics of disputes, and most participants accept this function.) The bidding now stands at one dollar. The person with the 95-cent bid realizes that he too may lose his bid with nothing to show for it, so he goes to $1.05. Usually at this point some participants drop out, although enough remain for active bidding to continue. The higher we go above the one-dollar bid, the greater are the increments between bids. We move from increasing in 5-cent increments to making 25-cent jumps, one-dollar jumps, and even three-dollar leaps.

At this point, of course, the game has become seemingly irrational. If someone were to enter the room and observe the exercise, they would marvel at a group of intelligent professionals yelling out bids of $15 and $18 for a mere one-dollar bill. At one seminar, two health care executives both decided they wanted the dollar. They became entangled in a bidding war that reached $31! Other par-

ticipants sat in wonderment as the two nervously moved the bidding beyond the bounds of the conceivable. It finally stopped when
the loser ran out of money: he had had $30 in his wallet.

The exercise is designed to illustrate the dynamics of conflict
and the role they play in building a motive to settle.

Conflict Costs

Conflict gobbles time and money, diverts attention from other activities, and consumes our ability to make rational decisions (see Blake
and Mouton, 1984). When we spend five work days engaged in a
battle, we are unable to retrieve the time lost. Just as we must pay
our last bid in the simulation exercise, we must pay the $100,000
legal bill we have accumulated on our $25,000 dispute, even if we
lose. And when a dispute plagues a health care practice, the toll on
staff morale lingers well beyond the last salvo of the fight.

The bidding simulation is called "Arms Race" because it illustrates an irrational pattern of competition similar to the Cold War
arms race between the United States and the Soviet Union.
Though each side could already destroy the other several times
over, when one nation developed a new weapons system, the other
felt compelled to further up the ante. We now recall that perilous
period with the hindsight and wisdom of history. The world was
subjected to enormous risk, cost, and diversion to build and maintain an ultimately unusable armament that voraciously threatened
our very survival.

The problem is that once we have acted irrationally, we feel
compelled to justify our madness. We do that by winning: "You see,
it made sense to pay $22, because in the end, I got the dollar!" The
terror is paying $21 and *not* getting the payoff. One can just imag-
ine the conversation with a spouse after a day of training: "Honey,
you see, there was an auction, and the instructor was selling a dollar. I paid $21, though in the end, I didn't get the dollar." Insult
compounds injury.

Picture yourself and a colleague in a bidding war. The price is likely to reach $10. You both can reduce your losses if you stop bidding at $3, $5, or even $8. And stopping before the one-dollar mark is reached allows at least one person, if not more, to actually benefit, since the total time, money, and investment is less than the value of the issue at hand. Similarly, if a difference over budgeting is settled before it becomes a time-consuming squabble, you are more likely to find a creative solution that shares costs and perhaps even provides mutual benefit.

You build a motive for resolving conflict by establishing and appropriating the dividends derived from reaching a resolution. Those dividends may be tangible, such as money, space, or equipment, or intangible, such as time, reputation, or satisfaction. Money not used in the battle can be split among the parties involved. Office space, for example, needed by one group in the first shift can be shared with a different group in the second shift, as can be the rental costs for both. Parties can share the kudos for resolving a dispute, combine the accomplishments of cooperation, and join in the benefits of good communication. If these benefits are known and mutually recognized, the potential itself may provide the motive to settle in and of itself.

Turning the Obsession

Bidders who climb beyond the one-dollar mark are often caught by the obsession to win. The dollar has taken on a new value. It is not a mere one hundred cents. It assumes grandiose symbolic meaning, enmeshing self-image, public humiliation, and personal objectives. To obtain the dollar is to achieve status, recognition, and power. To lose it is to risk ruin. Once the obsession to win prevails, jumping off the bandwagon becomes unthinkable.

Bidders captured by the obsession are quick to formulate a rationale for their bidding. They later explain that they were doing it for a "cause." They describe empathy for Jeremy's losing his dad. They want to give the kid some small compensation. They express their admiration for the charity and desire to make a contribution. The cause becomes a mask for their infatuation with getting the dollar.

This is a common human phenomenon. If we become convinced of the "rightness" of a purpose, there is little we are willing to withhold in its pursuit. The cause could be a moral principle, such as upholding a patient's right to determine the course of his or her care. It could be upholding your organization, especially if your professional survival depends on the plight of the institution. Or the cause could be on behalf of a profession or a larger affinity group, your country, ethnic persuasion, or religion. If the cause is right, we will sacrifice our life, risk arrest, or ruin our career in the name of the mission. Once we have made the first irrational leap—bidding $1.10 for a dollar bill—it is difficult to turn back. After all, how can we justify doing something that is clearly illogical? We march under the banner of our symbols—flags, professional prestige, or organizational purpose.

Anyone who opposes the cause is "the enemy." Overcoming the enemy assumes a virtue of its own, propelling the cause into a matter of personal pride or even survival. "If we don't shut them down first, our hospital and our jobs are gone." "It's a matter of professional pride. If everyone thinks they can do our work, soon there won't be a need for cardiologists." "We have to show the hospitals we can't be pushed around. Otherwise, why would the health commissioner want to keep our department funded?"

Conflict often is fueled by the "enemy" image. Only a few years ago, the president of the United States referred to the Soviet Union as "the evil empire." In the evil empire, there were no children in brightly colored cloths, no ballerinas or intellectuals. The predominant images were missiles parading through Red Square. This enemy image then justified increased spending for defense and further construction of weapons. Once the sides view each other as the enemy and their battle as the struggle for survival, conflict escalation becomes boundless.

In this way, the dollar assumes added value. I contribute to this inflation of value by noting several unremarkable features of the bill: "It's printed on both sides. It has a genuine picture of the first president of the United States. And it is suitable for framing." These facetious remarks somehow only fuel the fiction that this is a special dollar bill that you want in your possession.

Imagine a shift: the obsession to win transformed into the urge to settle. That obsession was fueled by its own momentum: it swelled so quickly that it became seemingly unstoppable. At that point, the momentum itself was frightening for the disputants, as they lost control of the acceleration and their role in it. Recognizing that ominous quality of obsession, the parties can be motivated to settle in order to avoid irreparable disaster and ruin. The dash toward victory pretended to be a plausible individual strategy for asserting control. Moving toward settlement is a way of regaining real, shared control. Tempering the pace not only reverses the obsession, it offers its own motive to settle. Achieving settlement becomes as righteous a purpose as the arguments that started the conflict in the first place.

Changing the Game

After the arms race simulation, several people observe that they entered the bidding because it was fun. Conflict can be fun. There is the thrill of taking a risk and wondering what will happen on the other side. There is a sense of engagement and participation that comes with being part of the action. There is the rush of victory.

Shortly after the Persian Gulf War, I spoke with close friends who had moved to Jerusalem. I asked them what it was like to retreat into their sealed rooms when the sirens signaled a Scud missile attack. They explained that while it was frightening, there was also a sense of excitement, especially in the beginning. There was a feeling that the whole country was pulling together, that they would overcome the Iraqis and that life would soon return to normal, with plenty of good stories to tell. Only after the threat had dragged on past a few weeks did the nights in the shelters become tedious.

A conflict between two departments in a hospital can offer the same thrills as playing a game of ball. There is the sensation of belonging to a team with a common purpose and a common enemy. There is the challenge to outdo the other side. There is the anticipation of victory and the anticipated delight of watching the other side fall in defeat. Sweet revenge.

A technique sometimes used in mediation can help parties in a dispute transform the character of the game. The parties enter the mediation room and naturally sit at opposite sides of the table. The mediator opens the session, describes the process, and asks each side to offer a brief explanation of the problem. After assessing points of disagreement and agreement and pinpointing the key problems, the mediator rearranges the disputants at the table. Asking them to sit together on one side, the mediator places the problems symbolically on the other side. The game is then reframed: it is now between the problems on one side and our collective capacity to solve them on the other. If the disputants can develop a mutual desire to move beyond the conflict, this conversion can help them turn the corner.

Turning the Temper

Placed together, cost, obsession, purpose, entanglement, and the pursuit of victory evoke strong emotions: anger, fear, joy, anxiety, pain, elation, and distress. These emotions of conflict assume an inertia of their own. When you are gripped by rage, mistrust, or animosity, forging a clear balance between what makes sense and what feels right becomes difficult, if not impossible. These emotions cloud our vision, inflame our passions, and forge walls between us and others. Passion is neither right nor wrong: it is simply there, and so it must be considered as you assess what is causing your conflict to escalate and what might turn it toward resolution.

At the end of the Arms Race exercise, we pass a hat around and people pay their last bid of the game. Once the hat has been around the room, someone adds up the collected money. I note that the dollar did not simply cost this group the amount of the last bid, $31. In fact, the real aggregate cost to the group was the total sum collected, $196!

The real cost of conflict is not merely our own legal bill, lost time, or frazzled emotions. For the HMO, nursing department, or medical practice, the real costs of conflict are the combined losses for each of the staff members: their time and morale, as well as the impact that the dispute has on the quality of patient care. For a community health project, the real price of infighting among coalition members is a loss of services and support for the people they intend to help. For the patient, a breakdown in communication with caregivers results in increased vulnerability and anxiety over interrupted care, and the negative impact that these emotions can have upon health status. Each of these have long-term implications that will negatively impact future interactions.

If you and your compatriot in conflict want to move toward resolution, someone needs to interrupt the process of escalation. It could be you, it could be the other person, or it could be someone else, perhaps a colleague who has watched the costs of the disagreement accumulate for both of you. After all, would it not be better to cease your bidding at $10, before it reaches $20, 25, or even more? What can be done to forge the motive to settle? What are the steps that will bring about an interruption of the escalation?

Step One: Accept Conflict

Step one in moving beyond conflict is to accept it as a given. If we acknowledge that in some form conflict is inevitable, then we can develop workable strategies to live and even thrive with it. Health care involves so many people, so many decisions, so many tasks, and so many problems. With overwhelming action happening so quickly, chances are that we will bump into one another at some point along the way. Not every bump need be fatal.

If professional disputes are expected as part of the lay of the land, they can be addressed for what they are. They can be anticipated, prevented, managed, assessed, and resolved. They are a part of doing business.

Several years ago, I spoke with a physician who was planning an innovative service for AIDS patients. Putting together the necessary network of insurers, providers, and community agencies demanded a complex and costly process of negotiation. I asked what would happen if a conflict emerged among these many groups once the service was in operation. The physician replied, "Well, then we'll just shut it down." While the response seems extreme, it is not uncommon. If one can't work with conflict, then the only available option is sacrifice of enormous work, investment, and opportunity.

Conflict, if functionally conceived, even can be seen as a plus: an expression we want to encourage. The willingness to assert a concern offers an important check and balance on health care. If a nurse believes an inappropriate medication has been prescribed, raising the issue will benefit both the patient and the physician who ordered the medication. The interchange can only be constructive if the nurse knows how and is prepared to raise it and the physician knows how and is able to accept it. If this balance does not work, an important piece of information will be lost.

The airline industry recognized the importance of conflict as a check and balance after the early 1980s Air Florida crash in Washington, D.C. It was a snowy day at National Airport, and flights were backed up for hours. After much delay, the Air Florida plane was finally de-iced and allowed to head for the runway. Sitting on the tarmac for over thirty minutes, more snow and ice accumulated on the wings, forcing the pilot to return to the terminal for another de-icing. Once again the plane headed for the runway, and after another delay it was cleared for takeoff. Just as the plane started to accelerate, the copilot observed a dangerous buildup of ice on the wings and mentioned it to the pilot. Impatient to finally get off the ground, the pilot ignored the warning and accelerated down the runway. Without proper lift, the plane barely got off the ground before crashing into the Potomac River. In reviewing the tragedy, investigators realized that the problem was not one of aerodynamics: it is known that airplanes can't fly with ice on their wings. Rather, this was a problem of conflict and communication. If the pilot ignores the copilot, a vital source of information and balance is lost to crucial decision making. Commercial pilots now are required to attend resource management courses, during which they are trained to better express and work with their differences.

A conflict does not exist between two people if not given some form of expression. The expression can be manifest in many forms: you can verbalize it; you can absent yourself from a planned meeting; you can file a lawsuit. In other words, if you are unhappy with someone and do not reveal your displeasure or disagreement in some way, then you have personal frustration and anxiety, though not conflict. The question becomes how the conflict is initially framed and presented. It could begin, "You jerk, you did it again!" or it could begin, "I think there is a problem here that negatively affects both of us and that we should discuss." Two very different ways to express the very same predicament. The first breeds a climate of antagonism and the second opens a door to resolution.

Conflict is a social phenomenon. It exists between two or more people. Even if the disagreement is not acknowledged or understood by the recipient of the frustration, once it is out in the open, the bidding has begun. The question is how to express disagreement—and how to hear it—so that the problem can receive some form of constructive attention. Without such an exchange, building progress toward a resolution is a formidable if not impossible task.

Step Two: Recognize the Consequences

The second step in moving beyond conflict and building motive is recognizing the costs of ignoring a shared problem. If two people work closely together and one becomes annoyed with the other, then both have a problem. By dodging fundamental issues, there is the risk that the matter will escalate. The tone of the conflict is shaped by initial expressions and reactions. Will it be a fight? Will it be a solution? What are the consequences?

Remember, the fact that one person disagrees with another is not inherently bad. Whether or not the disagreement becomes a problem depends on how it is handled. If the problem is ignored or dismissed or demeaned, then you have an even bigger problem.

The dangers of a fight unresolved are especially acute in health care. Clinicians function in close quarters, exchanging information and assisting one another in patient care. A standoff not only damages professional relationships, it invariably infects patient care, spreading the contamination well beyond the scope and cost of the origin of the dispute. Similarly, an unyielding attitude agitates the balance necessary for effective health care management. It interferes with the stability of relationships necessary to guide a steady course for the organization. Certainly, combat over health policy and regulation sends providers and patients scurrying to keep one step ahead of the next constraint by skipping into the nearest loophole. The cat and mouse game only distorts the cost and quality of care. Whatever the forum, the tasks of health care require uncommon interdependence. Unresolved conflict is a formidable obstacle.

◆ ◆ ◆ ◆ ◆ ◆ ◆ ◆

Forty-six-year-old Gail Godfried has spent the bulk of her nursing career in intensive care. She has always found ICU work to be the ultimate in nursing: helping the people who most need attention. It is exciting and challenging work, with something new to learn every day.

Heather Harriford, twenty-five, has been out of nursing school for three years, and has been working in intensive care for the past seven months. She is not sure she wants to stick with the ICU. The work is draining. Everyone is always in crisis mode. People seem to forget the basic courtesies of "please" and "thank you" when they are in the unit. She doesn't mind it from the patients—after all, since they are so very sick.

It's the families that really bug her. Families don't understand that the ICU staff have a job to do and that they can't do it if family members are constantly bothering them.

The charge nurse assigned Godfried and Harriford to set up Artie Ashwood in Room D of the unit.

"Ewing really wimped out with this one," Harriford complained as the two moved around the bed, setting up the equipment surrounding Ashwood. "I thought we were going to have a quiet night after he acted so uppity about that last patient. If Walker were still chief resident, this never would have happened."

Before she could think, Godfried blurted out, "It's not a matter of wimpy. This patient needs to be here." She immediately stopped herself. She hates it when a nurse or doctor talks about a patient while in the room. Harriford set the trap once again and she fell right into it. Godfried was furious at herself for responding. There was a stony silence as each of them hurriedly finished her work. The tension was palpable.

Harriford was the first out the door and on her way to the nurses' station. Godfried marched out shortly thereafter, and caught up to her at the desk. Two other nurses and a physician were quietly writing in the medical charts. "You never do that again, Harriford. I've told you this a million times. If you've got a complaint, do it out here, not in the patient's room. And Ewing wasn't a wimp! That patient is very sick. He's in the right place." She stomped off toward the hallway.

Harriford turned to the others, who had watched the exchange. "Bitch."

◆　◆　◆　◆　◆　◆　◆

Both Harriford and Godfried have a problem. Its expression poses danger for both of them. It also poses a danger for their patients, the hospital administration, and the other people working on the unit. What if their hostility spreads? What if other members of the staff take sides: the older nurses against the younger nurses? What if it gets in the way of the vigilance and cooperation necessary to keep the ICU operating at necessary efficiency and effectiveness?

Step Three: Formalize Motive

Step three in shifting toward resolution is declaring your desire to settle. This desire eventually must be expressed and known to all parties to the dispute.

I periodically receive calls from people interested in mediation. Sometimes the call comes from a member of a staff concerned about an escalating conflict that threatens his or her viability. Sometimes it comes from an attorney, prompted by a judge to find a settlement for a malpractice case without burdening the courtroom. Sometimes the call comes from a director, wishing to resolve conflict among subordinates without managerial dictate.

I ask the same question of all parties: "Are each of you interested in looking for settlement? If not, I'm not interested in mediating for the two of you."

The response is rarely an enthusiastic "Yes!" Their hesitation stems from both pain and strategy. If I am speaking directly to one of the disputants, he or she generally feels angry, vengeful, and bruised. The thought of settling is mixed with the desire to see the other side eliminated from the face of the planet. I acknowledge these feelings, given the usual nature and the emotion associated with conflict.

The other concern is one of appearance. They recognize that continuing the battle is costing them dearly. A total win is unlikely. Nonetheless, they do not want to appear to be giving in. They want to distinguish the desire to settle from the acceptance of defeat. I assure them that settlement in mediation is voluntary. If they are not pleased with the process or outcome, they can walk out at any time. Throughout the process, they remain in control of the negotiation.

An attorney once told me that the insurance company she represented did not believe a settlement was warranted in the malpractice case that we were discussing. I replied, "Fine, then we are not interested in mediating the case." She called back several weeks later. "The carrier reassessed the case and they are now ready to discuss settlement." Finding a resolution required little more than four hours of mediation.

In another case, the mediation discourse had descended into bitter feuding. One party turned to the other and proclaimed, "Before we sat down here, you said you were looking for settlement. You are not acting like someone looking for settlement." The other party calmed down. The reminder was helpful to both.

Whether it be a formal mediation or an informal discussion, if all parties do not share some desire to resolve the conflict, it is unlikely to end. If only one party wants settlement, the conflict is likely to continue. It may escalate to a win-lose situation, with one party eventually falling to defeat. Or one party may give up, resigning to a loss, leaving employment or surrendering the battle.

Between continuing to fight and beginning to settle, deciding to settle is often the better of the two bad choices. Though a reluctant framework for moving forward, it is nonetheless a legitimate way to weigh the options. Conflict is full of unpalatable choices. The key is whether the parties can begin to accept that they are unlikely to achieve an outright win. Recognizing this, their motives in the conflict shift toward exploring resolution.

Step Four: Begin the Learning Process

Step four in overcoming conflict is learning from it: not an easy task. The verbiage sent your way is laden with emotion and accusation. You hear it through your own filter of defensiveness and hurt feelings. Both sides are reactive.

Why struggle to learn? Because beneath the rhetoric, there is some measure of validity to what each of you is saying. The slurs and accusations you exchange may not be valid, though behind the aspersions you cast there are genuine feelings, concerns, convictions, and beliefs that lie at the heart of the dispute you share. In fact, you have much in common with the other person. There is much to be gained in understanding what are those points of commonality and difference. You discover that your different experiences, training, and beliefs have molded divergent approaches to everyday problems.

We often find this during a mediation. At the first mediation session, we seat the parties around a table. Each disputant opens with a brief explanation of how they see the conflict. While their adversaries listen, the disputants recount the words and events that led to the standoff. The talk is usually solemn and measured. At this stage of the process, disputants begin to hear each other, calmly, for the first time. They are learning about shared differences and commonalties. They discover their regard for one another, their frustrations with one another, and their common desire for settlement.

This learning process was key to the resolution of a dispute between two physicians that I mediated several years ago. In the course of the mediation, the two physicians were surprised to learn that they shared many of the same objectives for their joint practice. On the questions of money and management, the matters about which they battled, there was fundamental agreement. On the most important issue, whether they respected each other's clinical skills, there was complete congruence.

What then were the problems? The most important turned out to be differences in age, attitudes, and personality. One of the physicians was nearly fifty years old and preferred a hierarchical approach to decision making and authority. "When I was in his position, I paid my dues to my mentors. I've been paying my dues all my career, and now it's your turn to pay yours." The other physician, ten years his junior, was in college during the Vietnam protests and had no interest in a hierarchical decision-making structure—or in paying dues. He grew up to "question authority," and he felt that there was no need to submit to the demands of his colleague. With better understanding, they found that they could accept their personality and attitudinal differences in exchange for maintaining an important common objective: keeping their joint medical practice alive.

Step Five: Find the Logic

Step five is assessment. To listen and to agree are not the same. Is there some validity to what the other person is saying? What is the problem that underlies the words? Is the other person perhaps reacting to an experience separate from the immediate problem? Are you reacting to what the other person is actually saying, or rather are you reacting to the way or the time it is said?

◆ ◆ ◆ ◆ ◆ ◆ ◆

Gail Godfried always found a cup of yogurt to be her best source of relaxation. She sat alone in the nurses' lounge off the ICU. She needed to compose herself before she went back onto the floor.

She reminded herself of how she hates Harriford. Harriford is arrogant, inappropriate, and inexperienced. Gail hates Harriford's popularity. Perhaps that mouth will finally be her undoing, and create enough trouble that she is shown the door.

Despite those feelings, Godfried had to admit that she had the same reservations about the patient. He needed to be in the ICU, not because of his condition. No, he needed to be in the ICU because sending him to the medical floor would have been dangerous. Everyone in the hospital knows that the medical floors are so understaffed they can barely make it through the night. One sick patient needing close observation would overwhelm them: they have other patients needing care. It's true that the ICU isn't doing anything for this patient. Though if he weren't here, he would die before anyone on the med floors would notice.

And then there are the crazy reimbursement incentives. What if he is a Medicaid patient? It's always easier for the hospital to collect if it is shown that the patient was really sick.

That's the logic of the system: if he was not sick enough to go to the ICU, he was not sick enough for someone to pay the bill.

All these big questions are no matter, though, when it comes to Harriford. You don't create more stress for the patient by mentioning your concerns bedside. That was simply wrong. They should be teaching these young nurses good manners.

* * * * * * *

By its very nature, conflict is a process of polarization. When two people are in conflict, they characteristically move to opposite sides of the issue. They fortify their position by overstating their case, creating further distance between themselves. As the conflict escalates, they become more resolute in defending their position and destroying that of their opponent.

Conflict is also a process of simplification. We ignore the reasons, justifications, viewpoints, and concerns of the other side. We dismiss the texture of their statements, and we are blind to the weaknesses of our own. They are wrong and we are right. Their problem is without merit; ours is valid.

Given this common tendency to polarize and simplify the issues, accomplishing a balanced assessment of their concerns and yours is no easy matter. Ury (1991) suggests that you "go to the balcony": get a view of the conflict from a distance. Understand the dispute from the vantage of their experience: How might the responsibilities, training, and objectives of the hospital CEO affect her view of the staffing question? In light of their experience and salary expectations, how might we understand the unrelenting resistance of the medical staff to budget changes? How is their child's terminal illness affecting the parents' ability to cope with the requests of the staff? All of this is not to say that you must agree with those on the other side of your conflict. The CEO may be callous, the medical staff may be unreasonable, and the parents may be obnoxious. Yet, as we begin to grasp their rationale, we transform the conflict from

black and white to gray, from right and wrong to common ground,
and we begin to move from conflict toward resolution.

Step Six: Check the Choices

Often, people enveloped in a dispute assume only two choices: "I
win or I lose." Furthermore, "When I win, I want to inflict some
multiple of the pain and expense I suffered upon my opponent." In
these scenarios, even if there is a clear winner, both sides suffer
unrecoverable losses of time, money, and professional regard. The
hours spent plotting, the opportunities lost in the process, and the
discomfort shared among colleagues are endured by all sides in a
win-lose scenario. The winner gets to lick wounds in the comfort
of victory. The loser is left to ponder what might be the next line
of attack.

Finding common ground is a process of joint discovery. Step six
requires you and other disputants to embark together on that quest,
to develop options for settlement. It may be a compromise. It could
be an exchange. Perhaps an acknowledgment or an apology. As this
happens, the parties amplify their learning about one another. And
even more important, they begin learning about themselves. In portraying the other side as the villain, you have ignored your own contributions to the predicament. How have your behaviors or demands
polarized the dispute? What changes might you consider? What do
you really hope to achieve? What will satisfy those objectives? What
are you concerned about losing? What do you hope to retain? The
answers to these questions gradually become evident as you consider, accept, and reject newly discovered possibilities for agreement.

Step Seven: Ponder the Possibilities

Imagine what could be accomplished if we are really working
together. You have considered the consequences of continuing the
battle. What about the possibilities of making the unit work again?
What if we could get beyond the battle and share the rewards: there
is money, professional satisfaction, and loads of recognition waiting

on the other side. These are the rewards of making the system work. The peace of having the dispute behind you. The satisfaction of solving a challenging puzzle.

That sense of hope and resourcefulness can motivate disputants toward resolution. If consequences are the sticks, then possibilities are the carrots.

Finding the possibilities is elusive in a complex organization. The immediate parties to the conflict may not have the authority to change the operant variables.

◆ ◆ ◆ ◆ ◆ ◆ ◆

Iris Inkwater dreads these early-morning meetings. As chief executive officer of Oppidania General, she balances among the competing demands of too many departments. She sometimes feels her job is in the realm of the near-impossible, especially with all the changes now crossing her desk. On one side, she is negotiating with HMOs, government agencies, and insurers who expect more service for less money. On the other side, she has to make the hospital deliver with fewer dollars to spread around.

Last week Fred Fisher, the hospital's chief of medicine, asked for this morning's meeting. He requested three people in the room: Inkwater; Janice Johnson, the vice president for nursing; and himself. He wants to discuss staffing for the night shift on the medical floors.

Fisher and Johnson exchange the usual niceties as they enter the office. The mood turns serious when Inkwater turns to Fisher and asks, "What's on your mind?"

Fisher opens, "I've been talking with a number of the residents and chiefs. We have a major problem with staffing on the medical floors, especially at night. The nursing coverage is so poor that people are reluctant to admit onto those floors. There is an unspoken assumption that if patients are sick enough to be in the hospital, they're too sick to be on the medical floor. If we were confident of better coverage, we could reduce the number of people going into the ICU. I'm sure that would save a bundle in the long run. As it stands now, I think this is a dangerous and wasteful situation. I did mention this to Ms. Johnson a while ago, but there has been no improvement."

Johnson was seething. This was a setup, and she didn't like this accusation in front of her boss. She looked at Inkwater, made eye contact, and then turned to Fisher. She wanted to signal that she was taking the high ground in this discussion.

"Dr. Fisher, I recognize that this is a problem. I share many of your concerns. Each of our departments is working with a bare-bones staff. You only brought this to my attention two weeks ago. Since then, I have been meeting with my supervisors to see how we might shift people around. It's not only a matter of positions; it's also a question of who has the experience and the desire to go where. I know that you have people putting pressure on you. But you have to understand, this is a complicated problem that can't be solved overnight."

Johnson looked back at Inkwater. Inkwater was impressed. There was silence. Fisher was caught off guard and felt a rare moment of speechlessness.

Inkwater reopened the conversation. "There seem to be a number of issues here. Besides the general problems of staffing and money, there is also the question of timing. Dr. Fisher, I don't hear Janice saying that she doesn't want to respond to your request. It's just a matter of when."

"It's not that simple. We have patients coming in here every day. We can't tell them to hold off while the nursing department decides to do a reshuffle. I have the medical staff down my back. These guys are worried about liability. What if something happens to one of their patients while we are waiting to fix this mess? It has been in the making for more than just two weeks."

"Dr. Fisher, I do want to fix this problem, though I am going to need your help," Janice offered. "Unless Iris tells me differently, I cannot look forward to any expansion in the number of nursing positions in the department. The only department that is overstaffed right now is the ICU. I might be able to move someone from that unit down to the medical floors, and to do so, I'm going to need your support. They have gotten accustomed to a large staff up there and they're going to squawk. I'll still be up to code, so we don't have to worry about legal problems. It's more a matter of political problems with your staff."

Fisher was unprepared for this line of reasoning. He had hoped that Inkwater would submit to his argument and offer Johnson some room to maneuver in the budget. That's what always happened in the past.

Inkwater supported Johnson. "I am afraid Janice is right. We're going to need your help on this one."

Johnson added, "One of the young nurses on the ICU, Heather Harriford, has been talking about a transfer to another unit. She is only reluctant about a cut in pay. I think I could keep her at the same scale as a way to encourage her to move."

Fisher had heard of Harriford. Ken Kavanaugh, chief of the ICU, had mentioned her. He felt she was a good nurse, yet she didn't fit in well with the other ICU nurses, many of whom had been with the unit for many years. If Kavanaugh were to lose anyone, he would put up the least fuss about Harriford, especially if it were accompanied by a real effort by the rest of the medical staff to go easy on ICU admissions.

Fisher turned to Johnson with a smile, "OK, it's not ideal, but let's give it a try."

◆ ◆ ◆ ◆ ◆ ◆ ◆

Step Eight: Find Common Purpose

The turning point for Fisher came when he realized that he was in the same game as Johnson. He was even on the same side of the table.

◆ ◆ ◆ ◆ ◆ ◆ ◆

It's not merely nursing against medicine, or medicine against the hospital, Fisher thought to himself. It used to be like that. All you needed to do was ask and it was yours. Then things became tight. Now it's different. If you are going to get anything, you're going to have to give something up.

◆ ◆ ◆ ◆ ◆ ◆ ◆

Step eight in moving beyond conflict is finding a common purpose and common solutions. It's not one department against the other. Rather, if we view the hospital as a whole, then we share a common purpose in making the system work. Yes, that does sometimes mean giving to get. It is a perspective that implicitly acknowledges our interdependence as an institution and as a system. If we view health care as an interconnected mechanism, then we see that if one of the parts malfunctions, the whole machine breaks down. Common responsibility makes for common solutions.

Step Nine: Anticipate Conflict

If conflict is a known and anticipated phenomenon in health care organizations and relations, then we can prepare for it. As we plan a program, establish an organization, or reorganize our institution, we can ask a series of questions to help us prepare for conflict:

What are the potential disputes that we may encounter down the road?

How are we going to resolve those issues so they cause minimal disruption for operations and minimal drain on the budget?

What can we do to manage those conflicts that do occur?

How can we change or rearrange the organization to reduce the likelihood of conflict?

What will we do to learn from those disputes and then appropriately adjust our procedures to lessen the likelihood that the problem will reoccur?

With these questions on hand early in your planning process, and every day in your operational processes, the chances of conflict debilitating or destroying your operation is greatly reduced.

Step Ten: Move Beyond Conflict

We call this approach to moving beyond conflict "Whole Image Negotiation."

"Whole" points us to seek the big picture in our exchanges, to find our common purpose. If we are only looking after our own department, our own institution, or our own profession, the chances of making the system work as a whole will be greatly diminished. Building solutions based on our common interests and objectives will create outcomes that will work better in the long run for all of our interdependent units. That is the nature of health care.

"Image" requires us to see something that is not readily apparent. The health care system, by its very nature, is in a process of constant change. What emerges on the other side of each phase of transformation is only in our imagination. Our greatest discoveries emerge from that willingness to peer beyond our current realities to find innovative solutions. When we find opportunities and construct systems that best meet our common needs and interests — fairly balancing resources, services, and costs — our chances for constructing a health system that accommodates the full range of our aspirations are greatly enhanced.

The best negotiators are those who bring an imagination to the process. They can find solutions where they are not readily apparent. They can introduce processes that are otherwise unknown to the other parties. And they can reach outcomes that would otherwise elude the parties.

Whole image negotiation provides a W.I.N., a triumph that those who are part of the process can share.

3

Setting the Stage for Negotiation

Negotiation is a multidimensional process. Your understanding of the dimensions improves your negotiation style, strategies, and outcomes.

Negotiation is about exchange. Its purpose is to produce an action, outcome, or decision. You negotiate in order to gain something from someone else. In return, the other person likely will want to receive something of value. To get what you want, you must be willing to give that something or be certain the other person is getting it.

Negotiation is about discovery. It is how you learn what other people want to receive and give. It is how you inform them of the same.

Negotiation occurs in stages, over time. It begins with discovery. People define what they want or what they perceive. Information is exchanged. Through that exchange, the parties determine if they can find an agreement to satisfy their different desires. In so doing, they determine the outcome of the exchange. For people with an ongoing relationship, the outcome of one exchange influences what happens in the next round.

Negotiation is shaped by power. In the give-and-take of negotiation, the more power people have, the less they must give. Conversely, the less power people have, the more they must give. Because those with less power generally have less to give, they often find themselves dependent and vulnerable during negotiation.

These negotiation dimensions are dynamic: they constantly shift and change. As they change, they engender new balances and imbalances. The changes define and redefine relationships and actions.

Health care is shifting rapidly. These shifts affect each of these negotiation dimensions. To assume they are static is to significantly limit your negotiation effectiveness. To understand their dynamics is to influence the course of their evolution.

Negotiation as Exchange

Explicit Negotiation

We often think of negotiation as something we do when purchasing an item or service that has no fixed price. For example, in bargaining for an automobile, there is a back and forth about price, in which the condition of the car, how many extras it has, and the state of the market are all considered. A deal is either struck or declined. Likewise, we think of negotiation as something we do to reach or influence a decision about which there is a choice. There is negotiation about who gets what office space, for example, or when someone will be on duty.

We also think of negotiation as something that is used to settle a disagreement. Parties negotiate until a resolution is achieved or a stalemate blocks progress. If there is a deadlock and a decision must be finalized, such as in a legal suit or a personnel action, someone else will likely be asked to decide for the parties. This third party could be a judge or an organizational superior.

Negotiating a purchase and sale or settling a dispute are examples of explicit forms of negotiation. The terms of agreement are observable. The parties are clear about the nature of the process and the criteria for making the decision.

Implicit Negotiation

By contrast, implicit negotiation involves unspoken assumptions that frame the exchange. These assumptions are rarely discussed.

Implicit negotiation relies upon social convention to govern relationships and purposes. It is as if the parties have a script that defines their behaviors, relationship, and expectations. The script establishes the rules of exchange and the roles and status of the people involved.

We rarely consider the purchase of fixed-priced items as a matter of negotiation. When my son was six years old, he was fascinated by the back-and-forth of bargaining in Arab marketplaces during a trip to the Middle East. Upon our return, he suggested we try bargaining in the supermarket for a box of spaghetti. We explained that this sort of explicit dealing is unheard of for grocery items. I would be violating the "script" of appropriate supermarket behavior if I took a 99-cent box of spaghetti to the cashier and offered her 59 cents for it.

Though open bartering over the price of spaghetti is considered inappropriate, implicit negotiation does occur when you buy groceries. As long as I have the choice of shopping at another supermarket, I can go elsewhere to get a better price. Knowing this, the store is motivated to offer high-quality goods at competitive prices. This sort of implicit negotiation works only when there is another source of the desired goods. If there is no other source of spaghetti, my negotiation leverage works only if I am willing to forego pasta.

Similarly, implicit negotiation is at work in health care. However, it is problematic if there is only one health care provider in town and I require health service. Furthermore, if I am unable to discern what is good-quality from poor-quality health service, I am ill-equipped to effectively engage in implicit negotiation. This form of bargaining functions only when there is a choice available and criteria by which to exercise that choice knowledgeably.

Implicit negotiation is also the process by which we exchange intangibles: information and social status. Intangibles are constantly being traded in our clinics and between our health care institutions. These intangibles determine the substance and process of decision making and action. They are possessed by one person and desired by another.

Information Exchange

Information is the most commonly exchanged intangible. This category includes the knowledge, expertise, and data necessary for decision making. Knowledge encompasses everything from the psychosocial status of a patient to the clinical options for a particular disease category. Expertise incorporates the proficiency to apply knowledge to particular decisions and actions. While knowledge and expertise are cognitive capabilities resting with people, data are those dispassionate facts and figures that predict the likelihood of a particular medical outcome or trends affecting market share. When combined with experience, knowledge, expertise, and data spawn wisdom.

Given the scope of information necessary for good decision making, it is unlikely that one person alone can possess all the necessary wisdom. That is why health care is so social an enterprise: essential information must be gathered, exchanged, and circulated among numerous people involved in a case. This information is held by health professionals, researchers, administrators, and, very importantly, the patient himself or herself.

The outcome of care is only as good as the decisions directing the course of treatment. That decision-making process is dependent on the quality of information exchange.

Exchanging Social Status

The second and more perplexing category of intangible exchange is social status: authority, responsibility, and recognition. These shape our relationships with others and thereby frame our self-perception and affect our personal satisfaction.

Authority is about who decides. Who orders the medications? Who draws up the budget? Who determines whether the patient will be resuscitated? It also pertains to patients' rights. What is the system legally and morally allowed to decide for the patient? What set of decisions rests solely with the patient?

Who has the authority is determined by the social framework of decision making. It is assigned and delineated in job descriptions, laws, social mores, and other signals of behavior. In a changing system, the question of who decides is a moving target. This is now the case in health care. The problem of shifting authority is aggravated by the already complex and overlapping domains of jurisdiction. Current shifts blur the lines between what is in your complete control, what is in the realm of no control, and what is negotiable.

Insurance is a good example. A privately insured patient had substantial freedom in choosing physicians and hospitals in the days before managed care. Now many of those decisions are in the sphere of the negotiable or outside the patient's control. Likewise, in the past physicians were able to order procedures with little interference from a utilization review manager. Now many procedures must be approved through a process of negotiation, with the physician pleading the necessity of care. If the procedure is disapproved, the patient must choose whether to appeal to the insurer or pay for the treatment out of pocket. Similarly, if regulatory and insurance agencies rule that reimbursement rates are nonnegotiable, then providers find their compensation package in the zone of no control (see Figure 3.1).

The most rancorous debates about changes for the health system are essentially about shifting where these lines are drawn. What decisions are placed in what circle? Who decides the cost of drugs? Who prescribes those medications? And who is obligated to pick up the bill if the patient cannot pay?

Indeed, during a period of change, many decisions that were at either end of the spectrum are shifting to the middle circle, to that arena which is negotiable. Health care administrators concerned about balancing their books want to sway decisions, such as clinical decisions, toward the realm of the negotiable or complete control. Patients are apprehensive about weakened leverage, especially

Figure 3.1. Perspectives on Decision Making.

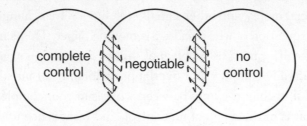

DECISIONS INVOLVING YOU AND SOMEONE ELSE
Do you agree on the circle in which the decision is located?

Shaded areas depict conflict in the decision-
making process.

if they have no control over when and from whom they receive care. Private practice physicians accustomed to entrepreneurial independence fear lost control of their earning capacity.

The "script" of health care decision making is being rewritten. During a period of change, everyone reads from a different draft that they presume will approximate the final version. In the process, colleagues read from unmatched scripts, using different assumptions and rules to define relations and decisions. Some, especially those who did well in the "good old days," cling to the old scripts. Others shift to a new script, certain that their associates will follow. And many are simply caught in the confusion, adjusting to the prevailing script for the day or occasion.

The very drawing of these lines is a matter of implicit negotiation. What do *you* decide? What do *I* decide? What do *we* decide? As it pertains to policy, the negotiation occurs in Washington and state capitals around the country. As it pertains to patient care decisions, it occurs in clinics, administrative offices, and hospital hallways every day, all the time. The pace and flavor of this negotiation are symptoms of the system's change. There will be conflict if consensus isn't reached on what decision is in what sphere.

These dynamics are intimately connected: authority is to control what responsibility is to consequences. In health care, both authority and responsibility are in constant motion. And as these shift, so too do consequences. The evolution of capitation, for example, has brought new clarity to the relationship of these dynamics: primary care physicians realize immediate financial effects for the care decisions they make for their patients. If they are able to render care inexpensively, they reap monetary gain. If their risks represent substandard care, they face legal liability. It is theirs to shape the balance.

The interpretation of responsibility is often limited to institutional or legal repercussions. When a budgetary decision flops, we point to the answerable administrators and expect them to bear the consequences. Likewise, if the outcome of surgery disappoints, the patient may turn to the surgeon and hospital and hold them accountable. Our society's obsession with litigation has turned finger-pointing into an industry.

Though we blame the administrator or surgeon who holds the smoking gun, the real burden is endured by a broader scope of people. If the new sports medicine clinic fails, the consequences are felt not only by the administrators: the repercussions are felt even more directly by the physical therapists and others who lose their jobs. Similarly, in spite of the elaborate system of compensation for victims of malpractice, ultimately it is the patient who bears the most awful consequences of an unfortunate surgical outcome.

In health care there is a daunting life-and-death or quality-of-life implication to decision making. And responsibility itself is very expensive. Because of the ethereal quality of health care responsibility, it is bartered and shifted to enhance protection, or at least perceived protection, for the many people who participate or who are affected by a decision. "I take the authority and you take the responsibility" is not an equitable split.

Especially as they pertain to fiduciary obligations or legal liability, responsibility and risk are constantly negotiated and exchanged. Nurse practitioners seeking greater authority to prescribe medication also bear an increased responsibility and liability for malpractice. Solo practice physicians recruited by managed care plans exchange some of their independent authority for a reduction in responsibility. While the elements of this exchange are actuated in insurance premiums and professional contracts, these are only one measure of the real meaning of these intangibles. Autonomy has great professional significance for those who work in the system, and it has great personal meaning for those served by it.

Certainly, recognition itself is the most perplexing element of intangible social status exchange. For those who work in the health system, "recognition" is the professional acknowledgment and fulfillment they derive from their work. For patients, it is a matter of the dignity and satisfaction experienced in receiving care from others. In his analysis of human needs, Abraham Maslow (1970) defines the highest meaning and accomplishment derived through social interaction as "self-actualization." Self-actualization is experienced in the acknowledgment received from others and from our own inner sense of purpose.

For health care professionals, there is particular significance to recognition. Their career choice was not intended only as a source of income. More importantly, a health care career offers the opportunity to constructively help other people. Saving a life, improving the lot of an ill person, and preventing disease are valued as exceptionally meaningful and prestigious social endeavors. The value of this work is either validated or invalidated by colleagues, patients, and the system that pays the bill.

Validation, therefore, is a particularly important currency of exchange for those involved in health care: we give it to others; we get it from others. Validation is derived from an appreciative comment, acknowledgment of important information, and the granting of decision-making authority. For example, "I am giving you an important piece of information about the patient. I do hope you will recognize its significance and therefore my contribution in sharing it with you." That feeling of validation itself can even replace financial reward: people are willing to work for lower wages if they derive a sense of social purpose from their employment.

Invalidation is marked by ignoring a remark, negating a piece of information, or excluding a colleague's participation on the basis of prejudice, hierarchical standing, or interpersonal relations. People are invalidated when their observations are ignored, only to be recognized when someone with higher status restates them and grabs the credit. This sort of invalidation is common in gender, interprofessional, and patient–provider relations. Sometimes it is explicit and intentional. More often it is unspoken though present. It is as if one person says to the other, "I purposely invalidate what you say to reinforce the fact that I am superior to you, and you must concede your place." This attitude is based on deep-seated assumptions and beliefs about relative value and relationships. Sexist remarks, even by well-intentioned men, fall into this category. The resentment, alienation, and desire for revenge resulting from invalidation is costly when it compromises the interdependent work needed in health care.

Exchange and Whole Image Negotiation

How does the premise of negotiation as exchange pertain to health care? When you negotiate the purchase of a car, the terms and nature of exchange are explicit. You give the dealer money and the dealer gives you a car.

In health care, the exchange is not as direct. One person receives the service, another pays for it, someone else regulates it, and a complex web of people deliver it. The pieces are circuitously connected, so that one person's action is not immediately reciprocated by another's reaction. When your colleagues are unhappy with their salary, though they may not have negotiated it with you, their dissatisfaction will affect you. Similarly, if one unit of the hospital is not working well—the pharmacy, for example—it will have ramifications throughout the institution. While you may not have the authority to change how the pharmacy operates, its delays could directly affect your work and responsibilities. Little control with full responsibility is a precarious and conflict-ridden mix. Therefore, your genuine interest is to have all the pieces function in balance so that your piece itself can thrive.

Among interdependent parties, your win against another department's loss eventually will ricochet back to you. Their resentment will provoke them to go for a win over you in the next round. Moreover, their weakness only diminishes your own vitality. If the whole picture does not work, your contribution becomes nothing more than scribbles.

Whole image negotiation is based on the premise of interdependent systems and interdependent work. If the aggregate is balanced—the big picture—then your work is more likely to be efficient and effective at the individual level—the pragmatic picture. These two pictures are intrinsically related. Therefore, by negotiating on the assumption of shared objectives, you also better your own lot.

Using whole image negotiation, you bargain for the shared balance just as vigorously as you promote your individual portion. When this premise permeates the culture of your institution, the system as a whole works better.

◆ ◆ ◆ ◆ ◆ ◆ ◆

Katherine Knight has been nurse manager of the intensive care unit for over five years, gaining the reputation as one of the best nurse managers in the hospital. Despite ups and downs in the nursing staff on other units, the ICU has maintained high morale and low turnover. The loyalty and support she gives her staff is repaid in hard work and a low absentee rate. The total quality management program implemented several years ago generated many new ideas that were integrated into the operation of the unit.

Knight was disappointed when Janice Johnson, the vice president for nursing, approached her about cutting one position on the ICU night shift. It felt as if she were being penalized for her very success. Up to this point, she had been able to hold off the staff cutbacks that plagued other units. Johnson explained that the move was part of a much larger picture. To remain competitive with managed care plans, the hospital is seeking ways to responsibly reduce patient care costs. A review of ICU patients found that many could have been transferred to one of the general medical floors, had proper staffing and expertise been available there. These managed care plans could become reluctant to continue referring sick patients to the hospital if there were overutilization of expensive care. If the hospital placed a better-trained nurse on the general medical floor at night, hospital physicians would be more willing to move patients into the less expensive general medical floor.

Knight decided to express her disappointment and not to resist the move. She did ask that the decision be reviewed in three months, to which Janice agreed. The next step was to talk with Heather Harriford. If Harriford accepted the move, Knight would meet with the entire staff to explain what was happening and why.

Knight opened the meeting with a question. "Heather, I know that you have several times expressed your desire to transfer out of the ICU. I have been asked to recommend someone for transfer to the general medical floors." Knight wanted Harriford to know that this was not a test of loyalty: it would be acceptable to take the transfer. She also wanted Harriford to know that she had not initiated the move, and that it was not done specifically to single out Harriford. "How are you feeling now about making such a transfer?"

Harriford hesitated. The answer was yes, though before jumping to respond she wanted to clarify and secure several things. It would be to her advantage to appear as if she needed some gentle persuasion.

"Before I answer, could I ask a few questions?" Knight nodded, and Nurse Harriford went on to ask about salary, promotion to supervisor, and flexibility of hours. Knight had checked with the nurse manager on the general medical floors and was able to answer affirmatively on all counts.

Knight wanted to clarify the reasons for the move. "You are a young, bright, and energetic member of this staff. If the hospital is to reduce utilization of the ICU, we are going to need someone up on general medical who can receive patients transferred from the ICU and the emergency department. Your knowledge and expertise will be an invaluable asset for the general medical staff. Your talents have been recognized here at the ICU and in other parts of the hospital as well."

Harriford smiled and placed her hand ready to shake Knight's. "It's a deal. When do I start?" Knight asked her to hold off telling anyone until that night's staff meeting.

◆ ◆ ◆ ◆ ◆ ◆ ◆

Health care is a uniquely social enterprise. It demands many people working closely together engaged in numerous and frequent transactions. The success of the enterprise depends on its capacity to enhance the fluidity of those exchanges.

Negotiation as Discovery

Your most effective negotiation tool is a good question.

People often enter negotiation focused on what they want to get. They expend great effort pushing their case. They concentrate attention on what they are going to say next rather than on what is being said. They ignore as distraction the concerns and desires of other people at the table.

This phenomenon is particularly evident when a person's relative self-perception is one of superiority. It is evident in the way men relate to women, doctors to nurses, administrators to clinicians, nurses to family members, and older people to younger people. This behavior reinforces the hierarchical nature of social ordering by demeaning the concerns and contributions of those considered less important. It frustrates those being silenced. And it wastes valuable knowledge and expertise. With significant information lost to the process of negotiation, the options at the table are limited.

Enter negotiation with the intention of learning. Learn about the other side. Learn about your options. And learn about yourself:

what do you want, why do you want it, and what options have you not considered? Allow for the possibility that in the process of learning about one another, you might discover options not imagined at the outset.

◆ ◆ ◆ ◆ ◆ ◆ ◆

When Larry Lumberg spotted Fred Fisher flying down the hallway toward him, he didn't know what to expect. Lumberg is the forty-one-year-old director of the emergency department. Fisher, the chief of the medical staff, is a generation older than him. Lumberg despises the paternalistic father-son relationship he must endure as a cost of the mentoring that Fisher bestows.

Fisher bypassed social niceties and got right to the point. "Larry, I want you to go heavy on ICU admissions at night. Inkwater is giving me a hard time about boning up the nursing staff for general medical. Until things change, we up the pressure on the ICU. That'll get some action. I'm off to a meeting at the medical school. Call me if there are problems. Carry on!"

Lumberg didn't know what hit him. That was classic Fisher. No questions, no reasons, no options. Just commands. Lumberg muttered out loud, "Of course, he proposes a solution that not only creates more problems: it also makes me look bad in the process."

Lumberg is a good friend of Melanie Melancourt, the chief of the surgical intensive care unit. He places a call to her. "Look, this is off the record, but Fisher just told me to go heavy on ICU night admissions. Do you know what's going on?"

Melancourt chuckled, "Yeah, Fisher's nose is out of joint. He just had a meeting with Inkwater and Johnson. He's as impatient as anyone with the problems the nursing staff's been having on the night shift in general medical. But I heard that Johnson just had it taken care of. The problem for Fisher is more one of who is running the ship. He doesn't like the fact that Johnson didn't jump immediately. This is probably his little revenge."

"His revenge, and I hold the smoking gun," Lumberg replied. "Does Fisher know about the change on the nursing staff?"

"No, it's being kept quiet until the nurse manager announces it to the staff tonight. I tell you, I'm not wild about this whole thing myself, though I think in the long run it's for the better. These are not the good old days anymore, and we're going to have to reduce the ICU census if we hope to keep those HMO contracts."

"Who is moving?"

"Heather Harriford. Even though she can be a loose cannon sometimes, she is a very good nurse. She has a lot of energy and will be a good addition over there."

"Do you think there is a problem if I share this with Fisher?"

"No, just as long as he doesn't get up on a soap box about it before tonight's staff meeting."

"I'll work on it. Thanks a lot, Melanie."

◆ ◆ ◆ ◆ ◆ ◆ ◆

By making negotiation a learning opportunity, you build the foundation for the next round.

Negotiation as Steps in a Process

There are those who regard negotiation as a direct linear process, with beginning, middle, and end. This notion prescribes a definitive objective which the negotiation intends to accomplish. Each transaction is a separate event, disconnected from what happens before and after.

Try another view of negotiation: beginning, middle, and end, though not necessarily in that order. The middle of one round may be the beginning of the next. The end of one negotiation may affect what occurs in the midst of a negotiation in the next room. Your ultimate objectives for the negotiation may be changed by new information learned during the process.

The linear perspective does not fit health care negotiation. With information and tasks so closely intertwined through professional systems, reimbursement, oversight, and regulation, each negotiation is implicitly connected to others. This is not only in the abstract, as it pertains to the exchange of one group to the next, such as nurses to doctors or patients to insurers; it also describes your negotiation with a particular individual or organization over time. In each round you gain information, experience, and feelings about others at the table. Your accomplishments influence your attitude and approach to the next round. Likewise, others create impressions of you. If the last round went smoothly, the parties return anticipating a repeat of their last, satisfactory outcome. If it was a battle with winner and loser, the former comes to regain victory and the latter comes to reap revenge.

With a long-term view of negotiation, you approach each round as an investment in the future and a payoff from the past. Each transaction fortifies the foundation upon which your professional relationships are constructed.

A systems view of negotiation acknowledges the interdependence of interaction. When you negotiate in a vacuum, nothing is connected. When you negotiate in a system, everything is interwoven. A change in one place demands an adjustment in the next. A solution in one section generates a reaction in another. The decision reached at your table affects negotiation tables far removed from your scene of action.

◆ ◆ ◆ ◆ ◆ ◆ ◆

Iris Inkwater considers her work with outside organizations to be the most important part of her job as CEO of OMC (Oppidania Medical Center). In particular, it is her contractual negotiations with health maintenance organizations and insurers that are most vital to the fiduciary welfare of the hospital. She likes to get to know the people with whom she will be working, and she usually lunches with the chief negotiator for the other side before serious numbers are placed on the table.

Nathaniel Norquist is chief financial officer (CFO) for Community Health Plan (CHP), the third-largest health maintenance organization (HMO) in the state. Because of a concentration of customers in the OMC neighborhood, CHP is the largest

HMO contract for the hospital, accounting for 19.5 percent of its business.

As lunch was drawing to a close, Iris placed the critical question on the table: "Well, how are we looking for next year?"

Norquist paused. "Iris, I tell you the truth, things are going to be tough. We are working in a very competitive market. There is a lot of pressure from our big users, especially the unionized manufacturers. They are putting the crunch on the numbers, and we have to keep low if we are going to stay in this business. Your shop is 14 percent above the costs coming in from other hospitals. We have had a good relationship in the past, and I have to be honest with you. If you can't come in line for us with the other hospitals in town, we just have to direct our people elsewhere."

"Nathaniel, what exactly do you see as the problem?"

"It's a matter of timing, Iris. Oppidania simply moves slower than the other hospitals. It takes you longer to get people in and out of the hospital. And when in doubt, you tend to opt for the more expensive course of care. I know there is a lot of pressure on liability. Nevertheless, other places seem to keep themselves covered without piling up costs."

Iris paused for a moment. She realized that she was in for some very rough sailing back home. "Nathaniel, we have had a long and productive relationship. If you stick with us, I know we can work this out."

As Iris drove back to the hospital, she planned her next step. The hospital would have to offer CHP concrete proof that they are serious about trimming costs. "We'll impress them with what we can do to turn this around," she thought to herself. "And if we can't, I'm sunk."

◆ ◆ ◆ ◆ ◆ ◆ ◆

The best negotiators recognize negotiation as a fluid process. With each round, style and strategy are adjusted to accommodate unforeseen contingencies and information. Flexibility, resilience, and tenacity accommodate these shifts and turn them into a plus.

Negotiation and Power

When it comes to negotiation and power, there are three types of people. The first are those who don't have power and want to get it. In their mind, their negotiation problems stem from a lack of power. The question we are most frequently asked is, "How do I negotiate if I don't have power?" The underlying assumption is that without power, I don't get to the negotiation table, and once there, I will be paid little attention. As long as this assumption persists, the underlying question really is, "How do I get power so I don't have to negotiate?"

The second type are those with power. They too ask about power, though in a far more circumspect way. Their concern is "How do I negotiate to keep the power?" They know that power is far more ephemeral a thing than it appears. You can have it in one room though not in another. You can have it one day and then see it slip away the next. One can create the perception that one has it. In fact, any number of culprits can steal it away in a moment. Once you've negotiated from a position of power, there is nothing more terrifying than having to live without it. It creates a sense of vulnerability that horrifies.

There is a third type. Those are negotiators who recognize that if power is the only currency of negotiation, then options and actions are severely limited. Why?

With so much energy invested in getting power and maintaining the power base, good options and decisions are rejected not because they are wrong; rather, they are rejected because they do not fortify the base of power for those in charge. Fortifying that base becomes an obsession. It has been so in health care for many years. If not changed, significant progress will elude us. All our positions will be insecure. And we will not accomplish what we presume to do: deliver good health care for our patients while enjoying satisfying careers.

Wise leaders are beginning to change their use of power and their processes of decision making. They recognize that by involving and incorporating a spectrum of ideas and people, their decisions and their support are strengthened. In so doing, they do not give power away. Empowerment, when done from a base of mutual respect and recognition, adds to the total sum of power. It does not mean giving in when there is disagreement, though it does mean extending acknowledgment. It does not necessarily mean sacrifice, though it does require sharing both the spoils and the struggles of collaboration. "Who is holding the power?" becomes less important than "What are we trying to accomplish?"

Can a type three emerge in health care? Is it possible for people to negotiate based on their common purpose rather than merely based on their comparative level of power? This book is based on the premise that such a breakthrough can be achieved in health care.

This third model does not naively suggest that power will go away or that it won't be an important currency in our negotiations. Rather, it proposes that power not be the central currency of good decision making. In its place there can emerge common interests, which better frame our endeavors. The uneven table at which we sat for so many years can be rebalanced so that robust ideas and resourceful options find room for sensible consideration.

◆ ◆ ◆ ◆ ◆ ◆ ◆

Fisher's secretary handed him a telephone message when he returned to his office: "URGENT! Inkwater wants you and other hospital leadership in her office 8:00 AM tomorrow for an important meeting!" Fisher smiled. The plan had worked before it even got off the ground. Inkwater finally realized that she is going to have to shift things around if this place is going to work. Victory!

When Fisher arrived the next morning, Inkwater, Johnson (nursing VP), the chief operating officer, and the chief financial officer were already huddled in Inkwater's office. Fisher likes to show up a few moments late because then he doesn't have to wait until others arrive.

Inkwater opened the meeting. "Thank you all for coming on such short notice. I know that some of you had to change your schedules, and it is appreciated. I got some bad news yesterday. I met with Nathaniel Norquist, the CFO at Community Health Plan. It seems they are under some very strong pressure from purchasers to hold down costs. It's a buyer's market out there, and Norquist knows that only the competitive health plans are going to survive. As it turns out, we stick out like a sore thumb on the expense side."

This is not what Fisher had expected. He looked around. There was silence. The others had a shocked, ghostlike expression on their faces. This was not good news.

Inkwater continued. "We all know that CHP could pull out of here and get away with it. They are our largest and most steady source of income. We can't depend on federal and state moneys, and other HMOs may follow if CHP leaves. Now, we have suffered belt-tightening before in this institution, and it's generally been a pretty bloody exercise. Every department has been out to protect their turf and keep the pain on someone else's territory. It's going to have to be different this time. If we can't pull together and come up with some imaginative ways to solve this problem, we could all find ourselves closing this place down. We've seen it happen elsewhere, and there is no reason why it can't happen here."

The meeting continued for another half hour. The chief financial officer and chief operating officer reported on their evaluations of the financial impact of losing CHP's business. Inkwater talked about new premises and new assumptions for framing the work of the hospital—a heightened culture of cooperation. She ended the meeting on an upbeat note. "If we really pull together, we can make this a win for the hospital as a whole. It's up to each of you to communicate this attitude to your staff. It has to pervade the way you think and act professionally. If it doesn't, you won't be able to effectively make it work for those you lead."

◆　◆　◆　◆　◆　◆　◆

There are many sources of power available to you in your work. There is certainly the power of position, based on your formal organizational status. And there is also the influence that comes from knowledge, expertise, and the capacity for discovering new ways to frame and conduct the business of your institution.

The problem with running your organization and your career from the basis of crude power is that it has the capacity to become an obsession. Because of its ephemeral quality, you have to continually reinforce power to be certain it is there for you.

There are other ingredients of effectiveness that can guide the efforts of people who work closely together. Interest-based negotiation offers a common framework and language for building a collaborative context for those endeavors. What is it, and how can you can make it intrinsic to your style and strategy?

Part II

Negotiation

4

. . . .

Interest-Based Negotiation

We bring a storehouse of hope to our negotiations. There are the ostensible objectives we aim to acquire, for example money, space, or equipment. Beneath those concrete foci, there is that sense of purpose that motivates our very reason for being at the table: a breadth of needs, concerns, ambitions, and fears. Interest-based negotiation evokes that range of human response. The intent is to engage in problem solving that elevates and responds to those interests, and in the process to invent added options for settlement. By attending to interests, parties are able to resolve a broader spectrum of desires, out of which can be woven a greater range of choices and a more fulfilling reach of mutual benefit (Fisher, Ury, and Patton, 1991).

Interest-based negotiation defines an approach to the exchange process. Rather than regarding each other as contestants, the parties associate as collaborators seeking overlapping objectives. Recognizing their interdependence, they discover that they each advance by enhancing the advancement of one another. In the process of building trust and opening communication, they derive genuine confidence which extends well beyond a specific transaction.

Interest-based negotiation is particularly appropriate when parties are engaged in tasks that elicit their underlying objectives—their sense of purpose—as is typical in the work of health care. It is also especially practical when there are limited resources to divide, as is often the case in health care organizations, because those limited resources can be most ingeniously extended through collaboration.

In spite of its inherent utility for health care, there are those who shun the model, preferring win-lose, competitive practices instead. This chapter compares the two approaches: the first being interest-based or integrative approaches intended to coalesce the parties, and the second being positional or distributive models that view the parties' interests as exclusive of one another. This and the next two chapters focus on methods and techniques of interest-based negotiation and how they can be integrated into your professional health care routines. Chapter Eleven considers circumstances in which a positional approach is in fact your wiser choice, and it offers recommendations on how to succeed when that is the case.

Setting Your Negotiation Tone

Using integrative approaches, your long-term negotiation effectiveness will be enhanced. By contrast, distributional methods not only reduce your immediate negotiation credibility, they also erode the necessary reputation and trust for constructive bargaining.

The following simple allegory illustrates the distinction between distributional and integrative negotiation:

Two people are in a rowboat in the middle of a lake. They are debating what type of music they will listen to. The dialogue becomes heated. One demands one style, the second demands another. Each insists that his style reign. It becomes a matter of principle and a test of power. The boat rocks as each flails his arms to make the point. Finally, in frustration, one grabs a drill, threatening to bore a hole in the bottom if his music isn't played.

The boat sinks.

In another boat, two people face the same dilemma. They discuss their different musical preferences. They develop options to cope with their dis-

tinct tastes: alternating each half hour, using earphones, enlightening one another to appreciate different musical styles. One does not feel he loses his power by engaging with the other.

They can't wait for the next excursion.

Using distributional bargaining, your only concern is to satisfy your desires and those of your constituency. Meeting the needs of the other side is unimportant. You want to take as big a slice of the pie as possible. In your mind, the size of the pie is fixed. Through negotiation, the bounty of goods is distributed. The more others get, the less you get. You want to control the cutting process to ensure that you get the portion you want. You yearn to win.

By contrast, when using integrative negotiation, you seek an arrangement assuring both sides of a fair measure of satisfaction. You want to achieve your own negotiation objectives. You likewise are concerned that the other side accomplishes theirs. You want to explain your interests, learn theirs, and in the process generate options to accommodate both sides. You view negotiation as an inventive process for integrating interests and generating new opportunities. These new opportunities invigorate and further inspire resourceful innovation. When it comes time to slice the pie, you want to hold the knife together to affirm your mutual trust and good faith. You want to achieve a gain-gain outcome.

Is the distinction one of selfishness and altruism? Is the distributional bargainer greedy and the integrative bargainer socially responsible? The answer is not that easy.

The difference is one of purview. The integrative bargainer understands that his or her lot is enhanced when the integrity of others is maintained. Especially when your survival is closely related to that of your partner, integrative bargaining is a strategy for self-preservation. The viability of your department ultimately depends on the viability of the organization as a whole. The effectiveness of the health system relies on the functioning of its many interdependent parts. Each component depends on the others' achievements.

Negotiation is viewed as a method for adjusting the balance to assure both fairness and mutual security.

The distributional bargainer demands immediate gratification. Oblivious to the destiny shared with negotiating partners, the distributional bargainer measures achievement by the standard of present good fortune. The distributional bargainer believes success rests upon the failure, or at least the submission, of others. Negotiating partners are competitors, ready to snatch the goods. What another department takes only diminishes your bounty. Your own success depends on your own bottom line, not that of adjacent departments. To claim triumph, the distributional bargainer intimidates, controls, and conquers.

For the distributional bargainer, the purpose is to win. The context is one of adversaries: the activity on the playing field distinguishes the winners from the losers. Truth is lost in the divisive process: a dangerous prescription for health care decision making.

The quandary is that in many health care circles, distributional bargaining is the predominant method of negotiation. Whether promoting professional, patient care, or organizational concerns, the inclination is to advance the cause through distributional negotiation. A nursing colleague recently recounted an example of this perspective that occurred at a national nursing conference. In a frenzy of "doctor bashing," the tone of discourse at the meeting turned to one of overcoming the rival force. The mood was "now it's our turn, and we're going to walk all over them." My colleague countered that as long as nursing adopts and reinforces distributional bargaining and does not use its emerging status to transform the rules of the game, then really nothing will have improved.

Similarly, rather than asking, "How can I adjust to better fit into a new health care reality?" doctors query us on how to negotiate to defend what little power they have left. Health managers cling to what they believe is good business, amplifying the importance of the "bottom line" as the singular measure of their success. Community health advocates are in such a frenzy to advance their cause that they don't remember to lay down their weapons amongst themselves. And patients are convinced that the only way to obtain service from their managed care plan is through belligerent demands.

A colleague recounts a meeting of engineers at a major American automobile manufacturer. The electrical systems department reported that new components proposed for the next year's model drew too much current from the system, threatening the battery with shutdown. Each division had proposed innovations requiring more electricity: air conditioning had a better cooling mechanism; the dashboard people had a more splendid display; and the directional light section had a more dramatic signal. Adding to the car's electrical capacity would boost its gas consumption unacceptably. There was no compromise at the table. Each representative was there only to advocate for the best air conditioner, dashboard, or light display. No one was there speaking for the overall operation of the car. My colleague lamented, "*That* attitude is the problem with the domestic auto industry. It is not an engineering problem. It is a human systems problem: we are not aspiring to make the whole machine synchronize to operate smoothly. We are building parts. No wonder the car breaks down."

That attitude pervades our health system. The assumption that professional and organizational behavior can be better controlled through competition illustrates the misconception.

The real question is not "How can we control the parts to reduce spending?" As long as that remains the primary consideration, the health system will not function effectively and efficiently to improve aggregate health status and costs.

Rather, two basic questions ought to frame our approach to health care and the negotiation that probes for answers:

1. *What are we trying to accomplish?* This question applies to all health care negotiations, from matters of national health policy to decisions regarding the operation of a clinic or the care of a patient.

2. *How do we work together to achieve those ends?* This question directs our attention to what we do and to whether we achieve our objectives.

The aim here is not to postulate specific answers to these questions. Rather, the purpose is to present them as opening points for everyday negotiation, whether about health policy, health administration, or clinical care.

Among health care colleagues who are working together, common ground does not emerge merely by dividing the spoils between what one gets and what the other gets. It emerges from congruence regarding shared purpose and interdependent activity. By engaging that shared purpose to formulate health care's common purposes, we achieve a system that evolves beyond our current predicaments.

There are those who will accuse this approach of being naive. It does not account for greed and avarice. One can point to the huge profits of pharmaceutical companies, the large salaries of physicians and executives, the malevolent workings of Medicaid fraud, or exclusive dominance of certain professionals as evidence that social accountability is extinct. One could build a health system based on apprehension of the worst of human traits.

On the other hand, remember that health care intends to improve upon the most fundamental aspects of the human condition: life and death and the quality of life. This common purpose can inspire shared objectives that extend beyond merely balancing greed with innocence, or exploitation with plunder. Rather, this shared purpose can be the premise upon which fair standards and socially acceptable outcomes are negotiated. Such an approach is a better fit for what it is we do in health care.

◆ ◆ ◆ ◆ ◆ ◆ ◆

By the time Artie Ashwood was finally settled into Room 624, he was a tangle of fear, frustration, and confusion. They still didn't know what was going on inside him. He knew he was feeling pain like he had never experienced before. They said they needed to do some more tests. They told him not to worry too much. The reassurance didn't help. He was still worried. He couldn't figure out why, with all this high-tech machinery and all these well-paid doctors, they couldn't figure out what was going on with him.

The other thing he doesn't like is the way this hospital is being run. They must be terribly overworked, or something. Everyone seems to be nagging at one another. He heard it two nights ago, when they first brought him in. The doctor in the emergency room lost her patience. Then the nurses in the ICU started bickering over his bed about one of the doctors. And the more he asked questions about what was going on inside him and when he would get out, the less information he got.

He read about this in one of his public policy courses at the university. There was a section on the health care system. He knew about costs going up, about the millions of people without insurance, and about what they are doing to cut back the system. Fortunately, he had health insurance through the university. But he was still worried. He'd never been sick before, and he hadn't paid much attention to what was and what wasn't covered.

What if they scrimped on his care? What if they kicked him out before they knew what was really going on? Maybe the reason they can't figure out his problem is because they are trying to save a few bucks. Wouldn't that be grounds for a lawsuit?

He felt vulnerable and dependent. He was labeled, depersonalized, and anonymous, except for the bracelet wrapped around his wrist. The woman who took his blood barely said hello before she removed four vials from his arm. Had she changed her gloves before she opened him up? What would all this mean for his career in architecture?

His gaze out the window was interrupted by footsteps coming around the old man in the bed next to him. Oscar O'Neill introduced himself.

"I'm sorry I wasn't here earlier to give you the formal welcome to Six West. I was tied up with another patient. I'll be your primary nurse. Let me know if you have any questions or concerns. I'll be with you through your stay here." The conversation continued on about Artie's anxieties, his questions, and their mutual interest in basketball. For the first time since he arrived at the hospital, Artie was starting to feel connected.

Things were changing for Artie. He was beginning to feel like a human being again.

❖ ❖ ❖ ❖ ❖ ❖ ❖

Integrative Negotiation: Finding Interests

You embark upon integrative negotiation by exploring interests: your interests, their interests, and your shared interests.

The difference between distributive and integrative negotiation is this concern for shared interests. Distributive bargainers are concerned about their own interests. They show little concern for the other side, and therefore they are unlikely to find shared interests and solutions to satisfy both sides.

Interests portray what you care about. What is of value to you? What do you hope to accomplish? And what do you hope to get? You are a unique combination of experience, values, and ambitions. You bring a distinct profile of interests to the negotiation table.

The challenge is not only to understand your own interests and how they affect what you do; you must also learn the unique interests of the other people involved. Just as what you do emerges from your interests, so too does what they do.

Using interest-based negotiation, you build agreement responsive to the needs, aspirations, and expectations of all the parties at the table. It is akin to assembling a puzzle. It requires discovery to find the pieces, ingenuity to put them together, and diplomacy to make them cohere. And, of course, it requires patience, imagination, and endurance.

Your starting point for interest-based negotiation is in learning those interests. This is detective work. Ask questions. Read. Observe. Find leads and follow them. And do not complacently assume that what you find is what it appears to be.

In the previous chapter, "a good question" was proposed as the most effective negotiation tool. The utility of this tool, though, is measured by what you do with the answer. You have opened the door to a wealth of information, some explicit and some implicit. Your objective is to sift through that information and learn what are the real interests of your negotiating partner. Survey not only what they say: assess also what they do, their body language, their attitude, and their anxieties. These are all important indicators of what you can offer to satisfy their interests.

When you enter a negotiation, you shoulder a profusion of expectations. On the surface, there is something of substance you want to get. It could be money or information, a piece of equipment, or a new office. Less apparent are the underlying gains you desire: recognition, professional fulfillment, and personal meaning. These hidden expectations play a vital role in the outcome of the negotiation. It is possible to achieve your substantive expectations, yet still feel unsatisfied because something was missing. Conversely, you may not realize all your substantive expectations, yet still leave the table feeling the outcome was a success. What is the hidden variable, and how can you discover and integrate it?

The most elusive interests to understand are your own. For example, is your interest *really* working out an arrangement to better handle patients? Or do you want to use the issue to get back at that administrator who was giving you a hard time last year? Revenge! Are you *really* worried about your patient's welfare upon discharge? Or are you advocating for the superiority of your own skills? One-upmanship! Are you *really* concerned about the quality of care on the unit? Or you are you demonstrating your authority over the staff? Control! At times, the easiest one to fool is yourself. When it's blatant, everyone in the room knows your number, except for you.

Beneath your substantive expectations and those of others are a multitude of process preferences and psychological needs that prompt your negotiation behavior. How do you find them?

Process Preferences

There is a process by which a decision or settlement is reached. Some people are included while others are not. Criteria are established to measure or distinguish the matters that must be decided. The decision may be reached by consensus, or perhaps against the will of those who are affected. The who, what, when, where, why, and how of a decision describes what is the process.

Why are process preferences important? We bring expectations for process. If it is a matter of vital concern to you, you resent being excluded from the decision making, even if the actual outcome of the negotiation is acceptable. Why were you excluded? Are your views not respected? Might you be losing your job? If you were excluded this time, what could happen in the future? The process by which the deal is made is imbued with meaning, in part because it affects the decision at hand, and in part because it predicts what may happen in the future.

My colleague David Matz tells the following story (May 1993):

A husband and wife fell in love with an antique clock they saw in a catalogue. At $1,000, they concluded it was extravagant and decided not to make the purchase.

While on a trip through New England, they stopped in a small-town antique store. To their delight they found the very same clock available for purchase. The problem was that the clock, in perfect condition, had no price tag. The husband whispered confidently to his wife, "Don't worry, I'll get that clock for $500."

Figuring he wanted to leave plenty of room to bargain up, the husband approached the store owner to say he would be willing to pay $150 for the timepiece. After a moment of silence, the owner replied, "That'll be fine."

How did the husband feel?

When I tell this story during training sessions, the responses to this question usually range from "cheated" to "sorry," "feeling like he got a good deal," and "confused."

The husband had an expectation. He was ready for the store owner to counter with a number near $1,000, the assumed value of the clock. He would then counter with $250, and this would continue until they reached a point of agreement. That this did not happen left the husband wondering. "Had his assumption of the clock's value been wrong? Is there something wrong with the clock? Could he have gotten the clock for less? Did he overpay for the antique? Is he guilty of shamelessly cheating the owner?" The negotiation process did not give him clues to answer these questions. He left the store with the merchandise in hand, though once home, these riddles haunted him every time he passed the clock.

Apply this simple story to the more complex negotiations typical of health care settings. You want to participate in decisions that affect you. You must be included when matters about which you have authority or expertise are decided. And you expect to be included when a decision is made about something for which you have responsibility. Others have the same expectations.

When process preferences are ignored, it is common to hear a variation on, "Hey, great decision. I would have gone along with it if I had been party to making it. Why was I excluded? Is someone trying to tell me something? Don't expect my cooperation in carrying it out!"

You incorporate process preferences into your negotiation by planning the decision-making strategy. You not only decide what you are hoping to accomplish, you also know how you might go about achieving it. Who should be involved? How should the question be presented? When should the discussions begin? And what might be the criteria to sway the decision in one direction or the other?

◆ ◆ ◆ ◆ ◆ ◆ ◆

Iris Inkwater calls them "think sessions." She and Perry Pratt, the chief operating officer for the hospital, sit in her office on the comfortable chairs, put their feet up, and with pads of paper on their laps, they think. Iris and Perry trust one another, and even long moments of silence are accepted between them.

Iris opened. "I don't think this is merely a dollars-and-cents exercise, Perry. We are already very lean. I think this is a matter of how we go about doing our business."

"What do you mean it's not a matter of dollars and cents? Norquist made it very clear. We cost too much."

"I know that," Iris countered, "though in the long run, this crisis is about more than just cutting costs. There is a difference between doing things better and doing things cheaper."

"I think Norquist was pretty clear about cheaper."

"Oh, I know that Norquist is concerned about money. He's a go-between, and his only currency is money. He's a salesman. The difference is that we're running a hospital here."

Pratt remained silent. Iris seemed to be formulating her thoughts as she spoke. She didn't seem certain herself what was coming next.

"For a whole lot of reasons, we've been willing to tolerate a surplus of inefficiencies in this place. Take the problem with the ICU and internal medicine. That's become a standoff and we've let it continue because there was no good reason to fix it. That's one of a half-dozen slipshod staffing problems that we've avoided. We've had problems in our billing department because we've been reluctant to spend the money to upgrade the system. And I think all these dangling problems eventually filter down to patients. I'm sure they don't inspire confidence. In the long run, that hurts us at our most vulnerable point, our census."

"You're going to have to disturb a lot of concrete cobwebs if you want to fix all those problems."

"Oh, I know, and I may not be around to tell the tale. Nevertheless, I really don't think we have a choice. People here have to know that we can no longer sustain waste. It's really a matter of survival."

"Well," Pratt challenged, "how do you intend to go about creating this metamorphosis?"

"That's a good question. I can easily think of a whole slew of ways *not* to do it." She paused and continued slowly. "I think there are two key principles. Attitude and involvement. If the staff approach this whole thing with the attitude that they want to make the hospital work better, and if they're all on board, I think we can do it. The key is that they have to be involved. They have to be a part of understanding the problems, and a part of formulating the changes. They have to understand that this is a matter of survival, and if the boat sinks, we all go down together."

"I think you'll have an easier time getting some people to go along than others."

"Yes, you're right. There'll be some who will stay away in the misconception that if they lay low, they won't be affected. They'll want to control by withholding their participation. In the long run, though, they'll have to see that their strategy can't work here anymore. And there will be some who don't want to engage in the give and take. That attitude won't make it either."

◆　◆　◆　◆　◆　◆　◆

Beyond the matter of *what* was decided during your negotiations, there is the question of *how* it was decided. Even if there is consensus on the correctness of the substance, when there is disagreement on the process by which the decision was reached, concurrence on the decision itself vanishes. The substance of a controversial decision, for example, may be accepted as *fair*. However, if there is dissatisfaction with the *fairness* of the process by which the decision itself was derived, then whatever consent there might have been turns into conflict. Process conflict can be confounding, because one party assumes that the decision itself is fine and meets acceptable criteria, while others may agree with the substance and really are protesting the process.

Attending to this question of process is vital to negotiation based on interests, since it speaks so visibly to the underlying concerns that people bring to the table.

What is said and done during the negotiation process, what can be seen, may in fact evoke a spectrum of emotions and needs that also affect what may or may not occur. Though not directly related to the substance of the discussions, these personal factors too influence the process and its outcome.

Psychological Needs

Negotiation is imbued with meaning.

When you negotiate your salary, the outcome is not only about pay. More importantly, the negotiation reflects something to you about your value to the organization and more generally to society. The bargaining implicitly appraises what you have done beforehand. It assigns you a social status. It is a benchmark that can either make you feel good or fill you with self-doubt, anger, and remorse. Similarly, when you negotiate for office space, the outcome is not only a matter of square footage. The location of your office situates you on the social map of the organization. The size, the number of windows, and the proximity to other people of influence publicly marks your own importance and prestige. And when you are included or excluded from an important policy meeting, it is not only a matter of scheduling, it also reveals something about the value of your knowledge and expertise to your colleagues.

If you view negotiation as simply about money, space, and scheduling, then you ignore the vital psychological significance of the process. This hidden dynamic prompts what you say and what you do. It motivates your reaction to viable proposals. It is the bag of emotions you bring to the table: fears, anxieties, mistrust, hope, anticipation, and aspiration. Some of these feelings are at the surface: they are known to you and to others. Others are known only to you. And lurking in your psychological underworld are a myriad of impenetrable emotions and constraints unknown even to you. They reflect your vulnerabilities and fears, just as they do your dreams and aspirations. They are an expression of what motivates and what satisfies you. They emanate from the core of who you are and what you believe.

Just as your underlying emotions pull on your behavior and the choices you make during negotiation, so too do they pull on others. What is totally logical to you may be rejected by the people across the table. Or they might offer a proposal that to you makes no sense at all. When your deliberation leaves the realm of the reasonable, you know that someone's psychological baggage is shifting the weight of discussion. These emotional signals may not make sense to you and may not even make sense to them.

When this happens, ask questions. *"What concerns does this plan raise for you?"* Listen carefully. Be empathic. *"This must be very disappointing for you."* Remember, you can acknowledge the other's feelings without agreeing with them. *"I appreciate why you might feel that way."* Reflect on what they are saying. Do not tell them what they are feeling. Give them permission and safety to reveal what is happening inside. *"Please know that I will keep this discussion in confidence."* Validate their expression by disclosing that you also have feelings on the matter. *"I know this is a tough issue for you. It uncovers many issues for me as well."* In so doing, you demonstrate that you are trying to understand.

When psychological needs enter the negotiation, you often find yourself in a reactive mode. You listen and respond to what the other party reveals.

However, if you can anticipate the psychological matters that will affect the negotiation, offer a proactive opening. Be explicit about the invitation, suggesting the topic early in the negotiation process. *"Before we get into the specifics about the merger proposal, I think it is fair to acknowledge that after being here so many years, this is a tough issue for all of us."* If the issues are sensitive, use an implicit approach, gently touching upon and acknowledging the subject. *"I imagine this must be difficult for you."* Yes, you may loosen a flood-gate. If it is done sensitively, however, this opening could offer opportunities to find solutions responsive to both their needs and yours. You are not sidestepping the issues. You are handling them directly (see Fisher, Kopelman, and Schneider, 1994).

In fact, psychological apprehensions are often formidable, unseen obstacles impeding negotiation progress. Even when they can't be resolved, merely acknowledging their presence can be significant for those affected.

Beyond acknowledgment, identifying psychological issues can guide your negotiation strategy. Learn what motivates the other side. Can you offer them something to satisfy their interests? What incentives can you create to respond to their needs? While the overt discussion may be about something as concrete as money or space, the underlying issues may be professional recognition, job security, or resentment about something that happened in the past. By addressing these underlying issues, you enhance the prospect of finding agreement.

This avenue is particularly valuable when what you have to divide is clearly limited or shrinking: money, space, or time. Attention to psychological interests will give you more to divide. If the topic on the table is assignment of office space, and the real, underlying issue is influence in the organization, then offer the needed assurances about influence. In fact, if you tender added influence in recognition of the person who takes the office without a window, you may find everyone on your staff requesting the undesirable space. You have created new elements for exchange, and the more you have to trade, the easier it is to achieve settlement.

Psychological interests are of particular importance in health care because of the nature of the work. The characteristic social purpose typifying the field accentuates the inherently weighty nature of negotiation. Staff working in particular sections, such as the oncology department, AIDS unit, or women's clinic, are particularly committed to defending the cause of their patients. An action or decision is particularly upsetting if perceived to compromise the quality of patient care. Addressing these interests by building safeguards or assurances into an agreement facilitates the process of reaching resolution.

* * * * * * * *

When Larry Lumberg (chief of the emergency department) heard the growl of Fred Fisher's "come in," he made his way into the medical director's office. Fisher was staring out the window when Lumberg entered and did not turn around to acknowledge his young colleague's arrival. This was not characteristic Fisher.

"Fred, is something wrong?" There was silence, and Lumberg prepared himself to hear of some personal or professional tragedy that had befallen his mentor. "What happened?"

"Nothing happened, Larry. Nothing happened and everything happened. I tell you, medicine is not what it was when I entered this profession. I think it's time I get out before this whole thing falls apart."

"Fred, what are you talking about?"

"You heard about this thing with the Community Health Plan. They are threatening to pull out of OMC. I tell you Larry, there is only so much blood to squeeze out of this hospital and out of this physician. It just doesn't seem worth it anymore."

"What are you saying?"

"I went into medicine forty years ago. It was a noble profession back then. We did good work for people, and we were treated with respect. We worked hard and we deserved every penny we got. We took pride and pleasure in what we did. It's not like that anymore. They are trying to manage us, squeeze us, and control us. It's simply not worth it anymore. I think it's time for me to pack it up and call it quits."

Larry spoke slowly. "Fred, there is no doubt about it. Medicine is not what it used to be. It doesn't even resemble what I got into some twenty years ago."

Lumberg knew Fred didn't need a lecture now about health

care economics or management. This is a man whose professional pride and authority were being abducted. In Fisher's mind, there was something sacred about the practice of medicine. The inviolable profession was being destroyed by far-off Washington policy wonks and cumbersome Oppidania efficiency engineers. Lumberg grew up in a different generation. He could understand what was happening. That understanding was beyond Fisher.

"Fred, I know these are trying times. We are all being tested. You've made an enormous contribution over your career. Your ingenuity has pulled patients through tough times. Now the medical staff needs your leadership to pull this hospital through tough times."

Fisher pondered what Lumberg said. It felt odd having Lumberg give him a lecture. It's usually the other way around. Larry, though, did a good job, he thought. Fisher pondered what Lumberg was saying. He reminisced briefly about patients, medical students, colleagues. Yes, Fisher old boy, you are still needed here. He turned around.

"Perhaps you're right, Lumberg. But I tell you, it's not going to be as much fun as it used to be."

"Maybe it'll just be a different kind of fun," Lumberg countered with a smile.

For Fisher, the changes in medicine are not so much a matter of money or even management. Lumberg understood his malaise to be more a matter of professional pride. That understanding framed his response.

Iris Inkwater would be wise to recognize Fisher's tribulation in her next meeting with him.

◆ ◆ ◆ ◆ ◆ ◆

Substantive Expectations

When you enter a negotiation, you likely have some sense of process preferences: how you want the decision to be made. You are less likely to be conscious of your psychological needs and those of others. You most likely are clearest about one thing: what you want to get out of the negotiation—your substantive expectations.

The matter of substantive expectations is really a two-sided question: what you want to get and what they want to get. On the other side: what you are willing to give and what they are willing to give. This is the get and give of negotiation. Strategically, you are concerned about both sides.

You negotiate because you don't have it all. You don't control it all. You need something from someone else. You and your negotiation partners balance narcissism (you get it all) with social responsibility (you share it) to reach agreement on the terms of your deal. If you cannot find a balance, the negotiation collapses and the transaction does not occur.

How do you reach agreement? And how do you conclude the negotiation so that your partner—perhaps a colleague, a patient, a representative from another health care organization—will choose to negotiate with you again?

To accomplish a gain-gain outcome, calibrate a standard of fairness to guide your negotiation. Construct that standard by assessing what is valuable to the negotiation at hand: time, expertise, money, effort, and outcome are examples. Agree on the value of what you propose to exchange by comparing what is on the table to similar commodities of established worth. This stage of the negotiation is arduous, since the appraisal process by nature is highly subjective. Your interpretation of merit may not be shared by others.

Having agreed on a standard of fairness, your next step is to propose an exchange. Compare what you are offering to what the other side offers. Determine if there is balance between the two sides of the scale. Inherent in the negotiation process is that you are giving one thing and getting something different in return. That is why relative value is important.

Once you have determined that the scale is in balance, consummate the exchange. You now hold something different from what you had before. You reassess the deal. Are you still satisfied? Is the other side still satisfied? If the answer is yes, conclude the transaction. You shake hands. If you both are pleased, you envision future transactions.

The problem with negotiation in health care is one of determining value. Real estate agents assess one property against "comparables" in the neighborhood. Car dealers pull out their blue book. There are no such golden standards in health care. Time is relative: what is the value of a physician's hour versus a nurse's? Outcome is relative: what is the value of an infant nutrition program serving thousands versus the outcome for a baby cared for at a neonatal intensive care unit? Opinion is relative: what is the value of a specialist versus that of a primary care practitioner? And given that the health care system is in transformation, an assessment of value one week may be altered by the next.

For this reason, careful attention is best given this appraisal phase of the negotiation process. If someone's or something's relative value is diminished, it likely will seriously offend some at the table. The offense assumes great professional, ethical, or personal meaning. When the identical opinion from one professional is weighed differently from that of another, it fuels bitter indignation. If the life of one person is placed above that of another, it provokes moral outrage. And if the equivalent legitimate concerns of a woman are belittled to elevate those of a man, it sparks valid personal animosity. In health care, you negotiate in these sensitive domains all the time.

The utility of interest-based negotiation is the adaptability to these inherently fluctuating circumstances. The starting point is exploration: questions, information, perceptions, and desires. This is a learning process that goes in both directions. It is through this process that you assemble the information necessary to assess value equitably. It is a tool that is particularly appropriate to the types of negotiation that occur daily in health care.

* * * * * * *

Before leaving for home, Larry Lumberg took a detour to the front of the emergency room. He wanted to touch base with Beatrice Benson, the attending physician on call for the night. Fortunately, she was standing at the triage desk looking over a chart with Charlotte Channing, the triage nurse. After exchanging greetings, he got to the point.

"You know they have added a nurse to the night shift on general medical. The intent is to shift as many admissions as possible away from the ICU."

"I know, I heard about it. Look, we'll give it a shot. It depends on what kind of traffic we get here tonight," Benson replied.

"With all these capitated plans, there's a lot of pressure to limit expenses when possible," Lumberg explained. "As long as we're not putting anyone in danger, we should get in line."

Channing chimed in. "Actually, general medical is in good shape. They transferred one of the star ICU nurses to Six West. They're much better able to handle cases on the fence."

"You're right," Benson added. "Quite honestly, I view this whole push as a matter of risk. I know one nurse is not going to change everything overnight. It is an important step, though, in giving us an alternative we can live with."

Lumberg left for the evening. Three hours later, Benson was on the phone to Eli Ewing, the chief resident in the CICU.

"I was hoping not to hear from you tonight," Ewing greeted Benson's call.

"Well, nothing personal, Eli. I was hoping not to talk to you, either. Actually, I think you might like this call."

"Okay, try me," Ewing replied.

"We have a fifty-six-year-old male here. He came in complaining of chest pains. We've pretty much ruled out a myocardial infarction. In any case, I think it wise to keep him here overnight for observation. A few weeks ago I would have sent him your way. I really don't think it's necessary, though. I ask just one favor."

"You got it," Ewing chimed.

"Would you be willing to come down and look over the charts? It's been a busy night, and I just want to be certain we didn't miss anything. If everything looks in order to you, we'll move him up to Six West, and save you an admission."

"You got it! Oh, and by the way, Benson," Ewing hesitated, "I think this whole arrangement may work out in the end."

"Well, we'll give it a shot. If we can slow down on you guys, it's in all our best interests."

◆ ◆ ◆ ◆ ◆ ◆ ◆

Forging a Common Language

Distributional bargaining positions negotiators against one another. When you negotiate on the basis of positions, you are rigid, uncompromising, and uninterested in other points of view. You are a contender, seeking conquest rather than congruence. You draw a line in the sand and hold firm on your demands.

In health care, numerous lines divide who we are and what we do. It is as if each of the professional groups speaks a distinct language to think and communicate amongst themselves. Nurses speak nurse. Doctors speak doctor. Health administrators speak administrator, and so on through the other disciplines. These languages refer not only to the distinct vocabulary of each specialty—the analogy also denotes the unique cognitive framework used to process information, make decisions, and assess value. Each has its own set of criteria. When presented with the same information, each deliberates differently. Departments, divisions, and disciplines have carved a place for themselves in the institution, promoting their perspective in what they do and the way they go about doing it.

That these differences exist is not a bad thing. In fact, these very differences invigorate what we do in health care: they inspire creativity, they serve as a check and balance on our work, and they are the avenue by which we assemble the vast knowledge and skills necessary to accomplish our objectives.

What binds us as a health care system are the shared interests and values that frame the work we do. We achieve common ground in our pursuit of these overlapping interests and expectations. As a tool, interest-based negotiation offers the integrative framework and common language necessary to tie the pieces together. By generating inventive options and new solutions, the method offers a potent resource to overcome our own stubborn obstacles.

. . . .

5

Framing to Generate Options

N egotiation is replete with conscious and subconscious decisions, trade-offs, experience, people, and repercussions. There
are facts and emotions to integrate. To elicit useful criteria, you need
to arrange this information into logical cognitive patterns: frames
and templates.

The frame helps you understand and organize information so it
is useful to you. The frame is your subjective lens, used to direct your
specific negotiation choices and decisions. It emerges out of your
template: the unique blend of philosophy, attitude, and belief that is
you. If you bear prejudice, bias, or intolerance, that part of your template colors your frame each time you negotiate, even if those feelings are buried deep inside. If your template brings openness,
compassion, and a willingness to learn, these principles characterize your negotiation (see Bazerman and Lewicki, 1983; Strauss,
1994).

Assessing Your Template

Each time you negotiate, your template shifts slightly. If experience
reinforces your preconception about the stubbornness of surgeons,
then that piece of your template becomes more rigid. So too are your
attitudes about race, gender, and professional competence swayed

by your everyday interactions. Positive experiences introduce new sentiments that shift your preconceptions. The surgeon who actually spends time to talk with you, and then even uses your recommendations, rebuts your notion about the limitations of the profession.

You consciously challenge and change your template when you incorporate new ideas into your persona. Through what you read, experience, and contemplate, you cautiously shift your underlying premises. Often these shifts are in response to changing mores and attitudes in your surroundings. Evolving societal sentiments about gender relations, professional interactions, and hierarchical ordering seep into your mind set, causing you to consider and reconsider your approaches to everyday decision making. Some ideas you welcome, and some you abhor. Some fit easily into who you are, and others seem to contradict your basic nature.

Active introspection is a constant companion of good negotiation. At the conclusion of a recent one-week negotiation training seminar, a hospital human relations vice president shared with me, "I came here thinking I was going to learn how to change other people. What I learned is that before I can hope to do that, I have to be willing to change myself." The fellow had discovered much about his attitudes on gender relations, his preconceived notions of people, and his blind spots, all of which had hampered his negotiation capabilities. He recognized that by ignoring the vital information his template deemed unimportant, he had offended women with casual remarks, ignored valuable suggestions from subordinates, and discounted worthy options that were outside his field of experience. His blinders wouldn't let him see.

When you study to be a carpenter, you learn how to use a hammer and saw, the tools of the trade. When you endeavor to be a better negotiator, the tool you learn to better wield is yourself. You are the negotiator, and your effectiveness results from what you think, say, and do. Taking inventory of your template and frame is the first step in that process.

Understanding Your Frame

Your template describes your general beliefs and attitudes. Your negotiation frame is specific to a particular negotiation, problem, or dispute.

Your frame is what you bring into the deliberations. It is your blueprint for assimilating information and taking action. To guide your negotiation strategy and choices, you want to understand your own frame and that of other negotiators. That understanding opens the door to generating creative options for resolution.

What are the elements of your frame? There are seven variables: people, problems, history, processes, outcomes, priorities, and stakes.

People

Health care decisions typically involve many people. There are those who make the decision. There are those who are affected by it. A supervisor decides that one member of the staff must be assigned to the night shift. A resident decides that a patient is ready to be discharged to a nursing home. An HMO administrator determines that it should no longer admit to one of the hospitals in town. The question is, who should participate in reaching the decision, and what should be each of their roles?

There are three categories of people involved in a negotiation. They are distinguished by their proximity to the negotiation table. The *primary players* are the people sitting directly at the table, participating in the give-and-take. They have an immediate interest in the decision, and they are visibly involved in the process of reaching it. The *secondary actors* metaphorically are standing just outside the door, being consulted and advised by the primary players. They are informed recipients of the decision more than they are involved players. While their opinions may sway the outcome, their influence is indirect. The *tertiary subjects* are not in the room. They are often unaware that the deliberations are occurring. They are the anonymous people affected by decisions: patients, staff, or the community. While they bear the consequences of what is decided, they have little role in shaping the outcomes.

Your negotiation frame assigns those involved in the issue to primary, secondary, and tertiary roles, based on your opinion about how the people and process should be ordered. Not everyone involved necessarily concurs: problems arise when there is dispute about who is assigned to which role. Consider the examples above. In the mind of the supervisor, she and her assistant are the primary actors, other supervisors are secondary players, and the staff member assigned to the night shift is a tertiary subject. What if the staff member expects to be a primary actor? After all, it is his schedule. The resident making the discharge assessment may consider the medical director a primary actor. The medical director, however, wants to see the young trainee assume greater independent responsibility. She prefers a secondary role in the decision. The HMO executive who wants to terminate the hospital contract considers the state's insurance commissioner a nonparticipant in the decision. Responding to consumer complaints, the commissioner nevertheless takes his authority to become an active, primary player in the negotiation.

If one of the involved parties has decision-making authority and uses a unilateral approach, then in his or her mind there is only one primary player. Staff members, colleagues, or patients affected by the dictate are excluded from the process. If they believe valid sentiments, information, and experience are being ignored, they naturally will resent the process, especially if it impacts negatively upon them.

As subtle as they may be, differences among parties about participation at the table are a common, though often hidden, source of negotiation conflict. It is advantageous to clarify this matter before negotiation begins in earnest. Otherwise, on top of your disagreement about the issues at hand, you will also be hindered by descensus regarding the process preferences of those involved.

Problems

The second element of your frame is your view of the problem. What is it that you want resolved, settled, or changed? In what ways is the current situation unacceptable to you? What caused the current impasse or situation, and how can conditions be changed to alleviate the problem? Other negotiators assess the same set of questions.

When people bring different views of problem and purpose to the table, they face a fundamental obstacle to negotiation progress. They are stuck until they recognize and acknowledge these differences in attitude and approach. It is as if they were trying to paddle the same canoe in different directions. No wonder they don't get anywhere.

Several years ago I mediated a dispute at a community health center. The center faced major budgetary and operational problems, crippling the capacity to provide good patient care. The problem was portrayed as an irreconcilable conflict between clinical and administrative personnel. The administrative people blamed the clinical people for being aloof and unconcerned about the overall welfare of the organization. The clinical people blamed the administrators for being blatantly incompetent. The flash point was the issue of supplies. Clinicians reported that teenage girls were coming to the clinic for pregnancy tests. When the clinicians went to the supply cabinet, the necessary supplies were absent. The girls were sent away, and they became reluctant to return, having lost their confidence in the clinic. The administrators complained that the reason for the shortage of supplies was the clinicians' unwillingness to properly complete insurance forms and make sure they were transferred to the billing office. As a result, the center was denied its rightful payment from insurers, and hence the budgetary crisis. The clinic had fallen into rampant finger-pointing.

It was learned during the course of mediation that the clinicians were sincerely unaware that they were supposed to send the forms

and finances to the administrative floor. They assumed it was someone else's responsibility. The administrators thought the clinicians
knew the required procedures; the clinicians, therefore, could not
understand the reason for the administrators' frustration. During the
deliberations, the problem was reframed from a personal problem
("It's his fault") to a systems matter ("Something isn't working
here"). It was discovered, in fact, that there was no mechanism to
transfer and trace the income from appointment to reimbursement.
The necessary organizational adjustment was made, and collaboration between the two groups was markedly improved.

This accord was achieved in part by pursuing the question
"What's the problem?" Without developing a common understanding, these groups would have remained in persistent conflict.
How can they solve "the problem" if they are, in essence, trying to
solve different problems? Having established consensus on the fundamental issues, it was possible for them to move together toward
a solution and a plan for implementing the agreement.

History

There is a pragmatic side to negotiation and conflict resolution. By
way of a simple formula, you can discern the problem and reach
consensus on options. In the process, you will find good choices and
lousy choices. The parties logically choose for the former.

In fact, real conflict and negotiation is rarely that simple. People bring an abundance of memory to the table. That memory is the
collection of good experiences and bad experiences that influence
their attitudes about others at the table. When that experience has
been positive and productive, the baggage enhances the negotiation. When that experience has been negative, the baggage consti-
tutes a formidable obstacle to progress.

When the parties are negatively predisposed to one another,
their negotiation choices may be motivated more by retribution
than by their own best interests. The parties are then more concerned with putting their trunk of stories on the table than they are

interested in talking about workable options. They are at the table to get even. That motive takes on greater meaning than apparent self-interest.

Old scores intermingle shades of fact with layers of illusion. What really happened is of secondary importance to what the parties believe happened. There is real guilt, and then there is guilt by association. Words and actions assume meaning that supersedes their intent. Emotion blurs objective assessment. The parties are compelled by perception and misperception.

Several years ago, I mediated a dispute between two high-ranking hospital administrators. After hours of exploring the issues and options, we finally reached a tentative agreement on a plan that would allow both to continue their employment at the medical center. Noticing the ambivalence of one of the parties, I asked him to remain in the room for a private caucus after the other left. Referring to the progress we had made, I remarked, "Alan, it seems that you got what you said you were looking for: the money, the quality, and the autonomy." Clenching his fists, gritting his teeth, and becoming red in the face, he clamored, "Yes, but I didn't get revenge. I can't let him get out of this room and go back to his job unscathed by this whole fiasco." He felt the other administrator had maliciously undermined his career and in the process condemned his personal life. Both Alan and John brought great antipathy into their negotiations, and during our meetings they reveled in recounting their stories of woe. My job as a mediator was to help them get beyond their bad history.

Alan's objective was to get even with the world, as he perceived it, by inflicting pain on his counterpart. This type of behavior is associated more with street gang violence than it is with the intricacies of health care professional relationships. And while actual physical violence is rare, the penchant for interdepartmental warfare is not. The result is decision making that offers only fleeting satisfaction.

Beware when "getting even" is a central ingredient of your frame or that of other negotiators. It is a warning: finding a mutually acceptable resolution will be difficult. Even if one of the parties is willing to acknowledge guilt and accept some pain—whether it be in the form of financial penalty, a public apology, or a professional sanction—it is unlikely to satisfy the other's appetite for revenge. If it is you who is motivated by a desire for retribution, carefully assess the reasons, review your *primary* motives and objectives, and determine whether revenge alone will suffice. Though you might revel in the fantasy, a totally wholesome diversion, you want to be careful about transforming your rage into reality. What sacrifice might you suffer for the short-term pleasure of seeing your counterpart writhe? And if others at the table are determined to occasion your demise, be cognizant of the limitations of the negotiation process. There is only so much you want to give in order for them to get even. (Techniques for handling these situations are discussed in Chapter Eleven.)

Processes

There are three types of negotiators: cooperators, collaborators, and contenders. The categories are distinguished by their preference in working relationships. How do you characterize your general working style? How does your general style translate into behavior during a specific activity? One's template describes general interpersonal tendencies. The approach assumed in a particular situation is one's frame.

Cooperators seek fair outcomes with clear parameters defining separate identities. When negotiating, cooperators emphasize the individual benefits that will accrue to each participant. They engage with others in order to achieve distinct gains: "I want to get mine; and because I want you to come back to the table in the future, I want you to get yours, too." Cooperators assess a decision or settlement based on balance: did everyone get their deserved slice of the pie? They are looking for the gain-gain.

Collaborators are more concerned with common purpose and

process than they are with dividing the pie. They emphasize over-lapping interests and rewards. To them, the very act of joining in a common effort offers important satisfaction in and of itself. They favor melding work, credit, and participation so the parties can evolve from separate entities into an aggregate unit sharing a common destiny. From the perspective of collaborators, your gain is our gain. They are looking to achieve a collective, mutual gain.

Contenders view others as discrete competitors, even others perceived to be on the same side. They emphasize conquest. For the contender, winning has meaning in and of itself. They strive for as large a portion of the pie as possible, and they justify their methods by reason of their higher purpose: triumph. The contender's concern for others is premised on how other parties' attitudes affect the potential for future wins. They give in order to get. Contenders crave to be on top of the win-lose.

There are pure versions of these categories—for example, the contender who is always in a contest, even with a spouse. For the most part, however, people's proclivities fall somewhere on the spectrum between collaborator, cooperator, and contender. The stimulus may be the circumstances of a particular negotiation. A contender might assume a collaborative strategy when impressed with the common purpose and the amiable nature of the other negotiators. Or someone may be influenced by experience in a previous negotiation: a cooperator becomes more contentious if recently burned in a negotiation. Or general, societal events may change attitudes. A collaborator becomes contentious when survival of a common mission is threatened. Your style adapts to your circumstances as you understand them.

Understanding your own template and frame for negotiation and that of others will help you plan your strategy. What approach do you generally use, and what approach do you favor in a particular negotiation? What approach are others using? How might their strategy affect the way you plan your own? Is yours adjustable? Is theirs?

◆ ◆ ◆ ◆ ◆ ◆ ◆

Iris Inkwater refers to Dr. Fred Fisher as "old school": white male, respected physician, early sixties, accustomed to being coddled.

Fred Fisher refers to Iris Inkwater as "young upstart": white female, well educated, mid-forties, overpaid.

Iris thinks of herself somewhere between cooperator and collaborator. When necessary, she can be a contender, though she feels that the costs of battle outweigh the benefits in the long run. In her mind, the board of trustees pays her to have the smarts and the guts to use the strategy necessary to get the job done.

Fred doesn't like touchy-feely, and he doesn't like mucking around a decision when he knows what needs to be done. He believes a bit of contention makes for creative tension: it keeps people on their toes. It turns the humdrum of work into sport. He finds meetings and group decision making boring. He is paid to *know* what needs to be done.

Iris called the meeting with Fred. She felt it was important to reframe their working relationship, given the predicament facing the hospital. He was impatient with the discussion before they had even begun talking. In his mind, he couldn't be part of a solution to a problem he didn't create.

"Fred, this hospital is facing a real threat to its survival. I want to be certain that you and I are working together. And just as important, I want to be certain that people who work here see the two of us working together."

Fred took Iris's opener as an accusation. "What are you suggesting, Iris, that we are not working together?"

"I am saying that our working relationship could be a lot better, and in fact has to be a lot better if we are going to pull through this."

"Look, Iris, you are paid to solve problems and to make sure those problems don't damage our capacity to take care of patients. If you have a problem, or if you have created a problem, don't expect us to solve it for you."

"That is just what I think we need to correct, Fred. I did not create this problem. You read the newspapers. You know the pressure the system is under. This problem was not invented by me or even by Community Health Plan. We'll get nowhere if we go around blaming one another."

Fisher was silent. Inkwater was making sense, and he didn't know what to do with it. "What are you suggesting?"

Iris hoped to reframe their working relationship and decided on a metaphor that Fisher would understand. "I suggest that we start playing as if we were on the same team."

Iris sensed Fred's discomfort at being one-upped. She recognized the need to help him save face. "Fred, you have more experience than anyone in this institution. The problem is, they are changing the ball game out there." Seeking to add a touch of humor, she added, "If we continue playing baseball when everyone out there is playing football, we're going to be laughed out of the stadium."

Fisher smiled. He began to appreciate that he and Iris in fact shared a common problem. She was not the "enemy administrator." He began to see her as just the opposite: she had the potential to rescue the ship. If she couldn't come up with a solution, the whole medical center might sink. Her analogy resonated for him. "Iris, I was never good at football." He paused. "You're right. I do believe we have to be working together. But it's going to take some adjustment on all our parts." Fisher did not want to retreat from his tried-and-true stance too quickly.

◆　◆　◆　◆　◆　◆　◆

A negotiation's outcome can only be as good as its process. Early discussion and agreement on process form and format shapes the size of the field in which agreement can be found: the further you move toward collaboration, the wider your possibilities. The more contentious you are, the fewer are your options. Though the parties may open with one frame, conceived from their template, that frame is adjustable. Reframing the process for conducting the negotiation creates new options for reaching settlement.

Outcomes

People enter negotiation anticipating what they will get. Indeed, the emphasis on "get" is seen in the literature and marketing of negotiation: Roger Fisher and William Ury titled their first book *Getting to Yes* (1991). Fisher went on to write *Getting Together* (1988), and Ury published *Getting Past No* (1991). In his airline seat-pocket advertising, Chester Karass (1970) pronounces, "In business, you don't get what you deserve, you get what you negotiate." Negotiation is achievement-oriented, and these slogans appeal to people's appetite for tangible and intangible dividends.

Your frame delineates what you expect to get, as does the frame of other negotiators. This is obviously an important ingredient, as it defines your very motive for being at the table. It becomes problematic, however, when getting is the only ingredient in the pie. If you are negotiating with someone whose sole objective is getting, it is unlikely that your own wishes will be satisfied.

Determining what you and other parties want to get is essential for understanding your frame and that of others in the negotiation. More consequential than understanding what you and others want to get is identifying what you are each prepared to give. This is where discovery becomes important. Negotiation requires learning what you are willing to offer, what the other side is willing to offer, and whether the exchange will satisfy both your interests. I have posed this question to parties involved in the process of health policy reform. Most of the rhetoric for change focuses on what each constituency wants to get. The key to resolution emerges as physicians, insurers, payers, consumers, and others articulate what they are willing to give and give up. Indeed, the process can be stalemated by the players' unwillingness to give up items of consequence.

Limiting what parties give and get simply to an exchange of what they already have is a lackluster approach. Creative negotiation requires the cultivation of new currencies; this way, everyone ends up getting more than they must give. This process of creating new options is termed "expanding the pie." How does expanding the pie work?

Imagine you are bargaining for the purchase of a used car. The discussion focuses on the price, condition, and value of the automobile. You are at a stalemate until you learn that the owner needs to use the car for two more weeks, at which time he is leaving the country. He cannot wait until the last minute to complete the sale. A new item is added to the exchange: time. Since you do not need the car immediately, you offer to complete the sale and wait for delivery, if the owner comes closer to your price. Recognizing that he has saved himself the cost of a rental car, the owner agrees, and you consummate the deal.

To think of negotiation only in terms of getting is to limit it to a unidimensional endeavor. Yes, we may harbor the fantasy of getting everything we want. Yet, it is not a constructive description or productive frame to engage in the process.

Rather, think of negotiation as three-dimensional. On one side there is getting. On another there is giving. The third dimension is the process for achieving the exchange, which links the getting and giving. "Giving to Yes" may not be a catchy proposition. Though face it: what you are willing to give is the enticement that ultimately consummates the deal.

Priorities

Negotiation is a process of relativity: there are no absolutes. Issues and concerns that are of paramount importance to one participant may be irrelevant to another. Values, emphases, and consequences are perceived and experienced quite differently. Your appraisal of these distinctions is essential for crafting a settlement.

Consider the car negotiation above. For the seller, gaining two more weeks with the car and concluding the sale was more important than getting the higher price. For the buyer, using the car for the next two weeks was less important than getting a lower price. They were able to consummate the deal by creating an exchange that meshed their two, relatively different priorities.

To analyze the parties' frames, discern the relative importance of each of their issues. For the seller, it was (1) concluding a sale, (2) use of the car, and (3) price. For the buyer, it was (1) price, (2) the condition of the car, and (3) time of delivery. In this case, their different priorities could be combined to create a fit.

Similarities in priorities also can be used to craft a settlement. When negotiating parties agree on vital principles, such as the importance of an AIDS clinic, institutional efforts to improve quality of care, or the very desire to settle a conflict, the recognition of their consensus increases the likelihood of bringing the parties to agreement. Completing the deal requires you to line up these matters of shared priorities and different priorities in order to accomplish a fit.

Each party brings to the negotiation process different purposes and priorities. Balancing the relative importance of the issues is what the negotiation process is all about. The frame is a constructive negotiation tool when it guides the parties to understanding, using, and adapting their differences and similarities.

Stakes

There are negotiation preferences: the rewards and benefits you hope to acquire. These represent your fiction of what will be achieved. Anticipating these benefits, you negotiate.

And then—good or bad, like it or not—there are negotiation realities. Stakes convey the tangible outcomes facing the parties. They reach a decision point when they seriously weigh these outcomes. "What will be the costs if I hold off? What can I get if we settle? What will I be required to give? Do I want to remain in this unresolved limbo?" The answers to these questions can offer an incentive when they reflect an expectation of rewards. They can become a threat when they signal fear of objectionable consequence, causing one or more parties to delay settlement to avoid a greater loss.

There are three kinds of stakes: good stakes, bad stakes, and opportunity stakes.

Good stakes are the bounty you reap from the deal: a well-priced piece of equipment, a few extra days of vacation, a lucrative contract. Agree to the terms of the offer, and these splendid prizes are yours. Other parties have placed inducements on the table to move you to agree, making it hard to walk from the table. Likewise, to encourage others to accept your offer, you sweetened it with inducements hard for them to refuse.

Bad stakes are the adversities that befall you on account of the deal: the loss of your job, the imposition of a fine, the closing of your department. Depending on your moves, these objectionable fates could be in store for you. In view of these circumstances, staying at the table when threatened with bad stakes is as painful as walking away. You confront a personal dilemma, choosing between bad options. One choice is to accept your fate. Another option is to retreat to your negotiation preferences, believing there is some way to forestall the outcome, defeat the opponent, and retrieve your illusion. This move propels the negotiation into another spiral of escalation.

Opportunity stakes are the undefined possibilities, for gain or loss, that could result from the deal. These are the "what could be" or "what could have been" questions that face the negotiators. Rather than "I'll give you $2,000 right now" or "Here is your program," an opportunity stake is conditional: "If we can develop the program, there is the likelihood that it will generate $2,000." Opportunity stakes are the calculated risks that you choose to accept or reject through the negotiation process. They mature with time, accruing value or disfavor as they evolve. You assess an opportunity stake for risk and reward: "What are the chances this transaction will generate my desired outcomes?"

There are two kinds of opportunity stakes: good and bad. Creating the program is a good opportunity. The demise of the program is a bad opportunity: "If only we had come to agreement, the program would still be operating." An opportunity stake, whether its outcome is good or bad, can only be judged in retrospect, and only with a taste of the hypothetical: "If only we had begun the program, we could have been holding $2,000 right now." Or, "We took a risk on the program, and it worked to benefit us all."

Stakes come packaged in mixed blends: a combination of good, bad, and opportunity stakes. You may be required to swallow bad stakes in order to secure the good ones you desire. Good and bad opportunities mix into the brew, barely seen though always influencing the willingness or reluctance of the parties to swallow the stakes. Seldom are the choices all good or all bad. Often they are arranged to form a combination that is only relatively better or relatively worse for each of the parties.

During the negotiation process, stakes are created, assessed, and exchanged. Creation resembles "If your department extends its hours, we will allot you additional office space." Assessment balances costs and benefits: "The stakes are the gain of added space, along with responsibility for a longer work day." And exchange establishes the deal: "We will extend the hours if you will also allot the department a new staff position." The other party balances the combined cost of the square footage and staff position against the increased revenues of evening hours to decide whether the exchange is reasonable.

How might the matter of stakes move the negotiation process forward? Stakes become real at the negotiation decision point. They are a spur to settlement. "Before the end of the week, we will either give your department the extra space or give it to someone else. Reject the extra time, and you loose the space." That is the choice. You accept or you reject the stakes on the table, good and bad. You assess the risks of the opportunity stakes: what are the odds that they will land in your favor, and what are the odds they won't?

Whether good or bad, there can be a reluctance to accept stakes. In your fantasies about what you hope to get, good stakes could be better and bad stakes could be avoided. The parties may need time to concede them, while they test the limits to determine if the stakes are real. There is an acceptance period, sometimes seconds and sometimes years, while the parties learn to live with their stakes as reality. The deal is consummated when both parties buy the stakes.

Negotiation, then, is a process of learning, molding, and accepting the stakes.

* * * * * * *

It was not a good meeting.

Iris Inkwater, Perry Pratt (the hospital's chief operating officer), and Ralph Richman (its chief financial officer) walked to a restaurant across the street from the Community Health Plan (CHP) offices to grab a cup of coffee and their breath. They had just finished their first round of negotiations with Nathaniel Norquist and his crew at CHP. They settled into the protective seclusion of a booth before they let go.

Ralph was steaming. "Damn, they've got us against the wall. There is simply no room to maneuver with what they've put on the table."

Iris was subdued, staring blankly at her cup. "There is no way we're going to come out of this looking anything like what we look like now."

Pratt echoed Iris's tone. "Yes, I believe 'reorganization' is a euphemism for 'layoffs.'"

"The problem," Ralph reasoned, "is that we're at a competitive disadvantage. Because of our location and our patient mix, our costs are simply higher than our competition's. Putting us on the same scale with the suburban outfits is simply comparing apples and oranges."

"Well, unfortunately," Iris observed, "community responsibility doesn't carry much weight these days, guys. If our rivals can do it for cheaper, then they're going to get the business."

"What's your sense of where we need to go, Iris?" Perry asked.

"We have to rethink the hospital. Obviously we're going to have to look at some major budget reductions. And no sacred cows anymore. We have to have the guts to face up to personnel cuts, and I mean a serious assessment of each department. And we're going to have to look into cooperative options with other hospitals as well. The problem is that, as an expensive inner-city hospital, we don't have much leverage in that ball game. That means that we're probably looking more at a takeover than a consolidation. In that case, the three of us can logically pack our bags and say good-bye. They'll have no need for us in that arrangement. After all, how many CEOs, COOs, and CFOs do you need in one organization? But that option will be up to the board. They'll have to be educated about the options."

Pratt saw his career, his aspirations, and his mortgage pass before his eyes. He had been on the hospital administration fast track. The move to Oppidania Medical Center had been a big leap for him, careerwise. And he had feared at the time that he might be investing his hopes in a sinking ship. It turns out that his worst fears may be realized. Still, he wasn't ready to give in yet. "I don't think we should throw in the towel yet, Iris," he offered hopefully.

"Oh, Perry, don't get me wrong. I'm not giving up. I'm just saying that this is serious business. OMC has to survive for a whole list of good reasons. And if we begin this process by excluding a set of reasonable options, then we're not going to find the key to the puzzle. That's scary. It's scary for the hospital, it's scary for our staff and the people we serve, and its scary for us. It's going to take a lot of courage and a lot of leadership on our part. In the long run, I believe that is how we are going to be judged. I just don't think we have any choice. We have to consider all the options."

"Such as?" Ralph queried.

"Such as, we come out 'leaner and greener,'" Iris countered with building confidence. "Ralph, in principle we have to turn around some of the numbers. We have to look at real costs and real production. That means we may have to become something less than a full-service hospital in order to be of service at all." Iris paused to ponder a new idea. "We have to reconsider what we do and how we go about doing it. We can contract out more services to reduce expenses: moving to vendors may help us stretch the budget. We'll have to renegotiate our fiduciary relationship with some of the physician groups. And if we are to have any credibility, we'll have to tighten our administrative ship.

"We may also have to seriously look at some of the medical departments in terms of volume, real costs, and income. The myth that we need to be a comprehensive medical center may have outlived its utility. We are not the only show in town. It may make sense to explore joint arrangements for high-tech procedures. We are dropping a lot of money into machines that get outmoded too quickly."

"Yes, although you don't want to throw away our big money-makers," Ralph reasoned. "Several of those high-tech procedures can keep us going for a long time. And the medical school is not going to like seeing you tinker with their tidy little house."

"Ralph, that's why we need your numbers. Many of the departments have survived on illusions about their income and expenses. And the medical school is going to have to live with a big chunk of us, which is much better than no chunk at all."

"Iris, what do you realistically see as the odds we're going to pull out of this?" Perry asked.

"If we buckle down, I think they're pretty good. If we don't, we can turn the building into artist lofts, and we'll all take up painting."

They left the restaurant and headed back to the hospital.

◆ ◆ ◆ ◆ ◆ ◆ ◆

Negotiation Claimers and Creators[1]

Consider a distinguishing characteristic of negotiators: those who are claimers and those who are creators.

Claimers engage in the negotiation process in order to grab whatever they can for themselves or their constituency. Sometimes it is a matter of gently taking whatever they are able to take. Other times it is more blatant, a game of seizing, appropriating, and plundering. In the mind of the claimer, negotiation is a means of accumulation. It is not about fairness, evenhandedness, or justice.

[1]The material in this section is derived from lectures of and discussions with Howard Raiffa (1982) and Phyllis Kritek (1994).

Negotiation is a sport of conquest, domination, and winning. It is distributional: "The more others get, the less I get; and I want to get as much as possible for myself."

Creators engage in the negotiation process as an inventive exercise. For them it is a means of forging connections between parties sharing a linked destiny. By building relationships, creators are able to share efforts, enhance resource expansion, and spur inventiveness. Negotiation becomes an entrepreneurial venture through which the parties discover that by working together, they each will have more to share and more to divide. Satisfaction with the process and with their relationship generates rewarding opportunities for future cooperation.

Whether creator or claimer, we negotiate in order to improve our lot: we want to get something. Our willingness to engage and remain in the process depends upon our belief that there is something to be gained for the effort.

How do these different approaches combine to affect negotiation outcomes: zero-sum, negative-sum, and positive-sum negotiations? Consider two negotiators, Tom and Bill.

What if Tom is a consistent claimer and Bill is a consistent creator? When a claimer and a creator negotiate, the creator tends to come out the loser. While Bill is naively building a relationship, Tom is plundering the stockpile. Tom does not care about relationships, and Bill eventually discovers that he attempted a meaningless relationship while losing his negotiation objectives. Tom reaps abundant spoils from the negotiation, and Bill is left with nothing. When a creator negotiates with a claimer—and the creator does not change his style—then he is likely to lose in the process.

What if Tom and Bill are both claimers? Then they each come out losers. Calculate total assets, including tangibles divided, such as money, space, and property, along with intangibles lost, such as time, opportunities, and satisfaction. They both invest tremendous effort in beating the other, and they both come out behind. In the process of claiming, the two expend time, energy, and resources that otherwise could be divided as the spoils of settlement. They both view the negotiation as a win-lose proposition, and they both invest abundant resources in ensuring their win. That combined investment, when measured against the total resources they could divide, represents their losses. The experience of the negotiation itself is a liability. The resentment and desire for revenge besieging both of them makes future accommodation less likely. This is particularly true if Tom and Bill are colleagues working in the same organization.

What if Tom and Bill are both creators? Then negotiation becomes an opportunity for valuable learning, discovery, and trust building. Their new relationship is an added dividend of the process. They cultivate new settlement options, discern hidden prospects, and devise otherwise unapparent solutions. The mutual satisfaction that results from each negotiation breakthrough spurs them to further resourcefulness. They build a synergy of ideas, solutions, and benefits.

The claimer-creator distinction reveals the negotiation template you bring to the process. It defines your fundamental approach to other people and the elements you are exchanging. Are you a giver, a taker, or a sharer? What values, code of conduct, and principles guide you?

So too, the claimer-creator distinction reveals the template your negotiation counterparts bring to the table. By understanding their negotiation style and strategy, you are able to analyze and even predict their approach and attitude to ideas and proposals. This insight is invaluable, particularly when you must frequently negotiate with the same people.

Negotiation Outcomes

Imagine that Tom and Bill are negotiating about a pie.

In the first scenario, Tom the claimer snatches the pie as Bill the creator tries to build a relationship. This is a win-lose scenario, with a zero-sum outcome: the overall size of the pie has not changed.

In the second scenario, claimers Tom and Bill expend so much time and effort fighting over the pie that much of it becomes inedible. This is a lose-lose situation, with a negative-sum outcome: there is less pie left to eat.

In the third scenario, creators Tom and Bill together bake a bigger pie. By multiplying their options and opportunities, they add to the yield. This is a gain-gain scenario, with a positive-sum outcome: there is more pie for both. Both parties have gained, though neither attained a victory over the other. If they perceive their destiny as interwoven, then together they have accomplished a win.

In zero-sum negotiation, nothing is gained or lost in the process: the sum of available resources remains the same. In negative-sum negotiation, the destructive process of bargaining causes a reduction in resources available. In positive-sum negotiation, the constructive process of learning allows for an increase in the use of and availability of resources.

How does one "expand the pie" in health care, especially when the popular perception is that the pie is already shrinking?

Generating Options

Trust is the foundation upon which negotiation rests. Relationships are the engine that keeps it going. And imaginations are the wings upon which it flies.

An inventive imagination is among the most important qualities of the very best negotiators. When two parties commence a negotiation, the actual result is yet a mystery: they could become frustrated and descend into bickering; they could achieve only a languid outcome; they might attain a solution exceeding their original expectations. The outcome is unknown. Their result derives from combined negotiation approaches and interpersonal skills, along with the resonance of their interactions. Without imagination, it is unlikely that they will conjure up more than the mundane and the self-evident. However, when they each bring their ingenuity, inspiration, and resourcefulness to the process, they encounter otherwise unanticipated solutions and opportunities. They combine intellectual and interpersonal risk taking with functional creativity to envision new solutions to old problems. They understand the possibilities and limits of what might be done and how to make it happen.

For those with an imagination, negotiation itself becomes a process of invention. Problems become puzzles waiting for solutions. The thrill of negotiation derives from the esprit de corps devoted to shifting the pieces so they better fit. Courage inspires the parties to ascend above the common thinking that the puzzle can't be effectively assembled. The importance of courage is particularly cogent for people or groups who are in conflict. It takes imagination to envision rapprochement, and it takes willpower to make it happen. When imaginative negotiation clicks, the reward is innovation of the highest order.

What negotiation methods can be used to prompt and validate imagination? Brainstorming is a useful and stimulating way to begin. When leading a brainstorming session, I place a clean sheet of paper on the table or on an easel and invite any and all ideas—the wilder and crazier the better. I instruct the participants not to comment or editorialize on the proposals: such judgments would inhibit unconfined thinking. Those who participate begin to contemplate ideas they had previously rejected or never considered because they were limited by the constraints of their situation, both real and imagined. Brainstorming is not only engaging, it is also fun and amusing, as different people naturally create options that seem incongruous at first. Even more entertaining is the prospect that some of these incongruous ideas could be transformed into workable solutions.

As you brainstorm, consider these aspects of the negotiation frame:

Which people might be included or excluded from the process?

How can the problem be defined or redefined to allow different approaches to resolution?

What history or old scores need to be settled, and what creative settlement approaches could be introduced?

How might new and productive processes be introduced into the negotiation?

What are the outcome expectations of the parties, and how can they be adjusted to find common ground?

How do the priorities of one group complement the different priorities of the other?

What alternative views can be brought in to expand the pie and sweeten everybody's stakes?

Use the results of the brainstorming to create a laundry list. The laundry list exercise moves the participants from free thinking into the realm of the plausible and the implausible. Analyze the points listed during the brainstorming session: put the ideas into categories; assess them for their feasibility, their merit, and their compatibility with other ideas and situations. The result of the laundry list exercise is a series of reasonable options for the parties to assess.

When the laundry list undertaking has been completed, the negotiators arrive at their decision point. For each participant, the question becomes, "What option or combination of options from the laundry list do I find acceptable?" They have progressed from brainstorming to laundry list assessment and now to settlement, with a greatly expanded scope of options. With a wider range of choices, it is easier to imagine and achieve a settlement. Furthermore, with so much to choose from, with so much invested in the process, and with so much inventive enthusiasm harnessed to make it happen, you will likely have accomplished a solution that is better suited to the interests of the parties at the table.

Generating negotiation options is about creating more choices from which to select a mutually acceptable settlement or outcome. When incorporated into the negotiation process, imagination sparks the resources of the human spirit to discover better solutions. It replaces the fear of losing with the hope of achievement. It is fear that provokes the claimer. It is hope that inspires the creator.

◆ ◆ ◆ ◆ ◆ ◆ ◆

Stuart Schilling has been with Oppidania General for nearly nine years. A philosopher by training, he translated his interest in applied philosophy and health care into a career in medical bioethics. He divides his time between teaching at the school and meeting as needed with staff, patients, and families at the hospital. He has gained the respect of the hospital staff as a good listener and problem solver.

The request for this afternoon's meeting came earlier in the day from Tanya Tarrington, head nurse on Nine West, a general medical floor. The problem, she explained, was a difference of opinion regarding a do-not-resuscitate (DNR) order for an elderly gentleman who has been on the floor for over two weeks. The internist and cardiologist who have been working with the patient disagree on whether a DNR is appropriate, and Tarrington is concerned about the family's getting mixed signals. She explained that both physicians agreed that a bioethics consult was a good idea. Shilling and Tarrington decided that, at this point, it would be best to include themselves, the two physicians, and the social worker who has been working with the family.

Victor Vining is a cardiologist who has been attending the patient, Mr. Ulrich, since he was admitted with a myocardial infarction. Wendell White is an internist. He has been following Mr. Ulrich since he was hospitalized two years ago with pneumonia. Ziva Zartman is a social worker who has been working with the patient and family from the start of this admission.

Dr. White spoke first. He explained that Mr. Ulrich, a seventy-eight-year old gentleman, is a patient with nine lives. When he had pneumonia, the staff thought he wouldn't make it, and he pulled through marvelously. Since then he has suffered an aneurysm and a severe infection in his foot. After each bout, he has recovered to return to his cherished game of golf. Dr. White concluded that he thinks it's simply too early to write this patient off.

Dr. Vining waited for his colleague to conclude and then presented his opinion on the case. He reported that Mr. Ulrich had been conscious though very weak for the first few days of his hospitalization. Vining quoted the patient's remarks: "Doctor, if this can't work, I don't want heroics. This could be it for me." Vining went on to delineate the patient's medical condition, which he concluded was grim. Given the circumstances of the case and the real costs for the hospital, Vining felt it was irresponsible not to recommend that the family sign a DNR order.

Ziva Zartman spoke next. She described the torment facing the family. She agreed with Dr. White. His miraculous recoveries have instilled a sense of hope for them. Yet they also sense that this illness is different. She went on to explain that they are so distraught and confused that they pleaded with her just to get a clear recommendation from the medical staff. Mr. Ulrich's daughter said that the family just couldn't bear to be left with an unclear set of choices. Mr. Ulrich, oddly enough, had no living will, and neither Mrs. Ulrich nor the children know what to do.

Tanya Tarrington spoke last. She agreed with Dr. White. Mr. Ulrich truly was the miracle patient who defied the odds. She remembers him from two years ago, and how at the time it had seemed unlikely that he would survive. She ordinarily wouldn't be optimistic about a patient as sick as Mr. Ulrich, though there are enough surprises in his medical chart to make her unusually cautious. The problem for the hospital, she explained, is that he is too sick to be discharged to a nursing home. In all honesty, she added, his continued hospitalization was a financial drain on the hospital. Realistically, she concluded, they couldn't ignore the financial consequences of their recommendation.

Shilling first asked for clarification on some points, and then began his work.

"Well, it seems to me that this is one of those difficult cases in which we end up making a decision even if we don't. If we can't decide on whether to recommend the DNR, then that is a decision with clear implications, as Tanya has explained. On one hand, we do not want to put the patient and family through unnecessary suffering and the hospital through unnecessary expense. On the other hand, if there is hope for recovery, we don't want to give up prematurely."

As a rule, Shilling doesn't tell people what to do. He sees his role as helping the responsible parties make their own decision.

He turned to Dr. White. "Wendell, as things stand right now, you are reluctant to recommend the DNR. What could happen, or what might you learn, that would change your mind?" The question reframed White's thinking, away from the stance that he was defending Mr. Ulrich's survival. He pointed to several clinical indicators, changes over a period of time, and a willingness from the family to call it quits. He noted that if the family wanted to give up, that would be an important factor for him — first because he would want to comply with their wishes, and second because it would relieve him of any concerns regarding a lawsuit down the road.

Shilling next turned to Vining. He asked, "Victor, what would convince you not to recommend the DNR?" Vining likewise reconsidered his position. He pointed to signs of clinical improvement over a specified period of time. He also wanted to be sensitive to the family's wishes and noted that they seemed to be reacting more to their grief than to the medical realities facing the patient. He also reminded the group that Mr. Ulrich may have realized that he had reached the end of his road. Tarrington, White, and Zartman each said that they were unaware of the patient's remark to Vining about giving up. Vining was surprised; he thought the patient had shared his sentiments with others at the hospital.

Schilling broke the silence as each of the people at the table rethought their approach to the case. "It seems that there are three factors here: time, clinical indicators, and the family." He went through each one individually. They agreed that twenty-four hours was a reasonable waiting period for clinical improvement. The clinical indicators they would watch for were acceptable to both White and Vining. If there was improvement, then a DNR order would not be recommended. If there was no

change or a decline in the patient's condition, they would recommend that the family sign a DNR order. The group agreed that
Ziva would discuss this decision with the family today, explaining that the hospital wants to feel certain that the most appropriate recommendation is being made. If the family wanted the
DNR decision before the waiting period was up, that was their
choice. If they wanted to hold out longer, an extension not to
exceed forty-eight hours would be acceptable.

Both White and Vining agreed that this was a reasonable
approach. Tarrington thanked Schilling for making himself
available on such short notice. Zartman headed back to Mr.
Ulrich's room to meet with the family.

◆ ◆ ◆ ◆ ◆ ◆ ◆

The multiparty decisions that face us in health care range from
the mundane to the monumental. The decision-making models
we utilize determine the quality of our choices. Collaborative models offer opportunities to build a wealth of constructive options,
from which we can select the best remedy for the problem. Especially when there is conflict, we improve outcomes by engaging
the parties to generate a range of settlement options from which
to cultivate resolution. This creative approach enhances both the
consequences of our endeavors as well as the processes for achieving them.

6

Reframing to Spur Momentum

You perform many roles as a negotiator: getter, giver, investigator, instigator, inquirer. And when the negotiation hits a standstill, there is another vital role to play: catalyst (see Bazerman and Neale, 1992; Stulberg, 1987).

Like good music, negotiation has rhythm and movement, from the slow adagios to the quick allegros. There is a cadence to negotiation: unspoken expectations about what can be accomplished and when it will happen. Without progress, the negotiation eventually fades or collapses.

That sluggishness and erosion results from perceived incongruity between the parties' frames. When there is basic disagreement about who should be at the table, then progress on other substantive issues is jeopardized. When irreconcilable suspicion about the history of the dispute remains, then veiled obstacles deter acceptance of new interpretations. And when the priorities of one party are incompatible with those of another, then each defends divergent purposes at the table. What can be done to overcome these predicaments?

The catalyst to revitalizing stagnant negotiation is reframing: reformulating pieces of the puzzle so they better fit. Through reframing, the parties transform fundamental elements of their outlook to find common ground. They reassess and adjust perceptions and attitudes about the people, problems, history, process, outcomes, priorities, and stakes of the negotiation. They seek compatibility.

The very process of reframing is an exercise that leads toward resolution. By devising fresh agreement on elements of their frames, the parties begin movement that nudges them toward settlement. In so doing, they discover that more complementary preferences, information, and hopes yield them better results. They needn't agree on each other's perceptions, though they can acknowledge their differences. They needn't abandon their objectives, though they might adjust them to enhance compatibility. They are creating a new balance between their distinct concerns.

How do you get the reframing process started? Interrupt the antagonism. Vary the rhythm of the negotiation: say something unexpected; bring in an outside neutral; place new consequences on the table; tell a joke; present a new offer for consideration; invite your enemy out to lunch.

If you are the catalyst, open with a question, an observation, or a concern. "What do you hope to accomplish?" "I think we're stuck." "Without some progress, we all lose."

◆ ◆ ◆ ◆ ◆ ◆ ◆

Oscar O'Neill knew there was a good deal of tension between Artie Ashwood's mother, Anna, and his girlfriend, Cindy Carrington. When he heard loud voices coming from Artie's room, he made his way to check what was going on.

When Oscar appeared at the door, the shouting suddenly stopped. He jumped into the silence. "Is there a problem?" Artie's mother and girlfriend exchanged icy glances and then looked away.

Artie opened the conversation. "There seems to be a bit of disagreement about where I go tomorrow when I'm discharged. Mom wants me to recover at home, and Cindy wants me at, well, our home. Quite frankly, I'm feeling torn."

"Well, you're already torn up enough, my friend. There's no need to do more damage," Oscar said, hoping his smile would lighten the mood. "Are we talking about where you're living long-term, or just for your recuperation?"

"I assume we're talking recuperation," Artie replied. Cindy and Anna both remained quiet, allowing this conversation to remain between patient and nurse. Artie turned toward the two women, looking for agreement. They both nodded reluctantly.

Oscar continued. "Having hung around this room quite a lot for the past few days, I've gotten the impression that there is not a lot that the two of you think you agree about." There was a pause, and Cindy meekly replied, "I guess you could say that."

"Well, in fact, I've found there is one very important thing that you do agree on." Oscar lit up with an ear-to-ear grin and pointed to Artie. "You both think this fellow here is the most lovable guy in the universe."

The two women sheepishly glanced at one another, and unable to restrain themselves, they both broke out in a smile. "Now, I do agree he's a nice guy, but I'm not sure I'd go to war over him." Oscar's dramatic gestures added an almost comic tone to the discussion.

There was suddenly a different feel in the room. The edge was off: there was a sense of relief. Oscar let the silence linger a few moments as everyone let it sink in.

"Artie's still quite sick. I mean, this guy gets applause for just getting out of bed and taking a hike around the nursing station. It's going to take him a week before he feels well enough to move around on his own. The question here is not where he's going to live for the rest of his life. The question is where he can get the best care for the next few days."

Artie wanted to jump in. He was afraid, though, that whatever he might say would refuel the fire. Finally Cindy opened up, addressing Oscar. "I guess the problem is that I just started a new job and don't have any time off. If he came back to our place, he would be alone for most of the day. Artie's mom has a lot of vacation time built up, so she could be with him during the day." Cindy turned toward Anna. "The problem is, I don't want to say good-bye to Artie for the week. I don't feel comfortable when I'm at your place."

With a warm smile, Anna placed her hand on Cindy's. "I want you to come, and I want you to feel comfortable."

Oscar had done just enough to turn things around. He got a thumbs-up from Artie as he left the room.

◆ ◆ ◆ ◆ ◆ ◆

Crafting a Fit

Negotiation and conflict resolution is the art of shaping congruity from incongruity.

Incongruity is a state of mind. It is rooted in the way we think. It eclipses our vision and our ability to imagine new options. It is the frustration we feel when our world doesn't make sense: when good people are mortal, when good health care is not available for people who need it, when others in the room don't appreciate the brilliance of what you propose. It is an apprehension that pieces of your life are supposed to be connected, and they are not. It is that discomfort we feel when logic disappears. It is the panic we experience when unfairness overwhelms.

When endured in private, incongruity is confusion. When it comes between people, it is conflict. We resist incongruity and the people who confront us with it. We fantasize away the confusion. We defeat the opposition.

How do you change your frame of mind? How do you move from fighting incongruity to living with it? How do you evolve from enduring incongruity to cultivating congruity? Required is a fundamental shift.

Rephrase to Reframe

Begin with a change of vocabulary that will induce a change in thinking. Take the word "but" out of your vocabulary. Replace it with "and." You will reframe what you say, what you think, and what you do.

For example, "I wanted to attend the staff meeting, *but* I couldn't" is an incongruous statement: first you say *yes* and then you say *no*.

There is a subtle difference in meaning when you say, "I wanted to attend the staff meeting, *and* I couldn't." Rather than expressing two opposing drives, you combine two desires that regrettably had to be balanced. You express two statements that coincide with one another. In place of a defense for your absence, you offer an explanation: "A new patient was admitted and there was no one else to do the workup." If your intention to otherwise attend the meeting is trusted, your "and" to connect the two obligations will prompt a much different reaction from your colleagues than a "but." Their anger and their disappointment will be allayed. They will more readily accept that you had a difficult set of expectations to balance.

Substituting "and" for "but" is subtle. Place it into your speech pattern. What you say "and," the reaction to it is transformed. You build connection between divergent statements. Try it in your negotiation. "I would love to give you additional office space, *and* I just don't have it." Follow the statement with an exploration of the other party's interests: is there a way to satisfy their needs within the limitations of your square footage? You reframe the negotiation from territorialism to a quest to satisfy legitimate interests. If these two phrases were attached by "but," there would be an implication of lesser worth, disregard, imbalance, and favoritism. The statement "But I just don't have it" has a ring of finality to it: the answer is "no."

It works both ways: "I do understand that you can't shift offices now, *and* that limits the productivity of our unit." You have acknowledged the limitations facing the other party as you reveal the consequences of those limitations. If there is mutual concern about reduced potential and productivity, then you have opened the door to finding solutions. You have reframed the discussion from a "no" to a common desire to find a solution for a shared problem. If instead of "and" you used "but," it would sound like you were posing a threat: "but that limits the productivity of our unit." The other party might react defensively.

Incorporating the word "and" into your speech reframes your

search for congruity. You balance pieces of your puzzle to seek compatibility in place of confrontation. You accept real limitations and creatively seek the field of available innovative options. You recognize that not all interests of all parties can be fully satisfied. You seek solutions that allow all the parties reasonable gains from the negotiation process.

Reframing Health Care

The move from framing on the basis of incongruity to reframing in search of congruity produces a pivotal shift in the negotiation process. It changes the premise for the conduct of working relationships. Rather than framing demands in order to compete, you discover solutions in order to satisfy. Rather than defeating the other side, you hear and respond to their legitimate interests. You reshape the assumptions for relating to one another. You seek connection, relationship, and fit among people and their problems.

Health care work bursts with incongruity. It operates in the realm of highly charged issues that often elude unambiguous solutions. The domain of one profession overlaps and sometimes conflicts with another. Money is not always spent in ways that maximize its effectiveness. Decision-making authority is grasped seemingly by people without the expertise to make good choices. There is concern for liability, reputation, and professional autonomy. And when the system is in the midst of change, unknowns and incongruities can suffocate.

These divisions often manifest as adversarial confrontations between eventual winners and losers. This pattern has been so ingrained in the operation of health care that some believe it is the best way to operate. Each piece fights to save itself, making the system as a whole more illogical, incongruous, and disjointed.

Devising a more compatible balance is essential to creating a better system. Our capacity to achieve that balance depends on the methods used to achieve it: product arises from process.

Listening and Responding

Negotiation is a form of expression. Through what is said and done, the negotiators reveal their objectives. They disclose their concerns. They signal consequences. They divulge information. They suggest alternatives. And they clarify misinterpretations.

There is a wealth of valuable information. Frequently it is lost. You are not listening. You are so taken with your next line, your overriding apprehension, and your compelling emotion, that you don't pay attention. You frustrate others who feel they can't get through to you. They expect a mindful response to what they are saying. You are preoccupied.

Negotiation is also a form of communication. It requires exchange of information. You become impatient when the other side disregards your offers, concerns, and suggestions. You feel belittled and disenfranchised, and you don't like it. You become reluctant to continue.

When the parties do not actively listen to one another, they reach an impasse. What is being said by one is not being heard by the other. It is not integrated. The parties are not building an exchange of information. Frustration grows. How can you better pay attention? Active listening.

Active listening is a dynamic process for hearing and responding. It requires some measure of repeating, reflecting, and reacting to what the other person says. You demonstrate to others that what they are saying is penetrating. You are working with the information they are sharing. Active listening requires effort on your part. You substantiate your interest in devising a workable solution by engaging with the other person.

Active listening means you integrate and synthesize what you are hearing. There is a range of possible responses, from agreement to acknowledgement to reflection.

Most satisfying is repetition and agreement. "Based on what you report, I must concur that knee surgery is the only option in this case." Agreement does not mean that you ignore your concerns. You can agree, and then add your "and" to specify what you need in return. Or you might simply agree, and by gracefully acknowledging what you learned from the other party, recover a measure of relationship and trust for your next negotiation.

If you do not want to signal agreement, demonstrate concern through acknowledgment. "I appreciate that there is a great deal of anxiety in your department regarding the budget crisis." Acknowledgment is an effective way to calm the other person without conceding your point of view. You demonstrate your attention to their concerns without admitting culpability. Likewise, you do not obligate yourself to their demands.

Finally, if your disagreement is too emphatic to show even acknowledgment, merely reflect what the other person says. "You seem very concerned about the new admitting procedures." Though you have neither agreed with the statement nor acknowledged it as legitimate, you have nonetheless actively responded to what was said. You have sent at least a signal of recognition.

Responding and Engaging

Communication involves both form and intent. Agreement, acknowledgment, and reflection describe your form: how you respond. Intent refers to the substance of your response: what you mean. Are you merely responding to their overt statements, or are you stretching further to explore their underlying interests? By attending to underlying interests, you open new avenues to resolution. You signal your intent to engage and satisfy some measure of their expectations.

When you respond to overt statements, you mirror what the other party requests. You clarify, reiterate, and signal your understanding. "You want the weekend off." "You are unhappy in your current position." "The department is not able to raise your salary." You have not submitted to the other person. With your response, you allay any concerns about whether you heard and understood.

Responding to underlying interests sends a more receptive, sympathetic, and potent signal. You demonstrate your concern for the breadth of what has been expressed, and you show that you are astute enough to figure it out.

You respond to the process preferences, psychological needs, and tangible expectations that motivate the other person. In response to a request for time off, you add, "You need time to prepare for your son's birthday." To the employee dissatisfied with his or her position, "You feel overstressed in the job." And to the boss who has turned down your request for a pay raise, "You would like to better compensate me, but the budget won't allow it." (Use "but" here because you have not yet accepted the congruity of these statements.)

Placing underlying interests on the table opens a new implicit question: is it possible to find a resolution that satisfies the interests of both sides? This question is particularly important if it is impossible to completely satisfy a request: "I can't give you the whole weekend off. I could give you a half day off on both Saturday and Sunday by extending the hours of two other people. I know that you have to shop and prepare, and obviously be there for the party. Which half of each of these days would be best for you?" You maintained your staffing level while you offered genuine understanding, concern, and choice to the other person. "The stress you now feel on the job wasn't there three months ago. What's changed, and what might we do to get ourselves back on track?" You have established your sincere attention and eagerness to uncover your employee's concerns and suggestions. "I understand that the department is short on cash. Would you be willing to explore other ways to adjust my remuneration?" You open the door to finding a solution while simultaneously addressing the constraints and hopes of both sides. In each case, you are seeking compatibility in order to balance different interests.

Active listening generates the cadence of negotiation. It sets the tempo and keeps the momentum. It engages the parties by moving them from exchanging information to exploring interests, until they finally consummate the deal. In so doing, they build momentum for developing an exchange based on mutual interests: it guides them to find integrative options and reach common-ground solutions.

A cautionary note. Active listening backfires when it is interpreted as patronizing, paternalistic, or pandering. If the other person perceives your response as trivial, incredulous, or erroneous, your efforts will only generate further suspicion. Negotiation technique, absent the essential ingredients of trust, sincerity, and integrity, is only a technique.

Negotiation Jujitsu

Active listening is relatively easy to practice during a civilized exchange of ideas, information, and requests. Conflict, however, often involves heated emotion and passion. The dialogue coming your way is rife with anger and aggression. You are assaulted with insult, disparagement, and scorn.

Your instinctual response is to shield yourself, to seek shelter from the onslaught. You may try to crush the offensive by outdoing it: throw them an even more scathing insult, craft an even more ghastly threat, or overpower with an even more outrageous act. Your impulse is to react, to defend and defeat. While this might provide some immediate gratification, in the process you only cause the conflict to escalate. What is the option?

Negotiation jujitsu (Fisher, Ury, and Patton, 1991). Imagine a fist coming at you. You could attempt to stop or crush it, causing shattering destruction as you collide. Or you could absorb it: grasp it, hold it, and gently slow it down. In so doing, there is no crash or explosion.

Metaphorically borrowed from the martial arts, negotiation jujitsu is a technique to diffuse the tensions and emotions that accompany conflict. It serves two purposes. First, negotiation jujitsu calms the other person, giving him or her a chance to release anger and frustration. The other person likely anticipates that you will strike back. Your response, to patiently listen and understand, surprises and calms down the other party. You have opened the door to reframing by doing something unexpected. You create a new frame in which there is regard and respect.

Second, negotiation jujitsu offers you a handy brace. It helps you maintain control of your own emotions and instincts when someone is shouting at you. Negotiation jujitsu helps you preserve your patience as the other person vents his or her feelings. Imagine using your left hand to absorb a blow directed at you. You may have to do this several times, repeating it as the person cools down. Finally, when the other party has witnessed your willingness to hear and respond, there is more openness to reframing.

After calming down the other side, you are able to offer an alternative frame, as if with your right hand, palm up and giving. You have signaled that you are amenable to considering their interests as well as your own. You demonstrate the legitimacy of their concerns as you implicitly ask them to do the same: "I hear you, and I hope you hear me." You have diffused the situation by finding a balance that looks for a mutually beneficial solution.

Negotiation jujitsu is a form of active listening. It is useful in health care situations, as emotions often do become impassioned. It calms a hysterical parent reacting to a child's illness, dissatisfied employees angry about their assignments, a disgruntled patient frustrated by the cold chicken soup. Instructing the parent to knock it off, telling the employees to get a job elsewhere, and informing the patient that you couldn't care less about the meal—these approaches only escalate the situation. You hope to cool passions by remaining cool yourself. An early measure of empathy and attention goes a long way toward preventing what could later become an onerous dispute.

◆ ◆ ◆ ◆ ◆ ◆ ◆

Katherine Knight, the nurse manager of the intensive care unit, knew there was a problem as soon as she entered Janice Johnson's office. Janice, the vice president of nursing, looked pensive and distracted as Katherine took a seat across the desk from her boss.

Janice opened the conversation, looking down at her desk as if she were reading reports as she spoke. "Katherine, I've been reviewing the budget figures for each of the departments. Your increase from last year on the salary line is 10 percent above other departments. Your overtime is way up from last year, and in reviewing your own time sheets, you personally seem to be spending much less time at the hospital." With that, she looked up and glared at Katherine.

Katherine was astounded. First, this was not Janice's usual style. Something appeared terribly wrong. Second, Janice had to know that the staffing issue on the ICU was not an isolated problem, and that it was being addressed with the transfer of Heather Harriford to the general medical floor. Finally, Janice knew that Katherine's mother had been ill this year and she had needed time off to take care of her. Janice had approved the leave time. Janice's attack was unjust micromanagement of a nursing unit. It was wrong.

Katherine sensed that something else might be going on. She wanted to learn what that might be. And more importantly, whatever it was, she did not want to escalate the situation by opening with a challenge to Janice's allegations.

"Janice, I know that our salary figures were up this year. This has been disappointing to me as well, especially given the financial crunch facing the hospital." Having shared a common concern for the problem, she wanted to gain a better understanding of the problem. Was it possible that there was something about which she was unaware? She continued. "Tell me, were there any particular surprises in the monthly reports that just came out?"

Janice's tone changed. "No, there were no surprises. It was just that, relatively speaking, your department sticks out like a sore thumb on these accounting sheets."

"That is not good," Katherine agreed. "Do you think that with the transfer of Heather Harriford to the medical floor, our salary and fringe line will improve?" She raised the matter gently, concerned about not embarrassing Janice if the problem was that she had overlooked a major staff shift that had not yet shown up on the accounting report.

"Oh, yes, I forgot Harriford. Well, that could bring you more in line."

Katherine sensed that Janice was reacting to the stresses of the hospital's financial crunch more than trying to micromanage the unit. With that in mind, Katherine decided to share some of her activities in order to assure Janice that the financial issues were being handled. "Janice, I am also concerned about the overtime issue. I met yesterday with Charlotte Channing, the triage nurse on the night shift in the emergency department. She is working with Dr. Lumberg and the other physicians in emergency to reassess their protocols for ICU admissions. If we can safely reduce the work load on the night shift, we will be much less dependent on overtime." She continued to fight the urge to tell Johnson not to micromanage her.

Janice sat back in her chair with a look of retreat. "That's good," she responded, now even more distracted.

Katherine continued. "You remember that my mother has been ill for the past few months. Obviously, it has been an enormous strain for me and my family, and it had to affect the department as well to some extent. People have been great, very supportive. Anyway, she's back home now, and my father is pretty much able to take care of her. I should be back on my regular schedule next week."

"Oh, yes, I forgot about your mother. She's feeling better?"

"Miraculously. She needed a total hip replacement, and she was quite depressed. She's doing better now, thanks."

Janice changed her tone. She became reflective. "I don't know what we are going to do, Katherine. I have to find someplace to cut our costs, I mean significantly. I am searching for some easy problems to fix. The department simply does not have much room to give. After our last round of cuts, we got pretty much down to bare bones."

"Janice, you have to know that your unit heads are behind you. This is tough for all of us. You can use us. If we each in our own little way can contribute something, the combination could be significant for the department as a whole."

The meeting ended on an upbeat note. Katherine had reframed the discussion from confrontation to reassurance, and in the process, the two reaped a mutual gain.

◆ ◆ ◆ ◆ ◆ ◆ ◆

Negotiation Face-Saving

One of the parties declares an ultimatum and draws a line in the sand. Preposterous conditions are demanded for any change in position: demands that are known to be untenable. The individual is tenacious, persistent, and unrelenting. There is seemingly no room for change. "This hospital will never accept another Medicaid patient!" "The chief of cardiology will now leave the premises, and with his department shall not set foot back in this hospital!" "From now on, absolutely no more evening hours!" "Kuwait has ceased to exist!"

This type of maneuver creates a standoff. Any progress toward a mutually satisfying solution ends. The conflict resembles a showdown at high noon: a macho duel. Negotiation turns into confrontation. The question becomes, who is going to conquer whom?

This is obviously a dangerous situation. First, the level of combat is disproportionate to the original issue. Information, events, and perceptions are distorted to justify the alleged menace. Such misrepresentations only cloud the real issues. Second, the destruction resulting from the confrontation will likely injure innocent bystanders. These bystanders are neither party to the original issue nor able to contribute to its resolution. Patients and staff members are common casualties of the feuds of hospital leadership.

What can be done to reframe this sort of stubbornness? The individual who made the statement is trapped in a box, with little room for escape. He or she has taken a rigid stance that is unlikely to be conceded. Demands are framed as win-lose choices. Whether you are one of the parties involved, a mediator, or even the perpetrator, there is a maneuver that can be helpful: negotiation face-saving.

Take the original statement and place it in a box: this is box one. Define the specific context and explain the statement within that frame: "When you said that the cardiology department must leave the hospital, you were under a great deal of pressure." Or, "You understood there were some financial improprieties, which turned out to be mistaken." Or, "You thought the head of cardiology was lobbying to have you fired by the board." Or, "You reacted to news of another malpractice suit being brought against one of their staff." Or, "You were unaware of how the community would react."

From these perspectives, the original, inflated declaration has a more logical ring to it. The statement is reasonable in its original context: box one made sense at the time. Now, create a new box, with different considerations: "Given your frustration at that time, you made a snap decision. Now there is new information that you did not have when you made that first decision." What you have done is legitimize a new context and therefore a modified statement. You have given the perpetrator a pragmatic justification to support the reframing. You have offered a graceful exit from a difficult trap. You have maintained the individual's dignity without compromising that of others. The new box, box two, is a sensible place to move into, now that the situation has been placed in a new light.

At the point when the parties are firing combative and destructive declarations (and hopefully the arrows are only spoken words), most are aware that dire consequences lie ahead for someone. They are caught in the spiral of their own escalation, outwardly confident though inwardly fearful of the consequences and humiliation of defeat. Reframing the dispute to allow a dignified return to the table is called *negotiation face-saving*. It is a magnificent maneuver, opening interest-based negotiation when most assume it is near impossible. You allow the parties to shift from box one to box two. You might even find at times that you can use the maneuver for yourself, when you realize that you have said something that on further thought you regret. Negotiation face-saving is a way to repair the damage without losing your dignity.

With the current pressures for change, one hears in the vocabulary of health care frequent reference to military metaphors: we are going to "attack" the market, "overcome" the other hospital, "quash" the competition, "undermine" the other department. These statements become the battle cry under which we cast our efforts. Given the necessity for coordination and connection of services among health care providers, this sort of mindset only obstructs good health service. Reframing the ultimatums that burden our negotiation is a step toward enhancing both the premises and the purposes of the system.

Negotiation Ripeness

Negotiation works on a time line. There is a cadence that measures tempo, sometimes in hours, sometimes in days, weeks, years, or decades. Like the punch line of a good joke, everything depends on timing.

Reaching agreement requires time to vent, think, consider, stew, consult, and ready oneself to settle. When you are ready, you are "ripe" for resolution. You want to reap the benefits of settlement. You want the pressure of the issue off your back. You want to move on to other business. Whatever it is, you want to get it over with.

Ripeness is a point in time. On either side of ripeness there is "too soon" and "too late."

When it is "too soon," you simply are not ready to settle. You may need more time to mull your emotions. If you are angry, you want to burn off steam before you encounter the other side. If you are perplexed, you want to gather more information to formulate a judicious choice. If there were parallel discussions elsewhere, you want to learn how they were settled, as a point of leverage. You become aggravated if someone forces the issue before you are ready.

If it is "too late," you are bitter about the costs and consequences of not settling. You are past ripeness and to the point of bitterness.

You know what you had hoped for. The opportunities are over and gone. Negotiation and settlement at this point are foregone. You are angry and disappointed about the original matters awaiting discussion, as well as about the fact that they have yet to be discussed. Your distrust of the other side is reinforced: they can't even get themselves to the table, to say nothing of getting themselves to settlement.

Ripeness is a problem if everyone is not ready at the same time. What is too soon for one person is too late for another. The "when" of settlement becomes a new bone of contention.

I know a couple who often fall into the ripeness trap when they have a disagreement. He wants to get the matter out and over with right away in order to return to a more pleasant rapport. She prefers to sit on it for a while, vent her anger and frustration, and only then get it over with. The husband, ripe for resolution, pushes the matter, further aggravating his wife. Getting nowhere, he gives up in frustration. By the time she is ready to settle, he is steaming about having wasted the day. His unwillingness to finally wrap up the matter further exasperates the problem.

They finally resolved to negotiate ripeness. After a disagreement, they would settle immediately on a time to talk: nothing more. This assures the wife that she will have time to vent. It also assures the husband that the day will not be lost. When they finally do talk, they are both ready for the process. Finding resolution on that original disagreement is greatly eased. They have negotiated ripeness.

The same principle applies to your professional work.

Compared to the complexity of a health care organization, the husband and wife have a simple problem to solve. The time is theirs, as are the consequences. In health care, time itself teems with significance. That importance affects the value and impact of time on your negotiations.

Income, costs, and quality in health care are calculated and perceived in measures of time: length of patient stay in the hospital, time spent in the surgical suite, number of patients seen per hour, and from the patients' perspective, "amount of time the doctor or nurse spent with me." Whether it be delay, indecision, or hustle, time translates into dollars and cents. Health professionals sell their time. If employed by someone else, their time is not all their own. If self-employed, their time is their money.

Time is also a variable in health service outcomes. The timing of when patients are seen may affect their health status, especially if their condition is serious. If the condition is not life-threatening and they wait, the delay adds to stress. Treatment and convalescence is measured in units of time: hours, days, months. Health care already works in a realm of stress and pressure. When time is not appropriately respected, that stress expands.

With time so valuable, descensus about negotiation timing seriously complicates the process of negotiation. When it causes what is perceived as an unnecessary delay in progress, that descensus builds resentment. Timing becomes a point of leverage if it is more important to one side than the other: "I'll discuss the matter now if you would be willing to . . ." Or, "I won't negotiate with you now unless you will . . ."

Attending to ripeness requires a balance of patience and perseverance. This is particularly important when negotiators are coping with different external pressures and staff priorities. Because substantive progress is more likely when there is agreement on ripeness, it is wise to frame and agree upon your time line early in your negotiations.

Your Negotiation Map

Patterns of clinical interaction set the tone for health care negotiation, even negotiations removed from the clinic. High-volume, brief though intense meetings of great consequence typify the culture of health care negotiation. In the course of a day, a clinician typically encounters numerous people, each different. Discussions ordinarily are for short periods of time. Decisions are quick. For the patient, the topic is of great significance. The professional must move efficiently from one conversation to the next, cognizant of the unique circumstances of each.

To do this, we use shortcuts: rapid cues to help us achieve a quick understanding of the problem and the person. Like a detective, we case the joint, we collect information, we draw a map to organize what we have learned. We assess people, placing them in categories and adjusting our interactions accordingly. There are two dimensions to this placement: position organizationally and characteristics personally. Our observations intermingle, leaving us with impressions that affect what we do: the information we exchange, the decisions we make, and the actions we take. Thanks to our quick assessments, we conduct our business without taking a detailed history of each individual.

Hopefully your diagnosis of the situation is accurate and your conclusions about the people and situation are valid. A quick journey through uncharted territory is helped by a good map. If the map is flawed, you encounter significant obstacles to negotiation progress. You misinterpret cues, neglect important information, and react inappropriately. Similarly, if other negotiators inaccurately appraise you, what you say and do will be misinterpreted. Your offers of conciliation are unheard, your concerns are ignored, and your efforts to settle are futile. To get back on track, all the parties must reframe their patterns of exchange.

The negotiation map is not merely a cerebral version of the organizational chart. That chart only partially describes the division of power and influence in the organization, since leverage is derived from more than just one's place in the hierarchy of the institution. What you know, whom you know, the value of what you have to offer, and the relationship of these to others contributes to your power and influence. The negotiation map constantly shifts, affected by and affecting the what, who, and why of bargaining. In part, negotiation is a learning process by which you assess the shifts and changes in the map.

Your understanding of the negotiation map is essential to your framing and reframing of solutions feasible across distinct organizational circumstances. Can you devise a policy for the medical staff that cardiology, surgery, and psychiatry can all accept? Can you reach agreement on a DNR (do-not-resuscitate) order that the patient's family, the medical staff, and the hospital's general counsel can all accept? Finding a balance between multiple constituencies with their different home teams is fundamental to accomplishing agreement in a large complex institution.

There are two dimensions to your organizational map. Representational negotiation describes its organizational aspects. Symbolic negotiation explains the personal aspects.

Representational Negotiation

Imagine you are negotiating the purchase and sale of a car. You have no spouse, colleague, or friend to whom you must report. No one will say, "You spent $15,000 for that junk heap!?" Likewise, the person selling the car has no one to whom they must answer. No one will say, "You sold the car for just $15,000!?" There are just two people involved in the exchange. The two own all the decisions, and they bear all the consequences. No one else is involved. This is called "simple negotiation."

Simple negotiation is rare in health care. Decisions and actions are integrally intertwined. The move of one person inevitably affects others. This is problematic when someone acts on the assumption of simple negotiation and others assume that person has a stake and say in what happens. You experience this problem when your staff, supervisor, or patient says, "You agreed to what!?" They are reacting to the effect your action has upon them. In your dealings, you represent them, and they bear the consequences of both your accomplishments and your shortcomings.

Representational negotiation typifies interaction in health care. When you speak to a patient about benefits and procedures, you represent the policies of the hospital. When you agree in a meeting to new functions for your staff, you represent their work and interests. When the board of directors assigns you to negotiate a consolidation agreement with another institution, you represent your hospital's objectives and concerns. Because of the integral connection of departments, functions, and people in health care, the actions of one person impose upon or enhance those of others. Information, reactions, and implications flow through the organization via everyday exchanges and negotiations. Recognizing and working with these formal and informal connections is the essence of systems thinking.

Your negotiation map helps you make sense of who influences you and whom you influence. It helps you assess the nature, power, and significance of that influence. You know that if you are at a task force meeting, about to agree on a change in staff policy, you must first check in with the head of your department, your supervisors, and your staff. Furthermore, you recognize the checkpoints of other people at the table. You each speak for constituencies that are best consulted before a decision is reached.

These constituencies, the people for whom you speak, are your home teams. If you work in a complex health center, you are likely to have many home teams. A male nurse has allegiances to the nursing department as a whole; to the other nurses; to the physicians, technicians, and assistants on Five West, where he works; to the overall medical center; and to the small group of male nurses who share his unique experiences. A female obstetrician likewise has allegiances to the OB department, to the medical staff as a whole, to her office staff, to the medical center, and to female physicians who likewise share her distinct experiences. You have an interdependent relationship with each of your home teams: you need them for support and encouragement, and they depend upon you for the same.

Therefore, when you negotiate, you attend to the effect of your actions and decisions on your constituencies. If you agree to an arrangement that is unacceptable to your staff, you will likely have a revolt on your hands. They will decry your disloyalty and wonder about your real allegiances: perhaps you are responding to a mandate from your own supervisor. They may not appreciate the onerous struggles and choices you faced during a meeting at which none of them were present.

Likewise, you want to understand the representational considerations brought to the table by others. Might they be anxious about the reaction of their home team to the agreement being crafted? "I would love to reduce the staff-to-patient ratio, though I am afraid that both our staff and our patients will walk out in protest." Is this a real concern or just a ploy?

Finally, you want to ensure your agreements do not disintegrate when they are presented to others' home teams. "I had wanted to join in the new project. The problem was that when I described it to my department, they were firmly against it." The wise negotiator is concerned not only about his or her own home team. Similar concern is shown to those of others. If the deal falls apart once it gets back to their home, then you are stuck. Put the question on the table. "How is your department going to react to this proposal?" "What has been your experience in bringing similar agreements back to your institution?" Reading between the lines, you will learn both about lines of authority within their home team as well as their influence therein. You can then craft an agreement that you believe will sell on their turf as well as on yours.

Symbolic Negotiation

At times, when I interact with someone else, I get the impression that they are not reacting to me, Lenny, for who I am and for what I value. Rather, they are responding to what I symbolize for them: white, male, slightly overweight, Anglo-Saxon, bearded, author. The possible categories and affinities are endless.

The quick interaction, negotiation, and decision making of health care requires that we use shorthand methods to comprehend and efficiently classify people. There is nothing right or wrong about this phenomenon: we do it all the time. The problem is when our assessment does not fit the person. When "white male" invariably equates to "insensitive, domineering, and narrow-minded," then real interpersonal interaction is hindered. Personal characteristics, race, employer, profession, gender, and culture likewise can produce rigid assessments damaging to meaningful negotiation.

Frequently we play out larger, unresolved, societal tensions on the personal level. Men and women struggle with readjustments of gender relations in their day-to-day interactions. Employees of different institutions shoulder the tensions between their organizations as they discuss the transfer of a patient. Similarly, patients vent general frustrations with their health care when they come to a clinic.

Given the nature of the work, symbolic negotiation takes on a particularly complex overtone in health care. For the terminal patient, the physician might symbolize "death." For distressed parents, the pediatric ward and everyone who works therein signify "hope." And for a laid-off employee, the supervisor symbolizes "rejection" and "calamity." What we do has extraordinary meaning. That meaning is ascribed to the people and institutions that convey the news, whether good or bad. I once spoke with a politician and identified myself as working at one of the large teaching hospitals in town. When he found out where I worked, he beamed. "You guys did a great job taking care of me when I was sick. I'd do anything for you." The fact that I am not a clinician was irrelevant to the discussion. Similarly, I was once introduced at a meeting as a faculty member of a large university. Someone at the meeting who had a bad experience with that institution began criticizing me as a symbol of the school, even though I had nothing to do with the source of her complaint.

The question is not only what you symbolize for others. The flip side is what they symbolize for you. Does that symbolic meaning limit your negotiation effectiveness? Are you overeager to agree with others simply because they are physically attractive? Are you reluctant to reach a mutually beneficial agreement with others when you're distracted by their poor taste in wardrobe? And most important, are there certain types of people, quirks, or character-istics that send you ballistic: people who are pushy, arrogant, timid, jerky, or under-qualified?

If certain characteristics do send you ballistic, it potentially com-promises your effectiveness. I sometimes come home and unleash a tirade of frustration about someone I met with during the day. My wife patiently listens and then observes, "She pressed your button, didn't she?"

People with those characteristics irksome to you hold and con-trol your buttons. Unless you understand and check your reactions, they will be pushed at the discretion of others. What you do and what you say will be out of your grasp. When you do not control your buttons, you likely will be impelled to do something counter to your own interests: make a comment you later regret, threaten in a way that escalates the conflict, or do something that damages you as much as it does others. Know your buttons. Ensure that no else presses them. When your button has been pushed, call a time out or do what is necessary to regain your composure and self-control.

What happens when the shorthand symbolic assessments don't fit the people with whom you are dealing? Then it is time to reframe. Get to know others for who they are and what they hope to achieve. Likewise, reveal yourself to them for who you are: let them know your own values and concerns. Reframe from stereo-types and symbols to individuals and relationships.

Humor: Negotiation Lubrication

A chapter on negotiation reframing would be incomplete without mention of humor. When it works, a well-placed joke, clever obser-vation, or quick-witted comment is the most potent way to in-vigorate a dormant negotiation. It offers perspective, a release of tension, and sense of togetherness. What is the relationship between humor and negotiation?

Laughter is our reaction to incongruity. Dan Quayle jokes were funny when there was the paradox of a sitting vice president making stupid remarks. Once he left office, the jokes were no longer humorous: there is nothing anomalous about stupid remarks by a private citizen. Jokes pose incongruous situations settled in an equally zany manner. Punch lines are funny because they are unexpected, timely, and clever.

Conflict resolution likewise reconciles incongruity. Two parties in a tense face-off confront one another with seemingly incompatible demands. It appears that nothing can bring them together. If found, compatibility will be applauded because it is unexpected, timely, and clever.

When it succeeds, humor confers a human quality to the negotiation process. And bottom line, good negotiation and good reframing are about bringing those human qualities to the table.

◆ ◆ ◆ ◆ ◆ ◆ ◆

Minutes after the morning paper arrived, Arlan Abbington, chairman of Oppidania Medical Center's board of trustees, called Iris Inkwater and instructed her to arrange an immediate, emergency meeting of the executive committee of the board. Every member of the committee was present for the noon meeting.

Abbington opened the session. "First, thank you all for coming on such short notice. I am sure that by now you have all read today's paper. Community Health Plan has signed a contract with Urbania Medical Center to direct all their patients there. They have constructed a feeder arrangement from two of the smaller community hospitals on the west side of the city. All CHP-covered patients will be directed to use Urbania."

Dr. Benjamin Bennington, a retired physician who has been on the board for two years, chimed in. "What about CHP patients who are being seen by physicians here at Oppidania?"

Iris responded, "This is an exclusive contract between CHP and Urbania. In exchange for lower rates of reimbursement, they get all the CHP patients. If those patients want their hospitalization covered, they must go there. If their physician doesn't have privileges there, and most of our staff don't, then they have to change physicians or change plans."

"But that's devastating for the medical staff," Bennington retorted to Iris, as if she had devised the new rules.

"Dr. Bennington, it's not only devastating for the physicians on our staff, it's also devastating for the hospital. We lost $15 million from our budget with this shift. We knew that CHP was contemplating some changes, and we were attempting to show them a good-faith effort to bring costs down. They never made a similar offer to us. Furthermore, the link between the two community hospitals and Urbania is a surprise. We had been talking to one of those sites, Perpetual Memorial. We also had been talking with two of the east side hospitals, and with this news, those discussions are going into high gear."

"Well, Iris, what are we going to do about this?" Catherine Cartwright chimed in. Cartwright is the resident character on the board, one of the blue-haired ladies who have been around longer than anyone else. "You know this means a lot of bake sales for the volunteers."

Iris smiled. "Yes, I know, Catherine, though I think we're talking about some very expensive cakes."

Abbington turned the conversation. "Iris, what is the picture as you see it?"

"There are several things to consider. First, there is no question that Oppidania retains a far better reputation than Urbania. I heard through the grapevine that CHP is catching hell from its members and from corporate benefits officers. People don't want to switch doctors or switch hospitals. Furthermore, the doctors at the community hospitals who have smooth relationships with members of our staff are outraged at having to change their referral patterns. The danger for CHP is that the loss may shift to them. With open enrollment time coming up, they may find that a lot of people in town switch to one of the other health plans."

Abbington listened intently and then asked, "Does it make any sense, though, to just sit and wait for that to happen? What if the allure of lower rates overcomes our patients?"

"We're not waiting. We have already begun preliminary discussions with Arena Health Plan. They also want an exclusive relationship with us, for which we will have to bargain hard to get a livable rate of reimbursement. They were thrilled with the CHP move, because they think they can draw patients away from CHP with only a marginally higher cost. Their premise is that patients' primary loyalty is to their physicians and to their hospital, and not to their managed care plan."

"Where does that leave our physicians?" Bennington jumped in.

"Most of our medical staff accept both CHP and AHP, and most employers in town also offer a choice, though AHP is slightly more expensive. If we are left only with AHP, it will be a different flow of patients, and there will be patients. The people at AHP think CHP made a strategic mistake that put too much emphasis on cost alone. AHP knows the reputation of our medical staff, and they believe our good reputation will rub off on their own public image."

Abbington picked up. "Iris, I think it is safe to say that the board is behind you in pursuing negotiations with AHP." He looked out at the other members, and they each nodded. "It seems you are taking the high ground on this matter and that is smart. We have quality and reputation on our side, and there is no use risking that for a bitter contest that will get us nowhere."

"I thank you," Iris answered. "It is comforting to know that our situation is not quite as dire as the morning papers would have us believe. We do have some tough times ahead, and AHP is going to want a tight budget to maintain their own competitiveness. We can pull through this one, and I think we can do it without adding another bake sale."

"Well, Iris, if you have that sale, you know I'll be there," Catherine reassured.

The meeting was adjourned with a sense of cautious hope.

◆ ◆ ◆ ◆ ◆ ◆ ◆

Renegotiating Health Care

Our working premises in health care are a balance of belief and reality: beliefs being the explanations we use to justify what actually happens in our day-to-day endeavors. The two are in synchrony when what we are doing accomplishes that to which we aspire. That fit bestows a genuine quality to our efforts. What we achieve in our professional life fulfills fundamental premises about people, relationships, rewards, and results. Our work is a principled means toward our mission.

When belief and reality do not mesh, what we do contends with what we believe. The pieces of our professional life are in contradiction: they do not fit. Our work is riddled with myth. We proclaim quality care when what we do is ration care. We affirm our commitment to patients even though our focus is an obsession with profits. Our actions are a cover for our intentions. We laud the wardrobe of the naked emperor.

The question is whether the health care community can achieve a new balance: new beliefs that mesh with new realities and worthy outcomes.

We refer to what we have in this country as a "health care system." In reality, what we have had is a "disease eradication system." We can do a remarkable job of saving a one-pound premature infant: our technological capabilities and willingness to spend have been nearly limitless. Yet we have been less willing to invest the same effort to maintain a square mile of infants in an inner city. We have been training our medical and nursing students to treat disease, with far less emphasis on promoting health. We reimburse for medical procedures delivered and not for those avoided. We reinforce the myth that machines, buildings, and treatment equate to good health care.

Many of those past realities are changing: new curricula, reimbursement systems, and funding streams are introducing a new set of assumptions and incentives into our work. These efforts to renegotiate the health care system reframe what we do along with our very purposes for doing it. These changes manifest at the system level through the policies, procedures, and regulations that govern us. In our organizations and practice, we negotiate and renegotiate this balance every day.

Because these changes threaten those who benefitted before, advancing through the obstacles of reframing is often an uncomfortable journey: the anger and frustration of their resistance is a loathsome though necessary step in the process. If you can progress from venting to learning, option building, resolution, and agreement, the journey will have been worthwhile.

There are numerous impediments along the way. These barriers are to be as expected as the very phenomenon of conflict itself. Like mice in a maze, those caught in conflict must find a common path to reach their bounty of settlement. It is a matter of adjusting and readjusting until the puzzle is unraveled and the resolution revealed.

Staying on board through this evolution requires reframing: shifting what you think, changing what you do, and modifying the methods by which you do it. Renegotiation based on common interests is a fitting manner by which to make the journey.

And what is the destination? A health system that keeps people healthy, thanks to an infrastructure and a wealth of collaborative professional expertise that facilitates the process.

Part III

. . . .

Health Care Practice

7

A Public Health and Health Policy Perspective

Velvet G. Miller

We speak of what we have had in this country as a "health system." In fact, what we have had is not really a system, and it has not been about health. The incongruity distorts our negotiation. The contradictions provoke conflict. And the misunderstandings confuse what it is we are doing.

A system is a coordinated, planned, and connected set of people, organizations, and functions. Actions follow goals, and interdependent connections obey ordered patterns. Procedures, methods, and formulas combine to routinize and regulate what is done. Those who are part of the system understand its operation and their responsibilities therein. When the system is changed, participants are involved in the process, or at least are informed of the shifts so they can adapt to the transition. People and functions are connected by a shared and focused purpose defining mission and appraising outcome.

Not a description of health and health care. Why?

No single, coordinating entity governs health in our country. Most hospitals, health maintenance organizations, and health care centers are operated independently by private boards or owners. They are affiliated with and accredited by nongovernmental organizations (such as the Joint Commission on the Accreditation of Hospitals and Healthcare Organizations) that oversee and sanction their work. Much of the money financing health care streams from employers and employees, not consumers; it is diverted through insurers before it reaches health care providers. Many practitioners—including physicians, nutritionists, and nurses—function as entrepreneurs, operating their own self-supporting businesses. Many people, vulnerable populations in particular, are excluded from care and prevention because little attention has been given to their health care needs. Each level of government provides a different mix of overlapping and sometimes contradictory services, financing, and regulations.

Then what is the problem in terming it a system?

We start with the wrong set of assumptions. "System" implies reason and control, when they do not exist. Without a unifying framework, we each devise our own goals and ground rules, perplexed that others do not share the same perspective. Rather than synthesizing, our different myths generate and augment our conflict and confusion.

The Cultural Context of Health

This "health system" has not been about health. The emphasis has been on sickness, pathology, diagnosis, and treatment, because that is where the money flows. Its priorities are reflected by its spending. It is a disease- and pathology-eradication framework, not a health promotion system. It has pursued the sensational and the spectacular in lieu of the common and the routine. Our data and our subsequent actions spotlight numbers sick, not people healthy.

If we truly had a system with health as its priority, we would turn our attention, invest our resources, train our students, construct our infrastructure, and measure our progress in terms of health, not illness, and in terms of services avoided rather than those provided. Dental care is a noteworthy illustration. Thanks to fluoride and the profession's emphasis on good dental hygiene, today's children have far better teeth, with fewer cavities, than did their parents. This model has not been the norm across the health care fields.

A true health system is more about promoting health than it is about treating sickness.

Our health care infrastructure is a derivative of our culture taken to its extreme. American culture can be distinguished from Eastern cultures in the relationship between humans and nature. In traditional Eastern culture, people are subservient to nature. It is therefore incumbent upon society to blend and conform to its surroundings. In Western culture, civilization is presumed to dominate its environment. We are therefore obliged to prevail over nature and surmount its limitations. We overcome rivers with our bridges, space with our explorations, and mortality with our health care. This is our inherent doctrine: no bounds should constrain us. We are overcome by nature when it exceeds our own capabilities. Death then is not only loss, it is defeat.

In our health care settings, we act as if mortality is the enemy. For example, the arduous emergence of the hospice movement reflects our discomfort with death and the culturally derived inability of our health care organizations to accept it. Hospice evolved as a counter-culture effort to save the process of death from the denial of health care providers. The movement created an alternative set of institutions to provide individuals with the kind of support, comfort, and care they need as they die. The initial resistance to the idea speaks to the cultural norms it challenged.

Confronted by this disposition to surmount our very mortality, we fixate on illness and death as if they were unnatural phenomena. We are impelled to act, to do something to overcome the obstacles of our own bodies. Our successes and illusions themselves have spawned the misperception of infallibility and mastery. Ironically, these illusions return to haunt medicine when they assume legal implications. The fallacy has become the basis for the legal premise of malpractice: if a problem occurs, it is presumed to result from the failures as opposed to the limitations of medicine.

This conviction translates into the moral imperative to never deny care, no matter the cost. In keeping with Judeo-Christian doctrine regarding the sanctity of life, we have been willing to spend limitless resources to save an imperiled life. The emphasis, though, is on peril and hazard: *that* is where we are most willing to spend, *and* that spending is expensive. Private insurance and public financing therefore grew to protect individuals from the financial risks of those costs and to ensure the availability, when needed, of that service.

In the process, the logic of health care was overcome by the logic of insurance, and the logic of insurance was overcome by the logic of health care.

Insurance intends to protect its policy holders from financial ruin in the event of disaster. Actuarial tables assess risk and price protection. Insurers focus on calamity and are therefore less interested in day-to-day events not associated with disaster. For example, we would not expect our auto insurance carrier to cover the cost of fixing our brakes. Auto insurance protects us in the event of an accident; it does not prevent the accident. Insurance logic motivated construction of a health system focused on disaster services and end-stage heroics because that was what public and private sources of insurance indemnified. Primary care, which should be at the heart of health service, was sidelined in favor of the pricey specialties. And prevention, the pragmatic approach to reducing costs and improving the quality of life, languished in the shadow of medical miracles. The result, of course, was that health costs inflated out of control, and health indicators revealed that we did far worse than other countries at far greater cost. Therein grew the paradox of health care.

That paradox translated into big business, attracting people, organizations, and professions to opulent opportunities. Sparkling career paths, abundant capitalization, growing budgets, bricks and mortar, expertise, and compensation emerged in the streams of health care funding.

Change those streams and expect resistance. Whether in training, financing, or building, investments expect a return. The individual who spends ten years in training and fifteen in growing a practice does not look kindly on a diminished payback for that effort. The company that underwrites a new venture expects a profit for their initial risk. And buildings and machines, once purchased, must pay off their debt and finance their maintenance. The premise of return on investment is ingrained in the business culture of our society.

So each constituency feels entitled and obligated to defend its turf, pushing and pulling to guarantee its place at the table. Noble purpose mixes with self-interest, and balanced reason is lost in the process. How can we remedy these disparities?

The Dilemmas of Health Policy

No service sector lives more at the cusp of public and private than does health care. While the sports industry depends on public buildings to hold its events, it is largely free of interference from the public sector, as is the entertainment business. Though the communication and transportation network is highly regulated by the public sector, it sustains itself primarily from revenue and investment financing. And while food production receives price supports from the government, the network of distribution and sales functions in the private sector and is largely consumer-driven. Why has health care developed so awkward a balance?

The explanations are many. First, the necessity for ponderous technical expertise excludes consumers, managers, and policy makers from the decision-making loop: clinicians decide what the patient requires. As a result, second, it is difficult to reliably assess the quality of care given. Third, when health care was recognized as a right with the entitlement acts of the early 1960s, public financing and entanglement in service was a necessary corollary, because, fourth, health service is expensive. As a function of that cost, fifth, the insurer generally serves as middleman between consumer and provider, insulating each from true market forces. Sixth, there is a moral dimension to health care—the life, death, and quality of life aspects—that takes health service outside the realm of other similar industries. Finally, medicine has a penchant for scientific validation of its work. This is a relatively recent development in its long history. Yet that history and accompanying mystery remain to influence health care practice to this day.

These unique factors become further complicated when imposed upon the pluralistic, democratic, incremental, and generally open policy-making process of this country. Together they combine as the fundamental sources of health policy conflict.

Until recently, the penchant for the status quo kept health care at a somewhat even keel. Those in control fought to stay there, and those who gained by the prevailing rules wanted the same. The known was better than the alternative, so health care was allowed to spend and operate with little restraint.

Enter the efforts at health reform, which intensified in 1993. Also add the naturally strong association between social change and the occurrence of conflict. Health care became embroiled in conflict. Old relationships were severed or sometimes renegotiated and realigned.

There has been little argument that the health infrastructure has been urgently in need of change. The changes occurring in health care, which will take several years to fully conceive, implement, and complete, offer a rare opportunity to tip the balance and renegotiate the premises.

Significantly, the process of change emerged more as an exercise in insurance and legal relief than as a transformation of health or health care. It left many of the basic tenets of health practice in place as it sought to change the insurance system. The premise was that once new incentives are imposed upon insurers, they will pass those measures on to practitioners, who in fact control the bulk of health decision making. Insurers, once controlled, will contain practitioners and patients. As originally posed, the question of health change was not how do we make people healthy, it was how do we get people health insurance. This was perhaps a necessary and appropriate starting point. We will have missed the opportunity, though, if we assume health change is accomplished merely by way of insurance reform.

True health care transformation demands that we reframe and challenge the assumptions that have led us to the conditions we want to change. Otherwise, we are going to end up with a health infrastructure that is not substantively different from where we began.

♦ ♦ ♦ ♦ ♦ ♦ ♦

With health reform high on the state agenda, the governor took the unprecedented move of appointing his lieutenant governor, Sarah Smith, to lead efforts to transform the system. She was a quick study, and she soon dazzled health experts, the state legislature, and the general public with her unwitting understanding of health care, health policy, and the political process. By design, the approach to change was framed as open and inclusive. A number of health care summits were held around the state. The lieutenant governor participated in many of these open forums, which included testimony from consumers, providers, the business community, and political leaders. The topic and the format caught the attention of the press, which maintained attention on the issue.

Before the health summit in Oppidania was even announced, Dr. Larry Lumberg, director of the Emergency Department at Oppidania Medical Center, was asked whether he would be willing to participate on the panel. Lumberg was outspoken and politically active on community health issues. He was pleased to have been invited, and he happily accepted the offer.

On the day of the summit, as he entered the civic auditorium with hordes of people streaming in, he passed the lineup of television vans, each with its microwave dish pointed skyward to offer live coverage of the event. He thought how fortunate he was to be at this point in his career now, when the system is in the midst of such important change. It was a rare opportunity to help shape what he believed would be a new health system. Sure, many of his colleagues only looked upon the process with disdain, worried about the independence, earnings, and status they would lose. He just didn't see it that way.

Bleachers rose on either side of the square table at the center of the auditorium. About thirty seats were set. The room was brightly lit to accommodate the bank of television cameras perched on a platform at the back of the room. Larry found his seat off to the right side of the lieutenant governor: "Lawrence Lumberg, M.D., Oppidania Medical Center." As he approached his place, an aide came over to brief him: his comments were to be short and to the point.

The lieutenant governor opened the forum with an articulate review of the need for health care change. Lumberg was impressed with the breadth of her knowledge and the spontaneity of her remarks. When Mrs. Smith was done, attention turned to the select participants at the table, as they each told their story. First came the laypeople, consumers who for the most part had been denied care because of insurance obstacles. Then came the providers. The moderator turned to Larry and quipped, "Dr. Lumberg, you work in a hospital emergency department here in Oppidania. What do you think needs to be changed?"

"Yes, thank you. I direct the emergency department at Oppidania Medical Center. Within one mile of our building are the affluent neighborhoods of Oppidania Heights and the low-income areas of the Crestview housing projects. When someone comes to our door for emergency care, they are each treated equally, no matter their socioeconomic status. Health and health care are the great levelers in our society. And in the emergency room, we see it all.

"In moments of frustration in the ER, there is a phrase often heard behind the desk or in the lounge among the nurses and doctors: 'Another preventable!' That phrase refers to another victim of violence, to a pregnant crack cocaine woman in crisis, to a vehicular accident fatality who wasn't wearing a seat belt, to a casualty of domestic abuse, and to a heart attack victim whose poor health habits made the tragedy almost inevitable. We know that the hospital will somehow get paid for our work with these people, either through Medicaid, insurers, or through the state's bad-debt pool. Nonetheless, we would all like to see fewer of these preventables in our ER and more of that money going to help keep these people alive and at home, where they belong. This is a human tragedy that is afflicting our society, and it undoubtedly can be avoided.

"We must remember that hospitals are businesses too. At the end of the month, they must pay their salaries, their electric bills, and their maintenance expenses. Just as we cannot treat people if we do not receive compensation to cover our costs, we cannot work with the community around us if that work is not supported. We have begun a number of programs already, with modest state support and in conjunction with several founda- tions supporting community groups. These programs have been welcomed in the community, and we are seeing very encourag- ing results. If expanded, I know that we would see far fewer preventables in our ER.

"Furthermore, I know our cardiology and nutrition depart- ments are currently being reimbursed by several HMOs for running health promotion workshops for their subscribers. Yes, these prevention programs do serve some people who would not otherwise have a heart attack, and you might argue that they are wasteful because they do not specifically pinpoint people for whom the program would save money. That is true. Though in any case, the programs do improve the quality of life of these people, and I believe that is a worthy outcome in and of itself. These programs require a copayment on a sliding scale, so their overall expense is modest compared to their overall benefit.

"To conclude, Mrs. Smith, I do hope that plans for changing

the system include not only shifts in the structure of health insurance—we also need a shift in our health care priorities, spending, and objectives. In our society, I believe we value life and a high quality of life. There is a price on that value, a reasonable one when compared to the real costs of illness and unnecessary death. There is much that we as health professionals can offer to keep this state healthier. I do hope that you and the other major players who affect health policy will help lead us in a positive shift in what we do and how we go about doing it."

The room was mesmerized by Lumberg's remarks. The moderator was taken off guard, and he turned to the lieutenant governor. "What do you think, Lieutenant Governor Smith?"

"First, Dr. Lumberg, thank you for those moving and important comments. I do agree with you. If we merely change *how* we finance health care, without also changing *what* we finance, we will have accomplished little. This is perhaps the most perplexing piece of this complex puzzle, because it is the most intangible. We have concrete numbers to calculate what needs to be changed in the insurance realm. What you describe is what we need to be attending to, and it is difficult because there we enter the unknown. What will it cost? What will it accomplish? How do we go about doing it wisely and efficiently? I hope we will continue prodding each other to ask these important questions and to continue searching for the answers, no matter how elusive. This is a historic moment for our health care system, and we would be cheating ourselves and our constituents if we did not take the challenge to re-create the system so that we can promote health and avoid what your colleagues aptly call 'preventables.'"

Dr. Lumberg and Mrs. Smith exchanged gestures of gratitude, and the summit moved on to the next speaker.

* * * * * * *

The formulation of balanced health policy is fraught with dilemmas: it must be uniformly broad enough to impact everyone, personalized enough to speak to the unique needs of each individual, secure enough to prevent abuse, and practical enough to make it feasible. Sculpting a configuration that will simultaneously accomplish all this is a monumental task. Your chances are enhanced if you begin with a well-suited frame.

Reframing Health Care

The most potent tool of a negotiator is a question, so let us begin the reframing with a potent question. Consider that each individual is responsible to ask him- or herself the following: "What can I do to promote health? My own; that of others for whom I am directly responsible, such as family members; and that of others, such as those affected by my professional work?" If we take the question seriously, it will likely change how we live our lives, relate to others, and practice our profession. It represents a shift in thinking and action.

Next, pose the question to our health care infrastructure: "How can you orient and reorient your work to promote health? How can you reorient the work of individual practitioners, health care organizations, and regulatory and funding agencies?" Imagine that every nurse, physician, social worker, therapist, and so on adopted this premise as the theme of their professional endeavors. It would turn health care upside down.

Now, you might think this approach is naive: "Health care is big business. Simply adding a new question to the stew is not going to change anything!"

Yes, that is the point. To state the obvious, health is big business. When people are sick or disabled, it costs business and taxpayers big dollars. Promoting health is a good investment, and it will reap bounteous rewards for our society. Business can be convinced to buy the theme because it saves them money. And business will reward health professionals who succeed in promoting health with their health care business.

Rather than opening health care insurance negotiations with "How will you lower the price of my employees' treatment?" business will begin with "How will you keep my employees healthy?" When that becomes an operative point of departure, we will have turned the corner on reframing and reorienting health care. The employer lowers the sick days of employees and their dependents, thereby enhancing productivity while reducing utilization of expensive treatment, thereby lowering costs. It makes good business sense because it makes good health sense. Health care organizations that can deliver these results deserve the business.

If this theme were to thrive, it would not only influence how we purchase and deliver health services, it would similarly influence environmental policies, food manufacturing, and even foreign policy, to the extent that no country lives in an insulated bubble on the planet.

A reframed health infrastructure that promotes health as its fundamental organizational premise will influence how resources are invested, how people are trained, and how outcomes are assessed. It would also guide our understanding of the limits of health care: what we should and should not do as a society, especially in the arena of expensive and marginally useful treatment. If we better understand what it is we are trying to accomplish, we can be more realistic about what we do and what we do not aspire to accomplish as a society.

How might this new theme help us regroup health care into what is truly a system? We might use our own body as a metaphor. We each have our own internal cardiology, neurology, orthopedic, and gastrointestinal departments. Thankfully, they all operate on the premise of interdependence and collaboration. If they began behaving like their outside counterparts in some of our health care organizations, we would be in real trouble. To the extent that parts of the system continue to compete, attempting to outdo and defeat one another, we will continue to pursue divergent and contradictory paths: our old ways.

Simply put, the system must be composed of interconnected parts that support and enhance one another. The emphasis is on what integrates, not what separates: our operational premises move from turf and hierarchy to integration. This method creates a far more logical arrangement of service and support from the patient's perspective, a more workable arrangement from the professional's perspective, and a more sensible prospect for the payer's pocketbook. People will know what they are getting, what they are doing, and what they are buying. Each of the pieces, whether they be different organizations, departments, or disciplines, brings a different piece of the whole picture to the table. With an eye on common purpose, each piece is better able to integrate its contributions and satisfy its requirements.

Integrated systems, such as managed care organizations, represent one possible step in the right direction. By linking services, creating economies of scale, and monitoring for unnecessary care, these systems can offer coordinated options for service delivery. They are able to leverage lower costs in exchange for higher volume, thereby securing less expensive contracts from providers. It is then in the financial best interest of the system to enhance the health of its insured, thereby creating incentives for health promotion and prevention. The problem with managed care arises when ends and means are confused. When it is allowed to become an institutional cover for excluding eligible though expensive people or illnesses, then managed care is bad health policy masquerading in the name of good profit-making business. And when integration is nothing more than a means to limit people to cheaper care, it becomes a formula for impersonal and sometimes inappropriate service.

Reformulating our health infrastructure into a health system requires us to reframe what we do and how we go about doing it. We begin with a new set of premises. And we negotiate and renegotiate constantly. A genuinely new health system is responsive: adapting, shifting, and changing resources and attention to promote good health. It simply makes sense: for our patients, for the businesses and taxpayers who support our work, and for our own professional satisfaction. The question becomes how to turn logical premise into workable policy.

Formulating Coherence: The Role of Health Policy

The title of this section may appear to be an oxymoron: placing "coherence" and "health policy" into the same phrase reads like a contradiction. Historically, our health policies have run behind the problems, filling in the unserved gaps and following the private sector pack. Health policy has been reactive, defined by its context. Public funding, regulation, and initiative embellished what was. The public sector has been reluctant to be proactive, to create its own public agenda.

It is unknown whether our country will ever adopt a single, centrally controlled system of health care, incorporating under one organizational roof everything from financing to service. Would such a network be an improvement on what we have now? In spite of what is maintained by advocates on both sides of this argument, we really cannot tell. Such a system, while perhaps evoking romantic images of a rational, fair, and comprehensive structure of service, could soon become a difficult-to-control behemoth. Its clumsiness could spawn the growth of alternatives, eventually undermining its original premise. Once such a system was in place, reformers might call for the return of a decentralized, personalized, and responsive organizational infrastructure similar to what we have now. The Veterans Administration hospital system, a chain of 172 hospitals operated by the federal government, has not earned a reputation to inspire replication for the entire population.

For now, therefore, the mixture of public and private organizations financed by a combination of public and private sources is likely in some form to endure. If well aligned, public and private agencies can balance and complement one another. Private companies, which tend to be relatively more consumer-driven, probably will set higher standards for service and responsiveness than public institutions. (Nothing did more to improve the operation of the U.S. Postal Service than the emergence of Federal Express.) The private sector tends to be more accommodating and adaptable because it is more proximate to patients and payers and because it is less encumbered by bureaucratic obstacles. The problem, of course, is that the private sector aims for the more attractive consumer, who pays costs plus a margin for profit.

Then what is an appropriate role for the public sector and health policy? What function can it play in shaping the health infrastructure so we derive a system that is responsive, reasonably coordinated, genuinely effective, and far more efficient? How can it advance the evolution of such a system on the theme of promoting health? Is it possible for health policy to lead the transition? What might such leadership foster?

The public sector can play two primary functions. First, it can set the theme. Prodded in large measure by business and labor, the public sector has propelled public debate on the issue of health spending. The problem of cost, which has excluded numerous working people from having health insurance, has elevated the ongoing problem of access to a new degree of importance. And just as concern for access has emerged from the problem of cost, so too can additional themes ensue to guide the process of health reform. "Promoting health" is an appropriate corollary to the initial issues, as it synthesizes concerns for cost, access, and quality. Making health promotion the primary focus of health policy initiatives is an appropriate starting point for the process of health care reform. It defines what the system does and appoints the measures for which it is accountable.

Second, the health policy and public sector can mediate between the distinct and autonomous components of the system. How can this objective be accomplished?

Good mediation begins with a good purpose. When the public

sector, whether it be the federal government, state agencies, or local health departments, conducts itself with a clear purpose, it enhances the focus and balance of the system. That fundamental purpose, promoting health, is different from the goals of the system's components. Hospitals are essentially concerned with providing service, insurers with accurately assessing risk, and vendors with marketing their products. The public sector, by design, blends these different elements into a unified mission.

Good questions are the tools of negotiation. These questions assess the intentions, actions, and effects of each of the parties. In the process, they promote understanding and clarify differences in order to construct compatible balance and resolution. In health care, these questions come in the form of policy analysis, research, outcome studies, program evaluation, quality of care measures, and peer review activities. In the past, this inquiry has been shaped by the overriding theme of the system: treating illness. Our questions have been directed at how well we are doing, not what we could be doing. This emphasis on treatment placed more attention on quality of care rather than quality of life, mortality rather than health, and spending rather than savings.

It is proper for the public sector to place questions of health promotion on the table and to keep them there, challenging and checking whether the system fulfills its mandate. It does so as a function of its public mission, in essence mediating between the concerns of constituent citizens and the system that serves them. As mediator, the policy sector balances the reasonable expectations of society with the likewise reasonable capacities of the health system. If either side becomes overindulgent, the policy mediator facilitates correction to restore equilibrium.

The health system cannot be a fountain of youth. As a nation, we must address and ensure reasonable individual entitlement. We must be willing to address limitations of that entitlement and service if the health system is to be accountable to the citizenry as a whole. This requires society to address difficult bioethical dilemmas through a reasoned process that accounts for individual needs, social equity, public accountability, and legal liability. By abdicating its responsibility to guide a principled examination of these issues, the public sector has allowed the health care system to make bad decisions, based more on fear of liability and repercussions than a desire to find reasonable solutions. Ultimately, the timidity of our public policy erodes both individual dignity and public responsibility. A family that is unwilling to allow the hospital treating their relative to suspend hopeless treatment exemplifies the problem.

Likewise, the health system must be confident that it will receive reasonable financial, legal, and regulatory support if it is to accomplish its mission. This is a difficult balance to achieve: creating it is a challenge for society as a whole. To guide this appraisal, the health policy forum must establish a respectable level of trust and accountability. This confidence derives from the quality of leadership of those elected and appointed and the principles they bring to their office. Government must demonstrate its proficiency at wading through difficult questions and finding reasonable, pragmatic answers. These answers can then guide balanced decision making for those at the front line. Without this guidance, the system is left in a quandary. The hospital reluctant to comply with a family's wishes to suspend futile treatment for fear of malpractice exemplifies the problem.

As the public sector engages its leadership, its enormous spending power, and its determination, it can advance congruency between the aspirations of our society for good health and the endeavors of our health system to make it happen. Mediating between the distinct pieces to mold a better whole system is one of the many functions the public sector can constructively perform.

· · · · · · ·

When Manuel Mendez was appointed city health commissioner last year, the media was abuzz with profiles of the new mayoral appointee. He did not fit the mold of previous commissioners. He was not a physician—he had a public health degree and served as director of a community health center. He was young, a member of a minority group, and energetic. He came into the position with a reputation as a "weaver." He had organized the neighborhood surrounding the health center, putting together an economic revitalization program to help local businesses, an antigang coalition to combat violence, and a new mothers' support group to ease access to public services and provide nutritional and child-rearing instruction. He had instilled a new-found pride into the Cityside area. Though he received countless honors and awards in his community, he was not known citywide until he assumed the commissioner position.

Mendez decided to study the job for six months before he became the public policy activist he had always aspired to be. He said to one of his aides, "For six months I'll manage the department. After that, I begin to lead it." He used the first half year to learn the agency's policies, to meet the people inside and outside the organizations that are part of its mission, and to develop trusting relationships. Mendez was well liked. He had the magnetic capacity to get people excited about conceiving a new vision for health and health care in Oppidania.

Nine months into his appointment, and after much study, consultation, and assessment, he decided on a banner under which the department would direct its work: "family health." He knew that it was a move not without political risk. Are homeless people excluded? The family is changing. Is he prescribing one form of family over another? And what about the gay community? Are they included or excluded?

He decided to define "family" as the sense of belonging that is vital for every human being. While people may belong to different types of clusters, it is through that belonging that we meet our vital needs, in particular those needs that are critical to keeping us healthy and well. Of homeless people, he said, "If they don't have their own sense of belonging to someone, then it is our responsibility as a community to give them that sense of dignity and respect." At the press conference announcing the new program, he made it clear that he was not proposing the answers. Rather, the city's family health project was about posing the questions and helping the community, the health system, and individuals themselves find the solutions together. The mayor was enthusiastically behind Mendez and made it clear that he would ensure that every department in city hall cooperated to make this program a success.

Mendez decided to pull together a representative group of fifteen movers and shakers in town to guide the program. This group was assembled to reflect the diversity of the community, the institutions that serve it, and the work that needed to be done. Mendez asked the CEO of Urbania Medical Center to sit on the steering committee. Mendez knew him well, since Urbania is located adjacent to Cityside, and the two had often collaborated. A representative from the Oppidania Medical Center was also needed, and Mendez decided to ask the hospital's medical director, Dr. Frederick Fisher, to join the project. Though Mendez noted that Fisher took a long time to decide whether to sit on the committee, he finally agreed in the days just before the first meeting.

As Fred Fisher stepped into his secretary's office to put his coat on, he seemed to be thinking out loud. "I'm off to this 'family meeting' that the new commissioner has put together. I have no idea what they wanted *me* there for. He probably wants a doctor in the room to make up for his own lack of credentials. Hopefully, I'll be back soon." He really did not want to be on this committee. Inkwater said it would be an embarrassment for the hospital if he said no or sent someone in his place. He has no liking for politicians, and he particularly hates their sloganeering. Iris gave him a pep talk before he headed off, and she reminded him of the many community projects the hospital had initiated. She also reminded him that it is the city that issues building permits. The hospital wants to be seen endorsing and supporting the mayor's new pet project.

◆ ◆ ◆ ◆ ◆ ◆ ◆

Negotiating New Policy Premises

To reform the system of health and health care in this country, we must reframe the fundamental premises used to negotiate what we do and what we are trying to achieve: the two must fit. If we agree that the mission of the health system is to promote health, then we should craft our institutions, payment incentives, and regulations to advance that mission. The negotiation process is about shaping congruity from incongruity.

Though it may sound easy and logical, we must be realistic about the obstacles facing so noble an objective. Efforts to create this shift will undoubtedly be met with, "But we've always done it this way." Objections, which are to be expected, will come from the troika of resistance: (1) For those who benefit by current arrangements, fear of losing power, prestige, or resources. They will wonder, "What will I lose?" (2) For those with little imagination, difficulty conceiving anything different than what already exists. They will ask, "What could be better than what we presently have?" (3) Finally, for some, fear of the unknown and untested. They will ask, "But can you be certain that it will work?"

This opposition will manifest as conflict between reformers and resisters. Such conflict is legitimate: it is one by-product of the creative process. If you work with the disagreement, recognizing it as an expression of apprehension by those who voice it, you will be in the best position to learn from it, adjust to it, and together reframe what you are doing. The quandary of conflict is that, fearing it, you run from the task at hand. The apprehension of innovation is that, dreading mistakes, you refrain from trying anything new. Those who raise the conflict will be the same who point out the mistakes in what you propose and pursue. True health policy reformers know that some conflict and some error are the inevitable baggage of true innovation. Wear your courage so others can see it.

Finding a new balance is a process of negotiation and reconciliation. Health reform will require us to delve into the unknown and ambiguous. There is little experience to guide us unmistakably to the right formula. Though we may learn from the health systems of other countries, what we develop here must ultimately emerge from the unique historical, sociopolitical, and economic context of this country. We will create new knowledge; we will commit errors and learn from them; and we will constantly adjust and readjust what we are doing in order to create a better system. It requires continuous negotiation jujitsu: active listening, integration of concerns, and reframing. This method of learning, listening, and inventing inspires mutual investment and support.

To create a workable balance, you need the right people at the table, representing the fundamental elements of reconstruction. Stacking the discussion with the same cast of characters that brought us the current system would be an exercise in futility. Alongside traditional constituencies, representatives of communities, vulnerable populations, consumers, employers, and others traditionally outside the health care decision-making loop must be incorporated into the transition. Attending to their concerns, responding to their questions, and integrating their ideas is essential. And remember that merely having the right people at the table is not enough: we must level the playing field to integrate the full range of legitimate interests. This calls for intentional and meaningful inclusion of women, people of color, the disabled, and other voices who may be ignored or so intimidated by the process that their concerns are not heard. Anything less would be imbalanced and incomplete.

If this process is to be a true exchange of insight, ideas, and solutions, it must be framed as one of both getting and giving. Too often, parties approach negotiation only as a means of obtaining what they want or protecting what they have. Such an opening premise frustrates the process. Participants must be as ready to identify what they can and will give to make the system work as they are quick to voice what they want from it. Short of such an exchange, our exercise in reforming the health system will be little more than a repeat of the feeding frenzy that characterized and stymied past efforts.

Building genuine reform is like devising and assembling a complex puzzle with many shapes and pieces that must ultimately align perfectly and simultaneously. Change one piece to make it fit better, and others are jostled out of place. There are numerous organizations, constituencies, and individuals involved. The timing, interests, and objectives of each vary. Getting them together requires a massive synthesis with constant negotiation and conflict resolution. Reform will happen incrementally, as one moving piece brings along the next. And as the system experiments with innovation, it will learn from its successes and its mistakes, replicating what works and avoiding the pitfalls. It is an exercise in framing, reframing, and reframing again.

Essential to the process of change is ripeness: readiness on the part of key constituents to engage in the process. We are now at a point of ripeness. Rising costs have prompted it. The political system has ignited it. Rarely do the conditions of ripeness coalesce so broadly and so decidedly. Many recognize that it is risky to withdraw from the table now: too much is happening, and it is happening too fast to be out of the loop. Ripeness offers a unique window of opportunity to reframe the basic premises that motivate the system.

In Chapter Six, there was brief mention of humor as a negotiation tool. I often wonder, is it possible to enjoy the process of reform? I watch many people stumble through it, fearing what they might lose. I also see many people who relish the process and are excited to be active and involved in what will be remembered as a historic moment in the evolution of our health system.

Go for the joy. This is an exciting time to be in health care. People are ready for new ideas. Put on your creative hat and give it a try.

Learn. Listen. Meet new people and expose yourself to new ideas that you never thought you'd discover. One day someone will ask you where you were when the health system shifted. Go for it. Great stories are being woven now. Put yourself into the cast of characters!

* * * * * * *

Fred Fisher did not want to be at this meeting. He crowded into the health department elevator with the masses of people going to various benefits offices in the building. He pressed the top floor for the commissioner's conference room. At each stop along the way, more crying babies and bratty children exited, until it finally quieted down for the last leg of the ascent.

Fisher had not met Mendez in person. He had only seen him on TV and spoken with him on the phone. He expected to dislike Mendez. Medicine would be better off without meddling politicians.

Fisher announced his arrival to the secretary in the commissioner's office. Within moments, Mendez appeared at his door and bounded out of his room. "Dr. Fisher, I am delighted that you are able to join us!" His welcome was warm, and he was well informed. Mendez had done his homework. From his comments it was clear Mendez knew about Fisher's background and career, and Fisher was impressed. As he took his assigned seat at the table, he noticed that Mendez gave the same greeting to each person that arrived for the meeting.

Sitting next to him was a young woman adorned in loud jewelry and wearing blue jeans. Had he known this was going to be a cookout, he thought, he would have come more appropriately dressed. The woman was talking with someone on her other side, and he had a chance to check out the others sitting around the conference table. He hoped this would be a short meeting.

Suddenly his neighbor turned around and placed her hand out to shake his. "Dr. Fisher, my name is Melinda Martin. It is a pleasure to finally meet you. I've really been looking forward to this."

"Well, it's a pleasure to meet you, Ms. Martin."

Melinda continued. "My mother, Pam Martin, has been a patient of yours for years. She talks about you all the time. She says she owes her life to you. I'll tell you a secret. She's a very spiritual woman. She says a prayer for you every morning. 'Praise Dr. Fisher!'" Melinda's arms raised into the air.

She was smiling ear to ear, and Fisher found it infectious. "Well, that's wonderful to hear, Melinda. Your mother is a wonderful woman. Please send her my regards. Tell me, what are you doing on this committee?"

"I direct the Harborside Youth Action League. We call ourselves 'Hi y'all.' I've been there about five years. We work in one of the roughest sections of town, and we have a lot of programs that are really making a difference in the community. Teenage pregnancy, AIDS education, violence, you name it, we have a project going." Though Melinda had once stood up without an ounce of fear to a kid who brought a submachine gun into the center, she was nervous talking to Dr. Fisher. She continued. "Our staff motto is 'We work *with* the kids.' The kids are involved in everything. We do a lot of leadership development, and the kids are responding. Believe it or not, we even have a college prep club. My kid brother is in it. He says he wants to get into med school and be a doctor just like you. So there you go, Dr. Fisher!"

"Well, that's wonderful. It sounds like you are doing splendid work. Where do you get the money to keep the League going?"

"We scrounge. I get a little money for one project over here, a little money for another project over there. The city gave us the building, though we had to put together the money to rehab it. Money is my big headache. The tragedy is that the kids and my staff have loads of great ideas they would like to get off the ground. I want to bring in a counselor who is an expert in helping kids get through tough times when they lose someone, especially if it was through violence. I want to start a photography workshop. I've got room for a nurse or doctor to sit in the center for a few hours a week — the kids asked for it. Great ideas, and without moolah, they're just great ideas."

Mendez took his place at the head of the table and called the meeting to order with a warm welcome, personally introducing each person at the table and describing each person's purpose on the committee. Fisher was touched by Mendez's comments, though he was wary of the commissioner's hope for the medical community's support and involvement in the family health initiative. Support is easy, though what does involvement mean? Our plates are already full. What more can we do? If Mendez wants money, he would be happy to write him out a personal check for $100 right on the spot. Maybe that could be his exit ticket.

The meeting itself was more intriguing and involving than Fisher ever imagined it would be. There were some captivating ideas, and Fisher became actively involved in the discussion. A recommendation to place nursing students and medical residents into the community was listed as one of the family health program's action plans. The King foundation was offering financing for community-based medical education. Fisher was particularly attracted to this idea. He thought it would be great to move some residency training into the community, especially into a place like HYAL. With the hospital census down, there had been comments about the residents' not being busy enough. It would be a good idea to expose them to health care experiences outside the hospital. The nursing school dean was also interested in the proposal. Nursing students could do some clinical work and also help with health education. He would talk it up at the next medical school department meeting.

Fisher was also captivated by the notion of a health professions' internship for neighborhood kids. For his own children and those of his friends, the thought of a medical career was not unusual, since they saw their parents or friends' parents in the profession. For the Harborside kids, though, health care work was out of their realm of experience. Yet, if they were to enter the medical field, with their background and experience, they would be an enormous help to the community. He promised to discuss the idea with Iris Inkwater.

After the meeting, Fisher rode down the elevator with Melinda Martin. Before they parted company, he again asked her to send his regards to her mother.

Settling into his car for the ride back to the medical center, he realized something changed for him during that meeting. He wasn't sure exactly what it was.

◆ ◆ ◆ ◆ ◆ ◆ ◆

Whole Image Negotiation

Chapter Two introduced the concept of whole image negotiation. This is the very approach now needed to transform what we have had before into a true health system for the future. *Whole:* A view of the big picture and common purpose—promoting health. *Image:* The imagination to devise, discuss, test, and implement new options, and the courage to accept both the failures and the successes of our innovations. *Negotiation:* An honest exchange of ideas, resources, and support, on a reasonably level playing field and in search of mutual gains.

Health is the great common denominator in our society. Any one of us could be Artie Ashwood, lying on an ER stretcher and wondering what is going to happen next. His fate is our fate. We are all born and we all die, and we share a common interest in the quality and length of the life that happens in between. It is in each of our interests to fashion a health system that truly promotes health as its great common denominator. We should construct a framework that invests the public's attention in the process.

Is it possible to construct such a health system? It will result from good public policy that encourages and rewards, through public dollars, the active promotion of health. Those of us in the field of health policy and public health must help to set the agenda by bringing the right questions and the right process to the table. What is our system expected to achieve? As long as we bring only sickness and disease prevention as our questions, then that is all the system will accomplish. We must advance from health insurance to health assurance. We must acknowledge and reward those who accomplish keeping people healthy: it is a truly challenging task.

Is it possible to construct such a system? Yes. And why should we make the attempt? Because to accept the alternative would be to sell ourselves short as a nation. And there is no good reason to do that.

. . . .

8

Health Care Management
Balancing Clinical and Business Perspectives

Janice B. Wyatt

B y virtue of the work they do, health care organizations embrace a formidable social mission. That unique purpose evokes a complicated set of expectations for both those employed and those served by these organizations. To meet those expectations, a manager must forge a delicate balance.

On the one hand, societal responsibility requires actions and decisions that are not always pragmatic from a strictly business perspective. For example, providing a high-cost and low-revenue service such as a trauma center may not make budgetary sense. The service must be fully operational around the clock, even at times when traffic is slow. Some customers run up large bills they are unable to pay. The financial and legal risks are not offset by adequate returns to make for a wise investment. Nevertheless, hospitals provide trauma centers as part of their community obligation.

On the other hand, at the end of the month the books must be balanced, the building must be maintained, the staff must be paid, and the patients must be satisfied. Achieving that satisfaction while realizing financial stability in uncertain times is the challenge of health care management.

Whenever a balance among so many different demands is this tenuous, there is certain to be abundant conflict. Each of the many constituencies with whom I interact—the board of trustees, the community, the insurers, the medical staff, the employees, the senior and middle managers—interpret the balance differently. There is constant tugging in multiple directions. The board demands fiduciary responsibility: that is their job. The medical staff lobbies for the latest equipment so they can provide patients the best care available: advocating for the patient is part of their mission. The nursing department makes the case for a competitive salary structure: they need it to attract a high-quality and stable staff. And insurers bargain to cut a deal that allows them to lower their premiums: they claim their role in controlling health care inflation.

My job is to maintain the equilibrium between expectation and reality, forging a congruity of purpose and endeavor. That job requires constant negotiation and a good deal of conflict resolution. I do a lot of listening and learning to understand the many distinct perspectives. Ultimately, though, it is my responsibility to run the organization. I must make decisions and take actions to guide it through these quickly changing times. And those actions and decisions may themselves cause conflict.

The Health Care Manager's Role

A health care organization thrives on movement: patients in and out, staff busily active, money coming and going, information efficiently available. As a health care manager, you oversee and orchestrate that movement. You maintain the dynamism of the action, adjusting the pieces so they better fit and coordinate. You assess problems and prompt solutions to achieve an acceptable pace.

To do so, you are first an *exchange agent*, moving information, decisions, and actions back and forth throughout the organization. You do that for the purpose of being a *change agent*, leading the organization's adaptation and adjustment to shifting internal and external realities. To chart the course of those shifts, you are a *visionary*, facilitating establishment of a vision, an "image," about which the organization develops appropriate strategies to achieve its objectives. With a view for the whole operational picture, you are a *coor-*

dinator, integrating functions, tasks, and responsibilities to ensure the job is being done and being done well. The organization is in constant motion. Your job is to guide that movement.

Charting the course has its many challenges. This is especially so when the health system itself is in flux. It used to be that success was measured simply by market share gains, long- and short-term financial results, and customer satisfaction. These are quantifiable benchmarks for which effective internal efforts can reap rewarding internal results. In the evolving health care system, success will also be measured by improvement in the health status of the population we serve. This shift in emphasis demands a total reorientation of the organization. Day-to-day work must change. Many of the variables that affect the health of the community are outside the realm of what health care organizations have traditionally viewed as their terrain and their burden. For example, hospitals will have a direct financial stake in whether patients quit smoking, whether a toxic dump is cleaned up, and whether violence is curbed. To accomplish these objectives, there must be constant exchange, focused change, a vision to guide the process, and ample coordination to make it work: in other words, efficient systems.

A health care manager is expected to know and understand a wide scope of activity: the work of the clinicians, the operation of the boiler, the status of the budget, and the satisfaction of the patients. And while the manager is neither physician, mechanic, accountant, nor patient care representative, there must be enough comprehension and insight to guide these many functions so they translate into a well-run organization. The common theme is negotiation and conflict resolution: facilitating a process whereby these different jobs, people, and responsibilities are effectively balanced into a coordinated system.

What is the unique domain of the health care manager? What tasks must be accomplished? How can negotiation and conflict resolution help in fulfilling management responsibilities? And how might we all adjust our training and purview to better integrate what we do as health care professionals?

The Manager as Exchange Agent

Central to negotiation is framing. For a health care manager, that framing process requires substantive questions and practical answers. What is it we hope to accomplish as an institution? What are our priorities? How can we integrate our work to accomplish those objectives? At times the answers come explicitly from staff, the board, or members of the community. Every day, though, answers arrive in more implicit form, such as through market analysis, the number of covered lives, a new state regulation, or a business deal gone sour. Your frame guides your actions. The reaction of others to your frame is your feedback. You integrate this information, consistently adjusting and adapting your frame.

Wise managers use flexible frames. This is particularly important at a time when so much is changing. The hospital executive who insists on having a stand-alone institution just like in the "good old days" will soon find himself or herself standing alone. The clinical practice that continually replaces outmoded technology with little-used equipment may soon find itself outmoded. And community health centers that do not accommodate the new needs of its clientele may soon find they are doing little of substance to maintain the health of the community. Inflexibility at a time of transition fosters a contradiction between purpose and practice.

Flexible frames are shaped by a continuous flow of information and an unceasing stream of work. Whether in a large medical center, a health maintenance organization, or a small medical group, the role of the health care manager is to guide the process of framing and reframing. To do so, you engage in constant exchange: a get-and-give of information, ideas, problems, and solutions.

There are the obvious places to get information: department reports, budget sheets, and external reviews of your organization. There are also more subtle though often more valuable sources. If you are reasonably accessible to the staff and patients inside and the constituents outside your organization, there is a wealth of important data to help in your decision making. Your reputation as a good listener presents opportunities to acquire that information. Such a reputation is gained by prudently using what others share and treating it with appropriate respect. You actively listen, properly respond, and, when necessary, use negotiation jujitsu to defuse anger thrust in your direction. This works when you are open, engaging, and receptive.

Certainly no one person can be the repository for such a wide range of information. Yet this knowledge is necessary to accurately adjust organizational decision making and activity. Problems need to surface. Opportunities need to be explored. And conflicts need to be heard and somehow addressed before they irreparably escalate.

Openness to this flow of information is established by organizational leadership. Management sets the precedent. If the leadership is available for learning, listening, and reframing, this behavior will extend throughout the organization. Your staff will treat others as they are treated themselves. Your manner of openness will filter through staff and on to patients, who will be more likely to voice their concerns and problems rather than silently taking their business elsewhere. As you influence the culture of the organization, you also affect its financial health.

How do you conduct listening so that it translates into productive negotiation and problem solving? You do not want your openness to become an invitation for endless and time-consuming whining. Rather, you desire reasonable venting followed by productive exchange. You cultivate this by framing the process as a solution-oriented transaction intended to address legitimate concerns before they become destructive. This transaction is one of mutual sharing. What can we give and get from one another to resolve these issues? Allow full expression of the problem: the listening itself is a step toward deescalation. Then redirect attention: what can be done to solve the problem? Brainstorm for options. Create laundry lists of viable choices. Open the door to reframing and resolution.

The other side of getting information is giving it. As a manager, you transmit a good deal of news. In what you do, what you say, and how you conduct yourself, you set the tone for your department, your staff, and your organization. You create the frame: the underlying premises, assumptions, and beliefs that implicitly govern your work and that of others. It is not only the substance of what is communicated, it is also the method. When, how, and with whom you communicate can be as important as the substance of what is disclosed. Whether the news is good or bad, a new contract or lay-offs, the meaning and reasoning you impose on the message will influence its interpretation and effect.

Information sharing is a series of judgement calls. For example, at times you withhold news because you do not have all the anticipated answers. You may feel compelled to keep staff motivation up during a difficult period, so you are guarded in what you reveal. Yet you disclose the information to other audiences, such as bond holders, community representatives, or regulatory bodies. And you are aware that this selective disclosure may backfire if one group resents not knowing what the other has learned. Since wisdom often lies in anticipation, you begin working toward resolution by carefully framing what you say and what you don't.

Ultimately, you create loops of knowledge to foster good organizational learning. What works well is maintained and strengthened, and what fails is fixed or avoided. Why is information exchange so important to this process, and why is the manager so central to making it work?

Consider the mouse in the maze. If there is just one mouse, it will eventually learn which passages lead to the cheese and which don't. The solitary mouse needs only to think, not to communicate. If there is a herd of mice, however, they can each explore different pathways, communicate which are the dead ends, which are the productive passages, and together find the most efficient and effective way to get everyone to the cheese. It is the manager's role to encourage and coordinate that communication. Furthermore, to maintain the confidence of staff, the manager must ensure an adequate supply of cheese at the end of the maze.

Information must not only flow through the organization, it must also be synthesized into a vision to guide essential strategic choices about priorities, services, and spending. That vision is developed through a collaborative process and then communicated so that it is understood and conveyed by each person who works with us. As a CEO, I work in conjunction with the board of trustees to develop that vision, which serves as both a strategy and a culture for the organization. The vision and values are the "glue" that bonds the organization's various constituents: the board, the medical staff, senior management, middle management, employees, and the community. These values are "lived," through words and actions, on a day-to-day basis. They are translated into what we do, how we treat one another, and how we behave toward the customers we serve.

Communicating Expectations

The end product of all this exchange, information, vision, and framing has direct personal meaning for everyone associated with the organization. That personal meaning is each person's set of expectations. Those expectations define the bounds of his or her "give and get" with the institution.

There are three kinds of expectation bounds. "In-bounds" expectations include what someone can reasonably expect to receive in exchange for their payment, labor, or expertise. "Out-of-bounds" expectations exceed what one can reasonably expect, given the operating procedures of the organization. And "negotiable bounds" expectations are those in-between and changing expectations that are mutually open to discussion. The rules and procedures of the organization define the bounds, as do the day-to-day relationships and experiences of those associated with it. At times the bounds are altered by factors outside the organization's control: shifts in reimbursement requirements, new regulations, or the changing marketplace. In a time of rapid change, what is in-bounds today may be out-of-bounds tomorrow.

For a health system's CEO, this question of bounds is a common theme. The methods of interest-based negotiation discussed in earlier chapters offer a constructive process for conducting these exchanges. When conflict does occur, frustration about unmet expectations is often at the heart of the matter. At those times, you hope all the parties are able to use interest-based approaches: the negotiation skills of those involved and their attitude toward constructively resolving conflict is what distinguishes organizations that function well from those that do not. How conflict is handled and negotiation conducted is one concrete manifestation of the organization's culture.

One way to reduce conflict is through clear communication about mutual expectations. A good job description, a clear contract, and a trusting relationship go a long way toward making this happen. Expectations can be further clarified by defining agreed-upon organizational, departmental, and individual goals and objectives; instituting an incentive system that materially supports collaboration; and providing an information system that provides timely, accurate, and useful information to people who make decisions.

Nonetheless, management realities dictate that in spite of all the careful planning, changing circumstances are likely to vary the conditions and means available to fulfill promised expectations. This is when the most sensitive negotiations are necessary.

◆ ◆ ◆ ◆ ◆ ◆ ◆

Iris Inkwater knew this was going to be a trying meeting, and she wanted no uncertainty about its purpose and tenor. Rather than convening privately with Janice Johnson, the vice president of nursing, she asked Perry Pratt (the hospital's chief operating officer) and Ralph Richman (its chief financial officer) to join the session in her office. Everyone knew this would be a somber meeting as they took their seats in the comfortable chairs at the far end of Inkwater's office.

Iris turned to Janice. "Janice, I have some disappointing news. Ralph has just put together a new report on the hospital's finances. Things now look worse than we anticipated, and they will probably get much worse before they get better. I know that you have been working on reengineering the patient care units and redefining roles for all the caregivers. That in turn has begun to reduce expenses. That effort has been appreciated. However, with the continuing decline in inpatient census as we sign more capitated contracts with managed care organizations, we need to reduce staff further on the inpatient side."

"What are we looking at now?" Janice asked with trepidation. Iris turned toward Ralph. That was planned. Iris wanted Ralph to deliver the bad news. That allows Iris to play the role of option builder and not mere tyrant.

Ralph spoke slowly. "Twenty percent."

"Twenty percent?" Janice looked to Iris for confirmation. "Twenty percent?" Iris nodded. "Twenty percent is too much change for the staff in too short a time frame. The process we established will allow us to get there, though it will take time." Iris had expected this reaction.

Ralph carefully explained the figures. Iris watched Janice as she stared at Ralph explaining the overall reduction in the current and projected census, the overcapacity of the nursing staff, and the hospital's dire financial straits. He placed the situation in the context of the hospital's reengineering, case management, and quality improvement efforts. Iris knew Janice was not interested in budget talk and administrative details at the moment.

Janice was pondering the painful human toll this would take on a dedicated and hard-working staff. This is not how to reward people for years of round-the-clock devotion. How would she decide who would go? How would she tell them? When would it all have to begin? Ralph ended his report and there was silence. Janice was almost in tears. It was hard for anyone in the room to make eye contact.

"Are other departments being asked to cut so severely?" Janice spoke as if she were looking for some justice in the news.

Iris explained that this was a day of bad news for many of the department heads. Janice asked if the 20 percent figure was negotiable. Perry explained that it wasn't. He added, though, that how the cuts would be achieved and the criteria for deciding what to cut would be open to discussion. He assured her that he and his staff in the human resources department would be available to help implement the directive.

Janice, with union rules on her mind, turned to Iris. "Iris, I have two concerns. I am concerned about the 20 percent who are leaving. Because of the union contract, these will be our youngest and most energetic nurses, and it will be a tragedy for them to start their nursing career with this kind of a beginning. If they are flexible, though, they will probably be OK. There are a number of jobs opening up in home care, and these nurses are probably better able to fill these positions than their older counterparts. It is the 80 percent who remain that worry me most. When we close down the designated units, we will be dislodging people who have been working together in the same place for years. We will have to rotate shifts for a lot of people now accustomed to the routine of a day shift. And they will all have to work harder because there will be no slack on the staff. What can we do for the 80 percent?"

Iris was impressed. All the other department heads had pleaded to keep the staff they were going to lose. Those meetings had turned into vain attempts to readjust Ralph's figures, which simply left little room for adjustment. Though upset, Janice recognized that would be a useless exercise.

"Janice, you raise a valid point, and I would like to work with you to address exactly that issue. We will do everything possible to make those who remain feel as comfortable as possible." A few plausible ideas to do just that were exchanged. The meeting concluded after forty-five minutes, and Janice returned to her office, pale and shaken, though confident that some reasonable solutions could be found.

* * * * * * *

The Manager as Messenger

The management perspective differs from the clinical perspective because of the balancing act that is brought to the job. Present needs weigh against an obligatory future orientation. Clinical preferences collide with financial constraints. One department disputes the space, budget, or status of another. These points of conflict typically push themselves to my doorstep. What does my typical day as a senior manager of a medical center look like? What are the issues on my plate, and with whom do I negotiate?

My first meeting of the morning is with representatives of the nursing, medical, legal, admitting, and accounting departments. I have been asked to attend a task force meeting assembled to address patient dissatisfaction with managed care. It seems that a number of patients making the transition from traditional fee-for-service to health maintenance organizations have been angered by the restrictions on their choice of physician and their access to high-technology diagnosis and treatment. While the restrictions originate from the managed care plan itself, it is often the local provider who must deliver the bad news. Our nurses and physicians, who are sympathetic to the patients' concerns, have complained that they are bearing the brunt of the anger, even though they are not to blame. The problem has depressed staff morale and created a public relations problem for the medical center.

A number of valuable ideas emerge from the meeting. I have agreed to speak about the issue on local-access cable television. I will also meet with staff to express our concern for the problem and recommend ways for them to cope with it. Finally, I will bring the matter to the executives of the managed care plans that serve our patients. I will suggest that they consider ways to improve their customers' awareness of these changes and their implications.

In each case, I will be cautious not to alienate those whom I address. My appearances before our patient constituency should not appear as finger-pointing. The community looks to us to take responsibility. I will explain general shifts occurring in health care and the hospital's role in mediating between our mandate to provide care and our requirement to control costs. I will emphasize that each insurer, hospital, and patient is part of the problem and part of the solution. I will suggest how they might express their frustration, reminding them to be cognizant of the limitations of those with whom they speak. I will encourage them to let their managed care plan know of their disappointment and their preferences. I will point out that managed care plans recognize that they must be responsive to their customers' wishes if they are to be successful, and that the plans are unaware of those wishes if members do not speak up. I will say that, while patients should share their frustrations with their providers, they should be aware of the restrictions placed upon them by insurers. Finally, I will tell them they should shop around, carefully assessing the benefits and costs of each plan available to them.

These changes reflect the realities of a capitated system in which providers, including physicians, are assuming the risks for patient care costs. This change has shifted the balance of incentives, rewards, and exposure for everyone, both consumers and providers.

In speaking with staff, I will express my awareness of their predicaments: they are at the point of the most profound conflict in the system. I will frame managed care as a series of choices: the consumer's choice of the plan; the plan's choice of services; and your choices as a provider. What you as a provider can offer each patient is limited by the patient's choice of plan and the benefits and restrictions the plan defines. I will assure them that I will do everything possible within those bounds to enhance the quality of care that they can offer their patients. Most importantly, I will tell them to be open to their patients' questions, responding to them openly and honestly.

My strategy with the managed care plans must balance concern with caution: they are an important source of business. I will do great damage to my institution if I alienate the plans, especially those with which we and our physicians prefer to continue working. I will first check with my counterparts at other hospitals to find if they have had similar problems and if those problems have been more serious with any particular company. Being careful not to violate antitrust restrictions, I will suggest that we raise these concerns together to those companies about which we have received the most complaints. Our message should be framed in a constructive, private manner. Our purpose will be to help the plans become more aware of their problems before they affect their own bottom line. I will suggest that they assess what they offer their clients, as well as how they deliver the message. Promising one thing and giving another causes customers to take their business elsewhere.

For patients, staff, and outsiders, I serve as messenger of news I do not create. As I offer perspective, insight, and information, my purpose is to help each constituency frame and reframe its views of a problem. I want to address this issue early to avoid a domino effect of destructive conflict. In fact, the current situation offers constructive opportunities for each of these groups to learn from one another. Health reform demands that everyone in the system adjust to a new set of realities. If this change process is to work, that adjustment must be part of an informed and collaborative process. My leadership purview allows me to move necessary information and to create the right environment for renegotiating positive working relationships.

After a few telephone calls back at my office, I am off to my next meeting.

The Manager as Boundary Spanner

To maintain a workable balance between the many competing forces internal and external to the medical center, I often assess and intervene on both sides of an issue. This requires me to understand a problem from multiple perspectives and then to realign perceptions and incentives to encourage all sides to find a feasible agreement on purpose and process. This is my challenge at the next meeting, with the chiefs of the medical services.

Physician recruitment is an ongoing activity that the hospital must pursue. It is one of the most controversial topics hospital executives and physicians must address to ensure the long-term vitality of the institution. Physicians already on staff tend to view the hospital's recruitment efforts as a direct source of competition, regardless of how busy they may be. They fear that new physicians will attract patients away from their practice. On the other hand, new physicians interested in joining the medical staff are interested in joining group practices and receiving a salary. From the perspective of physicians already in practice, these salaries provide recruits an unfair advantage.

I find myself caught between a number of opposing forces. First is the community's need to have an adequate number of physicians to ensure access and to offer them appropriate choice. There is the hospital's need to have more primary care physicians who can accept capitation from managed care organizations, thereby increasing the number of covered lives for which we are accountable. The board views its responsibility as ensuring that younger physicians are attracted to practice in the service area. They are also aware that funds expended on physician recruitment and employment represent a sizable institutional investment, and they expect those that are selected to contribute to the system's financial well-being. This dilemma comes to bear directly upon the medical leadership.

The medical chiefs express to me their ambivalence about the problem. They find that resistance is most severe among outspoken early-career physicians who perceive themselves as threatened by an erosion of their business. On the one hand, the medical chiefs want to be loyal and protective of their existing staff. To do anything less would undermine the credibility of their medical leadership. On the other hand, they look into the not-too-distant future to find a number of well-respected physicians departing into retirement. None of the chiefs are inclined to allow their departments to suffer from a scarcity of talent. They recognize that if the hospital is to maintain its reputation and increase its number of covered lives, it must have a sufficient number of primary care physicians and an adequate number of specialists who are efficient providers of care, all of whom can move into high-visibility practice. Preparation for that eventuality must begin now.

Members of the medical staff recognize that this problem has become more complex in recent years. In the past there was a reasonable supply of patients and plenty of reimbursement to keep physicians somewhat satisfied. Physician recruitment had been problematic though not traumatic. Now, cost pressures have prompted each physician to increase the size and pace of his or her practice: with decreased reimbursement, only by increasing patients per hour are physicians able to maintain a steady income. In addition, the emphasis on primary care has the specialists worried. They are torn between remaining specialists, which is what they love, or doing more primary care for economic reasons. Many physicians are splitting their practice between specialty work and primary care practice, especially in areas where there are too many specialists. HMOs, however,.take a less enthusiastic view of these hybrid specialist–primary care physicians, since they are less efficient than physicians who only do primary care. As a result, members of the medical staff question bringing on new physicians when the future promises less demand. They argue that in a time of rapid change, it is prudent to focus on current success and current staff, as only institutions that are strong now will survive into the future.

Both sides of the issue are persuasive. My contributions to the meeting are questions, not statements. My goal is to help them reframe the problem to find solutions compatible with the many interests affected by physician recruitment. Are there differences in need and capacity among the departments? Could we legitimately emphasize specific departments' needs rather than broad physician recruitment? What criteria might be used to determine which departments need to attract new physicians? Beside the long-term advantages, what other important functions do the new recruits offer? Are the needs of today's younger physicians different from those of their older counterparts? Using this strategy, I have not committed myself to a particular side, though I make it clear that we must find a workable solution.

The medical leadership agrees to collaborate on development of the criteria that they will support as a group. Attention will focus on those departments in most need of recruitment. OB/GYN hopes to add several female physicians and nurse midwives. Given the age of the cardiology staff, we likewise will augment that service. General primary care recruitment is a must.

This agreement allows the medical center to balance external realities with internal apprehensions. It resolves a growing conflict within the medical staff and between the medical staff and administration. While the issue will require constant attention and reassessment, the resolution assures all concerned that the legitimate interests of current staff, as well as the long-term concerns of the institution, are being addressed.

The Manager as Change Agent

One of my greatest challenges as a manager is to know what to change and what to leave alone. With the health system in such flux, it is only natural to keep every service on alert for adjustment. However, if a department is doing a sensible job, providing quality service with efficient operations in a stable market, we must carefully assess what can be improved, what could be changed, and what should remain the same. My first meeting after lunch focuses on this very question.

At teaching institutions, it is typical to have a regular schedule of external reviews for all departments. In our case it is done every five years. This afternoon, I welcome the external reviewer who will evaluate the department of obstetrics and gynecology. Joining us at the meeting are the chief of OB/GYN, the nurse manager, and the product line manager for women's and children's services. Everyone knows the evaluation is conducted at the behest of the administration and the board, on my budget, and to offer senior medical center management guidance in planning. I open the meeting by stating the evaluation objectives, trusting that the preparation of the report and the implementation of its findings will be accomplished through a collaborative process. A lively discussion ensues on questions of quality, cost, resources, and recommendations. The reviewer takes note of our objectives and then outlines what he intends to do. I know the department will accept the findings and recommendations of the reviewer only if they trust his competence and credibility. The meeting accomplishes that objective.

To complete his assessment, the outside consultant will interview members of the OB/GYN department as well as staff of other departments, such as surgery, anesthesiology, pediatrics, and nursing, that interact on a regular basis with OB/GYN. He will review utilization and volume trends over time, evaluate the clinical quality-of-care indicators used by the department, and assess the department's quality improvement process. In addition, he will analyze its operations in relation to the hospital's strategic objectives for managed care and cost-effective care delivery. He will look at other externally generated reports, including accreditation and insurer reports, along with other pertinent information from outside agencies.

We expect that the reviewer will identify a number of contentious issues. As more patients spend less than twenty-four hours in the hospital, there will be excess capacity and questions about whether our two maternity units at different sites should be consolidated. If quality-related problems are identified, discussions between physicians, nurses, and management will be arranged to address them. And if the department's direction must be adjusted to meet consumer needs, there may be an immediate impact on the income of private practitioners and the revenue of the hospital.

The results will undoubtedly be fertile ground for conflict, given the different perspectives, priorities, and preferences of those involved. We will address the issues with internal constituencies, our trustees, and representatives of the community. Each party will bring its own needs, perceptions, and interpretations to the table.

The report will provide us with objective criteria to assess and negotiate the questions. It will guide our formulation of options and choices. Eventually, we will decide what must change and what will remain the same, ideally in a manner that best represents the balance of interests at the table.

The Manager as Coordinator

By late afternoon, I am at a meeting with a small number of senior-level management. Its overriding purpose is to ensure that the strategy and structure of the organization are aligned so that we can successfully achieve our objectives.

The alignment of structure and strategy is a matter of great importance to me as CEO. An organization can only achieve its strategic objectives when lines of communication, responsibility, and authority are clearly devised. The less ambiguity, overlap, and competition incorporated into the design, the less conflict will occur in the organization. Accordingly, we chart what needs to be accomplished and assign each set of tasks to the appropriate department. The heads of these departments are given explicitly defined roles and responsibilities: they will make the final decisions for carrying out the tasks we give them, and they will be held accountable for the results. Information systems must provide the right information to the right people. Incentive formulas must be clearly understood so that appropriate behaviors are recognized and rewarded. Rather than butting heads, departments will integrate and coordinate their activities.

Today's meeting centers on negotiations with insurers. Under managed competition, insurers are asking providers to bid for patient care contracts. Because of the overcapacity in the system, insurers have the leverage to demand significant price concessions. In general, providers are willing to endure these deep discounts in order to maintain their market share. From the institution's perspective, these contracts are vital. Their importance as perceived by senior management may not conform to the perceptions of our medical staff, however. Physicians, in particular some of our well-known specialists, prefer to walk if the price is not right. Their practices are overflowing today, and given patient loyalty, they find little need to be "held hostage"—as some have described the negotiations—by the managed care market.

For those contracts for which we are still being paid on a discounted fee-for-service basis, almost every rate we get today is significantly lower than what we received before. That is why the question of the very control of the dollars is a major source of conflict now. Insurers are consolidating a deeply discounted inclusive price to reimburse the combined services of the physician and the hospital. This situation demands multidirectional negotiation: with the insurer regarding price and service, and with the physician to determine how this shrinking pie will be divided. Today we are discussing mechanisms to respond to these quandaries. We would prefer to maintain a collaborative atmosphere with our medical staff, and we want to avoid the appearance that one side is gaining at the expense of the other.

As I see it, we need to establish three mechanisms and get them in place and working well. The first is a coordinated procedure to prepare the bid, which usually must be assembled in a short period of time. The second is an established and accepted set of criteria for reaching agreement on provider fees. We can plan for these negotiations, devising formulas and clarifying expectations before the actual process is required. Finally, we must have a system to monitor patient care variations between systems, to ensure acceptable outcomes within the resource constraints imposed by the different insurers. Each of these items teems with potential conflict. Only through careful planning will the parties' interests be aligned. That we have to engage in this process is a given. My intent is to promote collaboration rather than competition between the players.

The Manager as Visionary

My day ends with an evening meeting of our board of trustees. These are the people for whom I work: they hired me, they decide whether to renew my contract, and they could fire me. Their confidence in me is critical to my ability to do my job.

These are demanding times to be a hospital board member. Many of our trustees sit on the boards of several organizations: they are an active, community-minded, philanthropic group of people. I know they compare their experience on this board with their involvement on other boards. The problem with hospital governance is that so much is shifting now. In the past, the trustees were accustomed to guiding the ship through relatively smooth waters. They are volunteers, and they do not always comprehend the operational complexities of managing a hospital. That is what they entrust me to do. Nonetheless, the many changes occurring in the health care industry have turned their responsibilities as board members into a formidable task.

Helping them understand these changes is an essential part of my job. Several years ago, the hospital I was then directing was looking forward to determine what the future health system might look like. A consolidation or merger was not absolutely necessary, though if the institution were to be a strong player in the newly evolving health care system, it would need to think about what it would take to get there. It was up to me to explain to the board why it was necessary to evaluate affiliation options at the time. The biggest challenge was helping them look beyond the hospital's immediate identity: this was a ninety-year-old, community-run institution named for a respected town elder whose wife had generously endowed the hospital in her will. The town took pride in the community hospital, which it identifies as its own, and the trustees felt it was their duty to protect this treasure. They had to understand that to do so they would have to reframe their view of the institution and their responsibilities therein.

After discussions with multiple potential partners, the most feasible option was consolidation with the larger hospital in our neighboring town. There was a psychological hurdle to overcome, as the two towns had a long-standing rivalry spanning everything from high school football to institutional pride. We needed to expand from a stand-alone community hospital to a multisite medical center with an overarching board. Our name would have to change. Because of specifications in the benefactor's will, the appointment of board members required a modification of the document by the state's attorney general. Such a radical adjustment of identity, governance, and affiliation was a tough sell for the trustees. They needed to begin thinking more broadly so that they would consider both the survival of the organization and the general health status and needs of the population.

How does a hospital manager pull this all together? The three essential ingredients are role clarity, information, and vision.

First, we all implicitly acknowledge that the board is not expert in hospital leadership. That is why they hired me. This is an important point. If a board and CEO do not have this understanding, the board may try to micromanage day-to-day operations. Because they do so without comprehension of the big picture, they tend to react and overreact to random problems collected from people in the community who know of their board membership. I welcome their reports, and we all recognize that I have to balance the compliments and the complaints. Anything else would be unhealthy for the organization, and the board understands this. This general clarity on roles and relationships eases resolution of the range of routine to formidable issues the trustees face.

Second, I want them to be appropriately apprised of what is happening locally in the hospital and generally in the health care field. A large part of my job is education. They perceive one of their roles to be students who turn their newfound information into effective decisions. The better the information, the better their decisions. They expect straightforward, objective, and clear data about both our failures and our successes. I make a distinction between quality of information and quantity of information. It is a mistake to pile reams of paper onto the trustees with the implied message that there is so much to know, they couldn't possibly make a reasonable assessment. Rather, I give them digestible facts. This works best for all sides. The board plays an essential communication role for the hospital, bringing perceptions from the community to the hospital and in turn educating the community about our changes and challenges. The better informed they are, the more satisfying and valuable this role is, both for them and for the public.

Finally, there is vision. I view leadership as a visionary process, engaging our board, our staff, and our community in creating and transforming the institution to balance our range of interests. It is the evolving vision that pulls us all together and keeps us together when disparate interests emerge. The board expects me to articulate, with them, a vision and values and then work toward achieving them in our daily operations. This vision helps them distinguish the hospital's direction amid all the changes in the health care world.

Our meeting tonight focuses on hospital finances. The board, with its fiduciary responsibility to the community, must establish the institution's short- and long-term financial parameters. In the past this annual discussion consisted of a complex though straightforward presentation, discussion, and process of budget approval. Now, as capitation is becoming the prevalent mode of hospital financing, we are forced to rethink our fiscal picture, in particular as it relates to our relations with the staff. One of the key points of discussion is a gain-sharing proposal, in which employee incentive payments are linked to the hospital's success in achieving short- and long-term financial, covered lives, and quality objectives. We also discuss the hospital's strategy for working with our physicians to share the risks and rewards of the health care marketplace. These proposals are driven by managed care, in which large purchasing groups are demanding concrete value from us. This catalyst places emphasis on the value of the services we provide and requires us to measure quality and satisfaction from the customer's perspective. We have built this perspective into the structure of the new budget. It is different from anything we have discussed in the past.

The board is ready and able to grapple with this novel approach because they have been prepared over time to think differently about the hospital, its budget, and its future. Most important, they recognize the real choices and the certain consequences for the institution and community. These choices are seen in the framework of a new future, not in the context of the way things were done in the past. The trustees also recognize that broad strategic issues are linked to specific budgetary decisions. They do not scrutinize each line item in the proposal. They ask good questions, offer valuable ideas and insights, and eventually approve an innovative budget.

Negotiation, Conflict Resolution, and Health Care Management

Managing a health care organization is a constant balancing act. As a manager, one of your primary functions is to set the negotiation table. You adjust it to fairly level the playing field, sometimes lifting up and sometimes toning down the wide range of people and their broad scope of interests. You ensure that legitimate aspirations and concerns are fairly heard and addressed and that workable solutions emerge from the process.

Often, parties approach the table with what they perceive to be competing objectives, especially when discussing the interface between clinical and administrative matters. If the organization is to function well, however, these objectives must be reframed from competing positions to collaborating interests. That reframing is essential to your job as manager and leader: it is a necessary ingredient for making the organization work.

How do you accomplish this feat? These diverse constituencies bring very different perspectives. These differences could be seen as a detriment. I reframe them as an absolute necessity: legitimate interests must be represented, and their voices must be heard. It is the way our organization learns about and corrects itself. We find out what is working, what needs to be fixed, and suggestions for how to make the corrections. The discovery is a two-way process. Parties must likewise be willing to learn the limitations and parameters of the organization. It is unlikely that they will leave the table fully satisfied. That message is more palatable if they realize a reasonable level of satisfaction. This approach frames the "give" and the "get" of the negotiation process and the leadership style that guides it. Managers establish the negotiation culture of their organization. I strive for negotiation and conflict resolution processes that are constructive and productive. I view the methods and techniques discussed in this book as a set of tools. When a decision has to be made, I want people to have the capacity to assemble the right information, develop an imaginative frame, and synthesize responsive and feasible options. If there is a problem, I want it suitably framed and addressed before it escalates to consume valuable time, before it ensnares more people, and before it creates further complications. And when we have made a mistake, I want us to address it, learn from it, solve it, and move beyond it.

Conflicts will occur. They are to be expected. What we do is very complex. The stakes are enormous for our own careers and for the people we serve. And our different personalities must rub together very closely. Rather than recoiling from disputes, we must respond to them. The fact that there is conflict is not necessarily bad: I sometimes refer to the presence of conflict as a sign of life. When there is a conflict, we put it on the table, deal with it, and move on. Nonetheless, there are parameters that must be followed. At times people are devastatingly stuck in their own conflict and circumstance. That is their choice. If they do not want to be part of a negotiated solution, then they will have to accept the imposed consequences. For a manager, knowing when to close the door is as important as knowing how to keep it open.

I prefer that differences be resolved as early as possible. For staff disputes, the hospital grievance process should be able to address problems effectively and efficiently. The process itself should be periodically reviewed and appropriately adjusted to ensure its proper functioning. And for interdepartmental disputes, I encourage a decorum of interaction to discourage tribal warfare within the institution. When we are truly aware of what is happening in our organization, we are able to be proactive in our problem solving.

❖ ❖ ❖ ❖ ❖ ❖ ❖

Rumors. David Dickenson hates rumors. Dickenson is the vice president of human resources at OMC. He has been there, moving up the ranks, for twenty years. It has been the last twelve months, though, that have given him gray hairs.

Dickenson is well liked and well respected at the hospital. His style is open, responsive, and helpful. Many on the hospital's management team regularly call upon him as a sounding board for human resource problems in their departments. He is solution-oriented. He believes most problems have the solution built into them. He asks questions—good questions. He offers perspective. He rarely gives outright advice. He prefers when he is able to help people discover a solution on their own.

He looks at the ten message slips on his table. Each call has the same theme. Employees have been hearing rumors about everything from the imminent closure of the hospital to a consolidation with another institution which could cut jobs in half. There was even a rumor that Inkwater herself had been fired. The problem with a good rumor, of course, is that there is usually an ounce of truth in it. And with the hospital in such visible external turmoil, with the contract surprise in the newspaper and the budget problems facing everyone, any rumor is easily ignited and spread. What to do about it?

He decided to call Iris Inkwater before he called anyone. It was a difficult, though constructive discussion. Iris was not surprised about the proliferation of rumors. They agreed that chances were good that something would appear in the next morning's papers. It was time to be proactive. Iris agreed that a letter should go out from her to the employees by the end of the day. Dickenson offered to prepare a draft. Iris outlined the main points: what could be said and what was not yet resolved. Dickenson quickly put it together and faxed it over to Iris's secretary.

Dickenson went back to the pile of messages. The one from Evelyn Edelman looked most urgent, so he called her first. Evelyn was the director of the dietary department, with overall responsibilities for both the clinical and the nutritional services sides. She asked for a quick meeting, and a half hour later she was sitting in Dickenson's office.

"David, it's awful what's happening. I'm afraid I may have a revolt on my hands. The food service employees' morale is very low. Many are earning a subsistence income, and the loss of their jobs would be catastrophic. It's one of those domino effects in which people believe they are going to be fired, so they act out as if to make it happen. The supervisors are having a really tough time keeping operations on track."

Dickenson saw the stress and tension written all over Evelyn's face. She went on for over five minutes, recounting stories and problems, before she even stopped to breathe. It was clear that the tension had taken its toll and she needed to vent with someone outside her department. She concluded with a question: "What should I do?"

Dickenson told her about Iris's letter and more or less what it would and would not say. "Do you think that will solve the problem?" he asked.

"That will solve one piece of the problem. For those people facing layoffs, the severance pay and outplacement service will probably offer some relief. For those staying, the anxiety will continue. I'm not sure what to do."

"What do you think would be helpful for people facing a job crisis in their lives?"

"Well, it probably would be helpful to talk it out with someone. I imagine it is difficult to bring this news home, since it will only unsettle the employees' families. Perhaps we can give them a chance to vent some of those feelings in the relatively safe haven of the workplace. If we combine that with whatever information Iris feels she can share, that might help things out. I know just talking with you about this has sure calmed me down."

Dickenson let the silence linger for a few moments. He talked quietly. "Evelyn, I've been in this hospital for almost a generation now. I've watched it go through some pretty tough times. Sometimes they were other people's problems, like that restaurant fire twelve years ago that stretched this place to the max for five days straight. Sometimes they were our own problems, like that budget scandal that hit the hospital just after I started working here. To be sure, this period is a really rough one. Yet, there is a vitality to this place. I think it is because we all believe in what we're doing—yes, even the people who deliver the food trays. Somehow, I trust we'll survive this one too. Probably we'll look a bit different afterward, perhaps smaller than we were in the past. I think we'll make it, though. Of course," he added with a smile, "if we don't believe we can make it, we certainly won't be able to pull it off."

Evelyn let the thought hang, and she too finally smiled. "Dave, once again you've been a real help. Thanks for your ear." Evelyn returned to her office, ready to do for someone else what Dave had just done for her.

◆ ◆ ◆ ◆ ◆ ◆ ◆

Changing Perspectives for a New Health System

One concluding plea.

The balancing responsibility performed by health care managers will be far more constructive when others recognize they are part of the equilibrium. Negotiation and conflict resolution training must be built into the preparation of all health care professionals. In their training, physicians, nurses, and other clinicians learn to focus on individual patients rather than broader system concerns. Rarely do we interact or learn how to work constructively with one another. Each profession emphasizes its unique perspectives and builds loyalty to the discipline, superseding a view of our task as a whole. This is a big part of the problem.

For each person involved with the health care system, a comprehensive perspective on the larger picture and an ability to effectively articulate and manage our differences are essential. This perspective should be incorporated into the initial training for health professionals, and it should be reinforced through continuing education.

Why is this perspective so important now? The current changes in health care are reshaping relationships and creating new premises. New health care policies, changed patterns of reimbursement, and new forms of information and clinical technology will change the landscape of human interactions in the evolving system. Our ability to adapt and adjust will not only determine the satisfaction we derive from our roles and responsibilities, it will also shape whether this new system can work to do what it is intended to do: improve people's health.

The health care system is undergoing dramatic changes. These changes can be expected to increase the levels of conflict for all of us. The rules are being rewritten. Working premises are being renegotiated. And old relationships are being realigned. Are we individually and collectively prepared to meet these challenges?

Ultimately, the vitality of our institutions will not depend on the strength of their bricks and mortar. Rather, our success depends on the vitality of our working relationships and our capacity to combine different expertise, resources, and talents to do the job. Those differences are essential to the process of health care work. By inspiring the tone, the manager sets the table, offers direction, and establishes the parameters for what can and cannot be achieved.

For me, the reward of health care management comes from the satisfaction of seeing different people in the organization working together to find creative solutions that can only be discovered through collaboration and mutual respect for one another. This capacity for achievement is central to what we do together as health care professionals.

9

Nursing

Negotiating at an Uneven Table

Phyllis Beck Kritek

N urses negotiate. It is their primary means of surviving on the job. It is the nature of their work. Most workdays for a nurse demand a complex series of negotiations.

The explicit expectation for nurses is that they provide for their patients excellent nursing care. To do so requires that they implicitly manage the context of that care, synchronizing the diverse components that impinge on outcomes, coordinating the people who provide nursing care, and integrating the multiple dimensions of quality patient care. Nurses blend the varied dimensions that operationalize the aggregate picture of health and healing for patients, their families, and their communities. For nurses, negotiation is so central that it has become an unstated assumption, an invisible skill. Ironically, it is most often unstated and invisible when it is done very well.

These negotiations are rarely recognized or valued. They are not charted in patients' records; they are not overtly included in personnel evaluations; they are not the topic of public discourse. When we coordinate the myriad forces that impinge on a smooth health care experience, combine the resources that enable healing in patients and their families, and guide communities through self-realizing health initiatives, the accomplishment is often assumed to have occurred automatically. This capacity to link needs to services, to intuit and discern necessary information and to be present for people through difficult choices and outcomes, is central to what we understand as nursing. Why is it so invisible?

By its nature, negotiation is relational. It occurs precisely so that we can attain the choices and outcomes we desire or prefer in our relationships. In health care, negotiation refers to the person-to-person aspects of our work, whether those persons are patients, other providers of care, family members, or community leaders. Since over 95 percent of all practicing nurses are women, this essential task of creating and sustaining vital linkages can be and often is devalued as "mere women's work." Yet these very relationships are central to the processes of healing, to seeking wholeness. Such everyday relationships ultimately are the basis for clinical effectiveness, administrative efficiency, and deep human satisfaction with a health care experience.

This dimension of our work is often noted only when it is done poorly or when it is not done at all. By not honoring this requisite dimension of our work, we risk not achieving the outcomes we desire. If negotiation is not recognized as something we do, we cannot learn how to do it better. We also fail to acknowledge when it is not working or when it is working to our detriment.

To attend to these negotiations is to unveil covert and unacknowledged power relationships that few are prepared to examine or alter. The expectation that we will perpetuate these power relations, even to our own disadvantage, is imposed without comment. "You will accommodate. You will negotiate. You will prevent conflict at all costs. When conflict emerges, you will resolve it. You will maintain the equilibrium of the patient's environment. You will prevail." These implicit assumptions are the source of much of what we euphemistically call "burnout" in nursing.

Thus, inviting nurses to one more discussion about the virtues of negotiation may not initially capture their interest or imagination. Is there really anything new to learn? And why? The temptation is to avoid the limitations of the negotiations in which we now engage. Instead, we focus upon the shifts in the health care delivery system and the new opportunities and challenges they offer nurses. After all, nurses, particularly those with advanced preparation, are experiencing significant increases in credibility, role responsibility, and formal power.

However, merely finding ourselves at tables we have not previously visited fails to capture the more compelling underlying issues. Indeed, the reactions of others to the changes in nurses' status and power are informative. Not everyone is thrilled with the changes, and many assume their license to dominate nurses will endure. In this unfortunate equation, simply inserting the skills of negotiation will not ensure satisfaction in our efforts to deliver quality health care.

There is thus a more compelling reason for pursuing a better understanding of negotiation and conflict resolution. These insights could bring us a more honest assessment of our place at these tables, and their impact on us and others. We nurses have paths of negotiation to walk that we have not yet walked, and confrontations with our current practices that could prove revealing. We might even find that we prefer to move beyond what we do now in favor of some more persuasive models of action.

The Current Context of Negotiation for Nurses

A starting point for this reappraisal is to acknowledge that there are a variety of ways for perceiving reality in health care delivery systems. A related acknowledgment emerges: almost no one other than nurses perceives the realities that nurses assimilate. This in itself can be quite troublesome and isolating for nurses. One of the most challenging aspects of nurses' reality is that they spend a considerable amount of their work effort studying the perceived reality of everyone else in the environment. This process is more subtle than is usually imagined by those who are not nurses. Nurses formulate substantive information systems to gather and share what is learned. They deliberately strive to understand and integrate the array of competing perceptions. The insights they garner, and often pass among themselves informally, are used to negotiate toward optimal patient outcomes.

Stated more directly, nurses' intellectual activity more often is silent and unobtrusive than it is overt and demonstrative. Based on that intellectual activity, nurses engage in actions. These actions often are experienced and viewed by others as less deliberate and reasoned than the more intrusive or dramatic dimensions of health care. They are even, on occasion, assumed not to exist. This distorted perception of nursing is commonly presented in the public media, reinforcing the distortion. Nurses' actions are embedded in relational negotiations. They respond to complex information sets about a variety of participants, each with unique interests. They often are mistaken, however, for "mere" informal communication.

An example clarifies the point. Most people have at one time or another had a nurse take their pulse. It seems like a modest and simple act, with a relatively clear outcome. Expert nurses, however, use this experience for a variety of other purposes. They establish communication with the patient first, assess eye contact and general emotional status and observe facial expressions and body language. They note the patient's skin temperature, tone, and degree of dryness or moistness. They check the degree of muscle tension, first in the wrist and then in other parts of the patient's body. They scan general body position to determine how the patient is currently feeling, if there is evidence of pain, discomfort, or anxiety.

They observe the environment to determine if anything is an aid or a deterrent to patient comfort and well-being: the accessibility of tissues or water or reading material or call button, the degree of lighting and ventilation, the position of the bed, the television, or the chairs for guests. They watch interactions with visitors or roommates and note whether the patient has received gifts, flowers, or cards. Based on these observations, they may elect to make one or more comments after the pulse has been taken: "My, you certainly have a stack of get-well cards there! " "You look a little tired this morning—how did you sleep?" They wait for a response, attending to what follows in the same fashion as their initial appraisal. All this to assure patient well-being.

To the outsider, what the nurse does while taking the pulse may appear as a simple set of friendly gestures that occupy the time as a part of contact for pulse taking. To the nurse these observations are a great deal more and are the basis for informed and responsible nursing practice. If a nursing student fails to develop these skills, we nurse educators do not believe the student is a safe practitioner. Which is to say, we take these "invisible" skills very seriously. It has been less important to us that others fully grasp the nature of our actions.

Nurses have learned over time that this seemingly informal model of negotiation, personalized and individualized, is more likely to yield the information they need and the outcomes they seek. Thus, the knowing and the acting of nurses, while often considered of marginal importance, has a substantial impact on patient outcomes.

Patient outcomes historically have been the central impetus to action for the nurse. These outcomes have never been conceptualized by nurses as the mere cure of disease or the tissue mending of fractures and incisions. When nurses set priorities for what can reasonably be done in a given situation, they do so by viewing the patient as a whole, with all the diverse responses people have to a health event. They perceive all dimensions of the patient's reality as important and germane. Nurses know that real healing for every patient involves a return to wholeness for this very specific and unique individual human. That is why nurses worry about the many elements of the patient's context and why they negotiate with so many people on the patient's behalf, addressing the human dimensions of health in all their interactive complexities. Often, when there is no science to guide them, they operate from a base of finely honed intuitive skills which the tools of science are inadequate to either describe or measure.

This holistic approach to people enduring a health experience is fundamental to how nurses understand nursing. An array of studies have demonstrated that nurses' job satisfactions are linked to patients and patient care. Conversely, nearly all their job dissatisfiers are linked to organizational practices and policies that disadvantage nurses. Making a difference for patients is gratifying and satisfying, and this is the primary impetus for nurses.

This holistic approach pertains to other service providers as well. Because the necessary linkages between patient needs, caregivers, and organizational practices is by nature a web of connected people, nurses recognize that quality care necessitates the effectiveness of those linkages. They view the system as a series of connections, not as separate and unrelated parts. Health care is not merely clinics, hospitals, long-term care facilities, home care agencies, and community care programs. It is also what the patient stores in the medicine cabinet, what the patient's mother fears, what the patient's boss demands, and what the patient's belief system portends. It is a view of each patient's reality that is one and that is connected, from the eyes of the patient. Understanding and relating these connections on behalf of the patient is an essential, albeit unrecognized, role of the nurse.

Just as nurses are a constant in the experience of health care, their negotiations are a constant in the process of making health care work. These negotiations are intended to foster sensitive and sensible work relationships. They emerge from a commitment to bringing people, information, and services together into a balance that ensures desired health care outcomes. While the invisibility of these negotiations may demonstrate their effectiveness, they can also become a serious liability, for nurses as well as for others involved in health care. In an era when changing health care delivery equates with elimination of portions of that care, what is invisible or undervalued can readily be eliminated. The impact on nurses is obvious; the impact on the needs of those for whom we care is more subtle and certainly more disturbing.

How Nurses Are Perceived

Several years ago I conducted a study with two nurse colleagues in which we interviewed patients after hospitalization. All our interviewed patients referred to physicians and various therapists and technicians with appropriate labels. These same patients also repeatedly referred to an unlabeled and unnamed "they." We asked who "they" were. "Oh, the nurses" was the consistent response. In exploring "they" with these patients more deeply, we learned that "they" obviously controlled, to a high degree, the quality of the patients' experiences, were critical to the patients' sense of well-being, did both noble and troublesome things, and nonetheless were a collective experience of "they."

We began to describe this phenomenon as "the great white nurturant cloud." We distilled from the interviews the message given to us about "they." "Nurses were very important to me during my hospitalization. I wanted a great deal from them. I often did not tell them what I wanted unless they asked. I wanted them to intuitively know what I wanted and to give it to me. When they did, I was happy. When they did not, I was very upset. They should know how to intuit all my needs, shouldn't they? They should meet them too, shouldn't they?" Nurses functioned almost as a substrate, a connective tissue in the patient's experiences, though only rarely as distinct or real persons with distinct or real needs, dreams, fears, hopes, drives, faults, and pain.

The environments in which nurses do nursing are structured to expect that nurses work in ways that are not self-serving or visible. The import or impact of the work is rarely acknowledged other than by other nurses. Platitudes, flattery, candy at the nurses' station from a grateful family may even deflect nurses from confrontations with the injustices they face in the process. In such environments, nurses are told that they have significant responsibilities in ensuring positive patient outcomes. They are advised that they take significant risks if they fail to meet these responsibilities. They are also told that they have little or no real authority in meeting these responsibilities. In management positions, they are told to dismantle significant nursing initiatives and then publicly claim that no serious losses to patients have occurred. They are told that fidelity to the organization is more important than fidelity to quality patient care. They learn to negotiate.

It is a strange starting point for complex decision making and competent intervention. Nurses are taught, along with the skills of giving an injection, how to deal with complex health care delivery systems in which their powerlessness and oppression are viewed as unchangeable givens that will not be taken seriously if challenged, and if confronted, could even cost them their job. They are taught how to achieve goals of quality nursing care in situations in which what they do may be ignored, ridiculed, denied, undercut, dismantled, attacked, or misunderstood with sudden ferocity or quiet, persistent erosion. It makes nurses very creative. It also makes them very durable. They learn to negotiate, though for them it is often not a conflict-resolving skill. It is a survival skill.

Nurses' Responses to Work Environment Challenges

It is the nature of these negotiations that warrant scrutiny. Often, nurses are involved in negotiations that presume to solve short-term problems. In the process, because they do not challenge the underlying assumptions that engendered these problems, the momentary solutions contribute to sustaining the overall system. The system itself is not questioned, because it seems immovable: the forces of inertia and power mongering appear too overwhelming. What is described then as negotiation is actually manipulation, the exercise of artifice and deceit to meet one's needs and goals. Manipulation, by definition, uses "artful, unfair, or insidious means to one's advantage." For nurses, that advantage is usually used on behalf of patient care. The manipulation may also be used to ensure simple survival in a nonsupportive and uncomprehending work environment. Despite these seeming laudable goals, it is still manipulation, and it is still an act of artifice and deceit.

These manipulations themselves are of concern because they may serve to sustain or exacerbate fundamental sources of conflict in health care environments. It may seem easier to simply flatter the physician with an overinflated ego as a way to get a necessary order for a patient, or to cajole the pharmacy to get a medication that is imperative. Conversely, assuming a role of the attacking shrew to take on the power players on their terms simply escalates the already problematic power relationships, increasing unease and distrust. Both options feel unsatisfactory.

A simple example illustrates the point. With the exception of some advanced-practice nursing authorizations, most nurses may not prescribe medications. Only physicians do this. Yet, nurses who work repeatedly with patients having the same conditions, for example those on a surgical specialty floor or in an intensive care unit, become very competent in understanding the effects of medications commonly used. Because of their repeated experience with these treatments, the nurses are able to identify, for some medications, secondary effects not indicated in the formal descriptions of these drugs.

Nurses administer medications, yet they do not prescribe them. This is a serious division of labor fraught with contradictions of power, status, and control. Why? Because nurses are present for patients on a twenty-four-hour basis, in hospitals, nursing homes, and hospices. They know their patients well. And they have witnessed more often the actual effects of these medications. Hence, one of the incongruous negotiation skills nurses master is how to talk a physician into ordering a necessary medication when the physician is disinclined to do so.

There are a variety of ways to do this. One may cajole or flatter, saying things such as "I knew you would want to increase his dosage when you heard of this." One may suggest the actual medication to be given, though this must be done subtly; the physician should not become anxious or offended so that the suggestion is resisted. If these approaches fail, nurses may take a firm stand and threaten to chart neglect of the patient, though this behavior is fraught with the risk of censure and possible loss of employment. The most ironic dimension of this predicament occurs when a nurse gives a formally prescribed medication to a patient that is either the wrong medication or the wrong dosage. The nurse is held legally accountable for this, even though the "offense" is simply carrying out precisely what were the "doctor's orders." It is instructive that these prescriptions are called "orders."

* * * * * * *

It was a particularly quiet Sunday evening on Six West. There were several empty beds on the floor and no new admissions. Heather Harriford realized that days like this probably did not help the hospital's budgetary crunch, though it made an evening shift easier to get through.

There were several patients who had been on the floor over a week now, and Heather was primary nurse for one of them, Mrs. Hayward. Mrs. Hayward, just a few months ago, was a robust seventy-eight years old. Suffering from colon cancer, she was now in a steady decline. Her family was taking her deterioration badly. Heather could tell that Mrs. Hayward had been a bubbling personality and was the lifeblood of the family. Heather had a very warm rapport with Mrs. Hayward and her children, and she found it rewarding to work with them.

Heather was at the far end of the nurses' station, making notations in Mrs. Hayward's chart, when Dr. Cummings nudged up beside her. At twenty-nine years, Chuck Cummings was in the last year of his residency and had an air of supercilious confidence about himself. He had that "I just popped out of a fashion magazine" look in the way he dressed and carried himself. Though he caught the eye of many of the nurses on the floor, Heather never found him to be her type. In fact, she rather disliked his macho arrogance and how he strutted about for both the staff and the patients.

Chuck Cummings loves a challenge. He also needs to know that any woman who meets him, adores him. Heather Harriford, for some reason, he had not captured. Because he found her the most attractive of the nurses on the shift, he was bothered by her coldness and wanted to fix this problem.

Cummings nudged up against Harriford as if he were reading the chart she was holding and whispered in a deep voice,

"Well, well. Aren't you loved by the Hayward family, Heather. They can't stop talking about you." Cummings's face was very close to her ear, and Heather could feel his breath as he talked. Heather pulled away and focused on the chart, continuing to write as she moved out of Cummings's range. She no longer felt him touching her.

This Cummings didn't like. He tried to get her attention. She remained icy. He liked to be in charge when it came to women.

He decided to change the topic to one that Heather couldn't ignore. Maybe this would win her over.

"You know, Mrs. Hayward is in a lot of pain. I want to double her morphine drip. Heath, I want you to take care of it, now." He lowered his head, mockingly trying to get her attention, and continued. "Please," he said like a little boy begging for candy.

Heather turned around and then stepped back to create a more comfortable distance. She kept her composure and, one word at a time, spoke in measured tones to Cummings. "We tried upping her morphine last night, and she became nauseous and very ill. I don't think it would be a good idea to try that again."

Cummings was getting very bothered. He was just about to start into a nurse-doctor lecture when he realized that there was a far better way to handle this little tiff. He extended both arms and placed them on Harriford's shoulders. "Heather," he started with a tone of clear condescension, "you have to remember who is the doctor here, and who is the nurse. Now, there is no reason to play hard to get." At this point, his hands were firmly massaging her, and she could feel his fingers playing with her bra straps. "I want Mrs. Hayward to get the morphine, and you are her primary nurse. Now, would you do that for me, sweets?" Cummings's hands pulled her toward him, as if he wanted to hug and make up. He was feeling a wonderful sense of victory.

Harriford was burning up inside. One moment suddenly turned into her entire career. Everything she knew and believed seemed to flash in front of her eyes as she stared at Cummings. And she knew that whatever she did next could be her entire career as well. She had no chance standing up to this macho icon. The whole medical staff would stand behind him. On the other hand, it was here and in public, and maybe she just had to take a stand right now.

She felt Cummings's hands caressing her arms. Then he glanced down seductively at her breasts and back to her eyes with an ever-so-slight smile of approval. That was it. She told herself to be calm. "First, I want you to take your hands off me." She was firm. Cummings pulled back, slowly. A shocked expression overtook his face. He lost his color and seemed momentarily speechless. Heather had a sense that this was an unusual event for this animal. "I want you to know that you are not to touch me, or for that matter, anyone else here who does not want to be touched. Do you understand?"

"I wasn't touching you. I was just being friendly, that's all." Cummings looked like someone had just punched him and his wind was knocked out. He was trying to keep his composure and it wasn't working.

"Second, Mrs. Hayward will have a violent reaction if you load her up with morphine. I think it is medically inadvisable. I refuse to administer the drug because I know it would be harmful. I watched it happen last night when you weren't here."

Cummings caught her. There was a sense of relief that she was turning what could have been a somewhat uncomfortable matter into something easier for him to handle. "Look, *Nurse* Harriford. Whoever you might think you are outside of this hospital, here I am the doctor and you are the nurse. Patients change their condition every day, and what happened yesterday will not necessarily happen again today. My orders are for you to administer morphine, and I expect that done right now."

"Well, Dr. Cummings. You might as well know now that I am filing two complaints against you. First for sexual harassment, and second for prescribing an inappropriate medication. If you had only spent more time looking at Mrs. Hayward's chart here and less time playing games with me, maybe you wouldn't have gotten yourself into this mess. It's written down right here in black and white." Though Heather was fuming, she was careful to keep the volume of her voice down so no one else could hear what was going on.

"Well, Ms. Harriford. You can do whatever you want. I just want to remind you of one cold, hard fact." He was whispering forcefully. "I am the doctor. And you are the nurse. And in the long run, my years of medical training are far more valuable to this floor, and to these patients, and to this hospital, than all your pretty little nursing combined. It's not even a contest. So the only one you're hurting with this little outburst is you, Heather. The only one you're hurting is you." He wanted her intimidated. Maybe a bit of reality would shut her up.

With that, Heather turned around and walked straight for the nurse's lounge. Fortunately, it was empty and quiet when she got there. She was trembling with fright. She was shocked at what he had said. And she was even more shocked by what she had said. She fell on the couch in the corner and broke down in tears.

◆ ◆ ◆ ◆ ◆ ◆ ◆

The Subtle Costs of Collusion

I have never believed that the injustices facing nurses should be sustained. Nonetheless, I was, during my own initial preparation for professional nursing, taught how to work the system with every manipulative maneuver imaginable. The most prevalent formula was flattery: never cross a physician or a health care administrator; appeal to their denied sense of vulnerability; speak to their inability to face their own human limitations; flatter their fragile egos and feed their vanities. These behaviors were taught with as much focus as the more compelling behaviors that assured me that I had given my patients excellent nursing care, both competent and compassionate. I was taught that nurses use complex communication skills to assuage the anxiety of the preoperative patient as well as the anxiety of the preoperative surgeon.

In teaching and reinforcing these behaviors, nursing has played a subtle though significant role in fostering some of the most troublesome aspects of a conflict-riddled health care system. They have contributed to the insatiability of the egos affected, the need of some participants to prevail and conquer, to always be right and to appear invulnerable. It is this inflated sense of ego that has made it most difficult for many persons with status and power in health care to attend to conflict. They are, in reality, unduly vulnerable and insecure because they have become emotionally dependent on this aggrandizement. They then begin to believe that they can demand this of nurses, that nurses are required to nurture vanity as an implicit part of nursing practice, that nurses should give the appearance of being submissive, docile, quiescent, obedient, and far less knowledgeable and competent than they actually are. The self-perpetuating nature of this predicament is obvious, and it opens the door to nurses' becoming acquiescent.

I have always believed that nurses should receive a fair salary, adequate compensation in benefits, and viable working conditions and securities. The manipulative maneuvers taught nurses, however, fail to confront the presence of injustices in these matters, and in effect make nurses part of the problem: the persons willing to sustain systems that abuse them. The denial of legitimate equity to nurses makes such inequities more prevalent for everyone in health care. These affronts allow the forces of avarice to more readily prevail. Hence, in spite of the fact that nurses are indispensable to quality health care, the working conditions and job stability of nurses shift dramatically with market swings.

Forays into cost savings in hospitals, nursing homes, home care, and hospices chronically focus on cutting nursing personnel. These cuts are explained as acceptable without acknowledging that far less competent persons will replace nurses. The impact on patient care is never addressed, and the public is rarely advised or aware of the losses they experience. Nurses, however, not only participate in these processes, they sometimes provide leadership in making them happen. In addition, nurses often stay in situations where they become exploited to the detriment of patient care, with severe patterns of understaffing or staffing with persons who are not prepared to give the care patients believe they will receive. Patients then perceive these care inadequacies as the failure of nurses. Most nurses would say they did it for the patients, some would say they did it so they would have a job, though few would openly acknowledge that they participated in continuing the oppression of nurses and the compromise of nursing care with their presence and collusion.

Where do we begin to confront the premises that contradict what we believe and to challenge the obstacles that impede what we hope to achieve?

I have never believed that health care is an industry. I believe it is a human right. The United States is the only "developed" country where it is not recognized as a right. The implicit dehumanization of this premise is actually embarrassing for me. How can the most wealthy nation on the planet justify its refusal to attend to the fundamental right to health? Certainly, health care delivery systems would be well served by the utilization of the best and brightest policies and procedures for cost-effectiveness and efficiency mastered by those who manage and study the lives of complex organizations. However, to make health care an industry in this country, without first making it a human right, is to make it a capitalistic system for profit. The fiscal gains for hyperspecialized physicians, for insurers, for complex health care networks, for equipment vendors, for pharmaceutical manufacturers: these are difficult to ignore. When you are suffering from an illness or pain, these realities are even more confounding.

Nurses who commit first to patient well-being need to confront this dilemma. Too often, we merely adapt to the shifts and vagaries of the market, assuming that someone else controls all this avarice. We may judge these others harshly, look with disdain on their blatant self-serving behavior, or become saddened by the inherent injustices. Nonetheless, to challenge these systems is an entirely different proposition. Though we may not believe that health care is an industry, we have accommodated and acquiesced to the changes swirling about us. To practice competent managerial skills and provide leadership, it is reasoned, does not mean collusion with those who view profiting from the pain of others as acceptable. We have not been willing to raise the uncomfortable questions evoked by these assumptions.

It can be very disturbing to consider the tacit contributions we have made to the creation and sustenance of conditions that we find reprehensible in health care systems and in our working environments. It can be even more disturbing to try to imagine how we might play a role in addressing these conditions constructively, and even altering them. Given the historically prescribed role of nurses, how can we hope to become a significant force in restructuring the table to better achieve our desired outcomes?

◆ ◆ ◆ ◆ ◆ ◆ ◆

Janice Johnson lives for the annual meetings of the regional nurse executive association. Over the past ten years, she worked her way up the ranks of the organization and earned the place of a respected old-timer. She enjoys the camaraderie at the meeting and the chance to share war stories. She always feels she can comfortably let go here, far from her public leadership stage at Oppidania.

Her favorite part of the meeting is connecting with longtime, comfortable friends, especially Patty Pinkerton. Janice and Patty go back to nursing school and have stayed in close touch ever since. Patty directs a nursing department in a large urban hospital about five hundred miles from Oppidania. In size and complexity, it resembles Janice's shop. Janice has a tremendous respect, and sometimes a touch of jealousy, for Patty's professionalism and her inspired thinking. Patty is able to take risks, to try new ideas and then make them work. Janice has never left a discussion with Patty without some new insight or approach that was both innovative and very practical. That combination is Patty's genius.

They both were eager to talk and planned to rendezvous in the hotel lounge after the opening plenary session reception.

They sat in the corner of the room on two comfortable chairs, each with their glass of wine. A bowl of nuts sat invitingly perched on the small table between them. They talked about family, birthday parties, vacations, and the work Patty was doing on her house.

Patty eventually changed the topic. "So, what's happening at your place, Janice?" This continuing discussion had been going on for so long that Patty felt she knew the people working at Oppidania, even though she had only met a few of them.

"We just got the mega-ax thrown at us, and it's turning into a bloody mess. Our biggest HMO contract walked, and a bad situation suddenly turned into a tragic one. I was just given a 20 percent marching order. It is not a pleasant scene." Janice stared down at her wine glass and paused before looking up at Patty. "If I have to think twice before coming here to this getaway, you know that the picture is pretty rotten back home. I was afraid to leave."

"So what are you going to do?"

"What can I do? I either go along or quit. I'll have to go through each department and tell the supervisors how many people they have to remove. Then we'll issue the pink slips and have the supervisors make the actual delivery."

"Are you going to be delivering any pink slips?"

"No, I think it's better for the department heads and supervisors to do that." She gave Patty a look of incredulity. "I don't think a nursing VP should be running around the floors handing out pink slips."

"That's not what I meant." Patty was speaking gently. "I mean, are you going to be eliminating any administrative or supervisory positions?"

"No, I have to keep my infrastructure in place. It's going to be hard enough to run the shop with fewer people around. I'll need those people to keep the ship afloat."

"*You'll* need those people, Janice. The question is whether those people are really needed."

"What do you mean?" There was a touch of annoyance in Janice's voice.

"I think sometimes we get stuck on keeping our own nest feathered, that's all. You know, there is another way to do this."

"What's that?" Janice was feeling both defensive and intrigued.

"I got just about the same message from my CEO. Our situation was a bit different, though. Rather than losing an HMO contract, we got one. The problem was that it became a do-or-die situation. There was some pretty heavy-handed bargaining going on, and to make a long story short, we ended up with a steady stream of patients and a meager stream of money. I mean, we're talking bare bones. Our CEO made a convincing argument that in the long run this was a better solution than losing the contract and starving. I mean, at least we're alive. I was told we had to 'readjust' to a 20 percent cut in nursing staff."

"So what did you do?"

"I cut my administrative staff and pretty much left everybody else in place."

"You flattened the organization?"

"Exactly. I have to admit, it shocked a lot of people. But once they came around, it made a lot of sense. The hospital has a great nursing reputation in the community, which I did not want to compromise. I had two meetings with each shift, so I personally saw just about every nurse in the hospital. I told them that our commitment to patient care and quality nursing would not be jeopardized. I talked with them about professional autonomy, and trust, and their doing their jobs. And I said that in the bigger picture, this approach would be better for us all. I thought this was the way we had to go."

"So you're suggesting that I trim my administrative people over my staff nurses?"

"Janice, you know I never make stock recommendations and I never make administrative calls for somebody else—it's just too risky for a good friendship if they don't work. What I am saying, though, is that there are some options other than cutting across the board. With a leaner administrative staff you can still get the job done, and you place your marbles on maintaining the quality of your patient care staff. It takes some restructuring and rethinking, and it's still very viable."

"I can imagine two groups that wouldn't like this kind of proposal," Janice mused. "Obviously my managers would go into shock. I think, though, that even the staff nurses would hate it. They count on an ever-present supervisory infrastructure as well."

"Janice, there is a good deal of talk at these plenary sessions about professionalizing nursing. Well, if that's ever going to happen, nurses are going to have to get used to working a bit more independently than we were used to in the old models. I have faith in what the nursing schools are giving us, at least back home. I think there are a lot of people out there who not only can handle a bit more independence—they thrive on it. Mind you, I am not talking about no supervisory staff, I am just suggesting a leaner one."

"But Patty, your situation is a bit different than mine. You have too many patients with too little money. I have too few patients, on top of too little money."

"Janice, bottom line, what I am suggesting is not about patients and money. It is about your thinking and strategy and priorities. And it is about letting the people in the hospital see how you work. All that I am saying is that you be clear about the choices you are making in the crunch. There are the obvious answers, and they get you obvious results. Just try rethinking those old assumptions, that's all."

The conversation continued on to what Patty was doing in her shop and finally got back to family, birthday parties, and vacations. Patty commented that there seemed to be less cigarette smoke at the meeting this year. Janice wondered whether it meant that people were quitting or just that a new generation was coming into the organization. They stayed talking in the lounge too late for both of them and finally called it quits when they remembered the 7:30 A.M. leadership breakfast the next morning. Janice returned to her room and dozed off, wondering what she would do with Patty's fanciful ideas.

◆ ◆ ◆ ◆ ◆ ◆ ◆

A New Role for Nurses

It is unsettling to realize that many in the health care delivery system hope that nurses will "just go along." I am proposing that we not do so. The implicit and explicit injustice toward nurses creates a climate where injustices can prevail. To force a nurse to act against her moral judgment invites the same behavior toward other persons. It creates a climate in which rights are not respected, with obvious implications for patients. The vagaries of informed consent are an example: the capacity for injustice is created not only by its perpetrators. It is just as much fostered by those who accept and accommodate it for secondary gains. Some forms of injustice are not safer or more acceptable than other forms of injustice.

For most nurses, the immediate dilemma is where to begin. First, that which is inherently wrong about health care needs to be named, confronted, challenged, and corrected. Nurses are the most numerous, and in some respects the most informed, group of providers. They witness daily the true costs of health care on a human dimension. Even more important, they witness daily the true costs of the lack of health care on a human dimension. When that care is more responsive to the desires of those giving it than it is to the real needs of those receiving it, nurses perceive what is wrong and what could fix it. Nurses recognize that healing is not the same as curing, that casting a broken leg for nine weeks ensures little for the person who has to live out a complex, unique, personal life with that cast for those nine weeks. We all want the cast when we have a broken leg, though that is merely the beginning of healing and often the least complex facet of the process.

In most sectors of our society, competent nurses continue to be a credible voice for the voiceless patient. To walk away from that role and responsibility is to implicitly participate in the duplicity we find so troublesome in health care. To tell the truth about the practices that implicitly threaten the quality of patient care could create a dramatic impact. It could also create new conflicts, unveiling what many know and few are willing to acknowledge.

Which of course is a very different yet still compelling reason for struggling to master the concepts and skills of conflict resolution. We may have once believed that simple compassion was enough to make a difference in the well-being of our patients. Today, it is imperative to face that conflictual environment, navigating the waters of conflict and generating resolutions that better attend to the needs of our patients while honoring the needs of others. It is no longer enough to claim naivete or provincialism. Nor is it acceptable to deny the realities in which we are embedded by engaging in mindless and self-absorbed rebellion or reactionary attack. If we want to solve the conflicts of health care, we must become active players in the conflict, naming our own hard truths and embracing the process for the good that might emerge in its resolution.

The temptation is to use the old tools, the manipulative maneuvers. They will not do. They have proven themselves untrustworthy in the larger scheme of things, prone to perpetuate conflicts best confronted and resolved. We will need to study and shape a negotiation that takes us beyond simple manipulation to a more creative set of outcomes. Our altruism may now lie in the ability to forego the secondary gains of manipulation in order to face the more compelling threats to the well-being of our patients. We perhaps have been silent too long.

There is something unnerving about this prospect. I was anxious enough about all of this to spend considerable time and energy clarifying just what my proposition might mean for myself and for others. I have summarized this very simply as the ability to negotiate at an uneven table. I have written a book about it, and describe there, in more detail, and from my personal experiences, the meaning and impact of manipulative maneuvers posing as negotiation (Kritek, 1994).

I also have described there new ways of being at such uneven tables. This is important since most nurses are virtual experts at being at uneven tables. They do so, however, in a fashion that does not alter the unevenness. Many of us are weary of these tables, and being invited to return again and again in time loses its appeal. To find new ways to be there, however, could substantially alter both our purposes and our outcomes.

Negotiating at an Uneven Table

Uneven tables are negotiation situations in which there is a structured and unacknowledged inequity among the participants. At such tables, participants assume that the inequity will continue to be unacknowledged and perpetuated. Thus, the negotiations are tainted before they begin. Outcomes of such a negotiation preserve at least one dimension of the conflict while purportedly attempting to address another.

All parties can choose to negotiate in a fashion that sustains the inequity of the uneven table: complicity implicates the advantaged parties as well as the disadvantaged parties. This tacit endorsement of the uneven table is most likely to occur when the participants who are viewed as disadvantaged find some mechanisms for acquiring their own advantages by perpetuating the inequity. Under these conditions, the negotiation becomes a place where a substantive conflict is avoided or denied.

The sustained inequities can then infect other relationships and decisions. Just as an uneven table can be structured on the basis of profession, it can also be predicated on the basis of gender, race, age, culture, or the status of the provider to the patient. If a patient, for example, is perceived as a helpless pawn in some larger power game, the patient's rights and dignity are at risk. One or another provider may believe that they know what is best or better for the patient than the patient can or will. Maintaining an uneven table that perpetuates the premise may unwittingly uphold this attitude and have a direct effect on the well-being of patients.

The decision to no longer accommodate the denial of inequity is a serious one. The option, carried out in action, often gives the impression that one is merely exacerbating the conflict rather than trying to resolve it. Yet, to negotiate toward solutions that have embedded in them the seeds of the next inevitable conflict is not only unproductive, it is unwise.

Negotiating constructively under these conditions, at uneven tables, is a valuable tool. It not only strengthens personal fulfillment and honesty, it also serves the purpose of transforming the health care delivery system. Current inequities diminish everyone. They are a drain of human energy into superficial and often destructive channels. Nurses have clearly and consistently positioned themselves as patient advocates. We cannot hope to contribute meaningfully to the evolution of health care delivery systems without concurrently assuming responsibility for moving beyond current ineffective patterns of conflict.

This role asks a good deal of nurses in terms of moral courage, truth telling, personal integrity, and compassion. We who are nurses need the skills and the knowledge that conflict resolution teaches us and helps us practice. We also need the support and assistance of other like-minded colleagues, people who would like to see a health care delivery system that is healthy.

The goal is not a simplistic illusion for the resolution of all conflict. Rather, the purpose is to introduce better ways for addressing this conflict, ways that move us all toward a more satisfying and satisfactory investment in our commitments to health care. One need not get grandiose about outcomes in such an endeavor. One does need, however, to craft an authentic personal agenda, a commitment to address conflict in the most constructive manner feasible, given the constraints of the situation.

Nurses can choose to accept this invitation and challenge. Our perspective gives us a creative awareness of how systems can be changed and managed. We can bring a rich array of interpersonal skills and competencies to conflict resolution, combined with a unique sensitivity to the concerns of patients. These relational perspectives are an untapped reservoir for a health care community seeking resolutions to the escalating conflicts that trouble us all.

A Precautionary Note

Effective change is more often organic and gradual than cataclysmic and revolutionary. Nature teaches us this repeatedly. Nonetheless, we humans seem prone to the cataclysmic and revolutionary more often than not, and this shapes our outcomes. Sometimes change that is not particularly dramatic is thus also perceived as revolutionary when it is merely disruptive of deeply ingrained patterns and expectations. Nurses who elect to alter their ways of being at an uneven table may find their efforts are perceived in ways quite contrary to the intentions that guided their choices.

The deeply ingrained power relationships in health care delivery systems assume the sustained powerlessness and oppression of nurses. Often, efforts at honest self-assertion are perceived as attempts to procure power from those who now believe they have such power. The habituation to power that dominates others can be so deeply ingrained that any effort to alter these relationships is perceived as a direct effort to appropriate power in order to exercise dominance over others. This distortion needs to be anticipated. It requires significant clarity in one's thinking and acting, both to stay grounded in the effort at conflict resolution and to avoid doing exactly what others fear: to access power merely for the purpose of dominating others.

There is no easy solution to this dilemma, though it needs to be acknowledged. Often it is the first and most potent response nurses receive from efforts at simple self-assertion of fundamental rights. It can lead nurses to withdraw from the challenge. Or, alternatively, it can evoke the equally ineffective response of fighting back and dominating others to gain ground. To state what is true about injustices perpetrated upon nurses can evoke defensive attacks; to say what is true about nurses' unique and considerable strengths can confuse persons embedded in hierarchic thinking, who believe that to assert the good in nurses is somehow to diminish others. I make these disclaimers simply because they are so familiar, and because they need

to be candidly acknowledged. The habituation in our culture to perceive power as necessarily power over another is so pervasive that
simply to assert personal power and self-agency is often assumed to
be an effort to assert power over others.

Ways of Being

In my book I attempt to explore this dilemma and others that relate
to being at uneven tables. I also have described there an alternative
to this habituation to viewing power as exclusively a dominance
over others. I call this alternative an "evolving" of "ways of being"
at an uneven table. They are called "ways of being" because they
speak to how we negotiate: how we think and behave toward others
when we negotiate. I believe these "ways" call for a substantive shift
beyond where we habitually find ourselves now.

My intent is to explore how anyone at an uneven table, and
I believe this is all of us, might function differently if guided by
integrative being rather than dualistic divisiveness; by both/and
thinking rather than either/or thinking; by the search for comple-
mentarity rather than competition. Negotiating from this "position"
creates a new set of emerging and attractive realities that capture
my imagination and energy more than any stale conflict ever has.
These new realities emanate from conscious acts of moral courage:
people willing to exercise leadership at tables where some participants would prefer their silence. To adopt these ways of being is to
become part of a much larger social evolution. Such evolution for
me is a continuous and active process in which I can choose to participate. It shapes my present and, at least in part, determines my
future.

Thus these ways of being describe a field of action, not a
sequence of events or skills or abilities, and certainly not a check-
list recipe. I summarize them here with trepidation, since I am sensitive to the tendency in our culture to want quick fixes. They are
not that, and they ask a great deal more of anyone interested in
attempting to be present at an uneven table. They all are mutually

interactive, each depending on the other. They arise from the personal moral character you have developed and not from the appearances you wish to sustain. And they are never complete.

With these disclaimers, I briefly summarize here the "ways of being." They intend to demonstrate that alternatives to our current habituations are available, and that these alternatives can be learned and adopted.

Find and Inhabit the Deepest and Surest Human Space That Your Capabilities Permit

To introduce alternatives to dominance power negotiations in health care conflicts, it is essential to identify those alternatives: the humanity of one another as colleagues, the central mission of quality patient care, the improved conditions for families and communities whom we serve. To introduce such alternatives, they first must be deeply embedded in oneself, grounded in self-awareness, self-honesty, and self-confrontation. To know and honor your values and capabilities builds confidence, heightens your peace of mind, and enhances your tolerance when you need it most. If you do not face your own vulnerabilities, if you tend to deny or ignore them, these apprehensions become the place where your fears are activated. This uncertainty makes it much easier to discount your ideas and contributions. You, of course, control the depth of your self-honesty and breadth of your convictions.

Be a Truth Teller

In any conflict, and in any negotiation, there is a complex mixture of truths and untruths. Humans struggle imperfectly with truth. To attempt to share one's own truth as candidly and clearly as feasible makes it possible for others to do so as well. It also calls upon us, as truth tellers, to first be deeply honest with ourselves. One must listen closely to find truth and to recognize untruth. Being a truth teller gives us the freedom to acknowledge an untruth placed on a negotiating table or to acknowledge a truth denied admission to the table. It also gives us the opportunity to support other truth tellers at the table.

Honor Your Integrity, Even at Great Cost

While one rarely is counseled that selling your soul is wise or clever, it is done repeatedly, in an indirect fashion, at uneven tables. The invitation is usually to "just go along," even when you know that what is proposed is counter to your moral convictions. When you go to the table honoring your integrity, you know that there will be times when you will stand alone. To do so requires clarity, wisdom, and abundant courage.

Find a Place for Compassion at the Table

Negotiation is a powerful and ultimately human process. It helps to invite compassion to the table, first for yourself and then for others. Having faced and acknowledged your own limits and failures, you are able to see, with greater compassion, the same in others. This does not diminish your capacity to be a truth teller or to honor your integrity. It can, however, temper it with the continued awareness that we are all vulnerable and limited humans. Rather than exploiting these limits and vulnerabilities, we acknowledge them as a reality that might help us all unveil our collective capacity for deeper human understanding.

Draw a Line in the Sand Without Cruelty

Uneven tables are created with an assumption that some forms of injustice will be sustained. Thus, others at such tables may elect to be destructive or avaricious when you choose not to sustain this injustice. You are faced with a decision. If you remain, you may open yourself to unacceptable compromise and manipulation. You can, however, make explicit your own position on these issues, as well as your intention to leave the table if these limits cannot be honored. Doing so clearly and candidly informs others of your boundaries and your intentions. In doing so without cruelty, you refuse to escalate a potential cycle of destruction. By drawing a line in the sand, you also mark the place to which the line can be changed, if change at the table becomes possible. If change is not possible, you have been clear that you will not participate in harm and will not encourage escalation of this harm through retaliation or greater exploitation.

Expand and Explicate the Context

While this seems a standard of all conflict resolution, it is dramatically altered when placed in the company of the other nine ways of being at an uneven table. Conflict, like all other human experiences, does not exist in a vacuum. If some aspects of reality are denied, bringing these into focus can offer a more comprehensive awareness of the nature of the conflict and can even reveal more useful options for resolution. Initially, however, such expansion can be resisted, so one needs to be both persistent and creative. If the context for defining the problem is constricted, the resolution will have a comparable constriction. Expansion assists not only you, it also assists others at the table who seek a comprehensive solution to the issue at hand.

Innovate

This is the most fun dimension of these ways of being. It taps into your diverse creativities. While all conflict resolution builds on innovation, it does so in a unique way at uneven tables. A light touch helps. You can ask for clarification about the rules: often the rules in place are designed to sustain dominant power and look silly when explained. Questioning them, and their incongruities, exposes the prevalent manner of being and the power relationships that underlie them. In doing this, illusions can be questioned and curiosity activated. You can then even decide to change the rules. Happily, innovation can apply both to the substance of what might be achieved as well as to the process for achieving it.

Know What You Do and Do Not Know

We come to a conflict ignorant in some aspects and informed in others. This is the human condition. Those accustomed to sitting at uneven tables as advantaged participants often do so while denying a substantial portion of other's realities. Their advantage is often framed as already knowing all that there is to know. Awareness that the table is uneven is for you a different kind of advantage, and it gives you opportunities to both learn and share what you know. If there is something you don't know, say so. This can create an environment where "not knowing" is acknowledged. It helps to make an "adult learner" commitment and live by it.

Stay in the Dialogue

If you are not at the table, you cannot change it. To make a difference, you have to be there. The challenge is to do so without sustaining the unevenness of the table, through co-optation or by being silenced. It is helpful to redefine what staying in the dialogue really entails. Being at uneven tables can be a drain and is sometimes hurtful. You can give yourself time-outs or change tables to ones more open to exploring unevenness and its implications. You can stay in the larger dialogue of health care conflict resolution without assuming that you must be only at this one table, or at this table at all times. Flexibility helps.

Know When and How to Leave the Table

The ways of being are interdependent: none work in isolation. When the other ways of being at the table cannot or will not be honored, this dismissal can serve as a useful indicator that it is wiser to leave this table. Leaving a table is never easy, though it is easier than staying at a table where you know you do not belong. In such cases, leaving is an act of self-worth and self-affirmation. Keeping these ways of being intact as you leave then enables you to approach other tables, keeping the dialogue active and hopeful.

While an admittedly cursory glance at the ways of being, this summary does serve to highlight the possibilities for alternate ways of being at an uneven table. Nurses who elect to honestly attend to conflict can thus choose to do so without first accepting the assumption that they must accommodate and collude in actions they do not want to further. These ways of being give us options. They ask a great deal of us, and they give us a great deal in return.

Taking the First Step

Nurses can play a meaningful role in better resolving conflicts in health care systems. They can be instrumental in addressing and reforming uneven tables. They might best begin by systematically mastering the skills of negotiation and conflict resolution. Study and practice in these skills are essential tools at all tables, including those where unevenness prevails.

We can also serve as models for those in search of options at uneven tables. We thus encourage more evenly balanced tables at which to work and live. It is not only a matter of devising new tables, it is also finding new ways for constructing tables sensitive to justice and injustice. It involves both processes and outcomes. Nurses, sensitive to these issues and competent in the communication skills needed to further these aims, are an invaluable resource in the resolution of disputes confronting health care systems.

Taking this first step can lead to a richer and more rewarding role for nurses and more constructive outcomes for patients and others who share nursing's values about health care.

10

The Evolving Doctor

Barry C. Dorn

There were the good old days.

We prospered in a relatively uncomplicated, straightforward, clearly defined system. Doctors, who were primarily male, took care of patients with the assistance of nurses and other ancillary personnel, most of whom were female. We were paid by some combination of patient fees and insurance reimbursement. Hospitals catered to us. We lived in an environment of plenty, as our work was compensated on a cost-plus basis: charges and reimbursement were not an issue. We cloistered within the mystique of our profession, and society was content to submit to the feats and embellishments we served them. The system was well defined, with a structured hierarchical order that seemed impenetrable. And we fought to keep it that way.

I call those the "bygone" days. There were many things right about that system: it certainly was a comfortable place for those of us in practice. We worked hard and gave good service. And there were also many things wrong about that system. Now, we and the system we have been a part of are being called to task.

We are in a period of transition. Why? No doubt, the call for change is in part a reaction to our costs, arrogance, and isolation. Moreover, society itself has changed: in the rubrics of access, legal rights, and interpersonal consideration, there is greater attention to the concerns of patients, consumers, women, and minorities. Efforts to control health costs have dislodged our preference for lucrative specialty care to a greater emphasis on primary care. Medicine, too, has changed: technology has redefined what we do and how we do it; AIDS has challenged the scope of our wonders; and malpractice has confined our willingness to explore and take risks. And just as there have been objections with medicine, so too have there been difficulties with insurers, hospitals, and other elements of the delicate balance we call our health care system.

My purpose is not to analyze the reasons for all these changes. That could take a lifetime, as the explanations no doubt vary by the specific circumstances and experiences of different people, organizations, and regions. The fact remains that change itself is now an ever-present topic of conversation for physicians.

Rather, my purpose is to offer physicians a constructive framework for understanding and working with these changes. This perspective views negotiation as central to who we are and what we are becoming. How are these changes reflected in shifting relationships and methods of communication? How do we as physicians become a part of the process rather than the mere object of its agenda? How can we engage in these shifts and still maintain our sense of both personal and professional confidence?

The Bygone Doctor

This is not a tale of good guys and bad guys. That would be too simple. Rather, it is a story of smart people growing into a profession that socialized them to a set of assumptions and premises that worked well for a time. It is a fable of status both earned and conferred, with a script written in part by those who played the leading roles. It was a career defined by a society in search of a fountain of youth and a well of immortality. It is a plot that jumbled fact and fantasy.

The bygone doctor, for the most part "he," lived in a world of "doctor's orders." Patients lived by our edicts, and nurses, managers, and other health care providers supported our central position. We were revered, and what we said and what we wanted was conceded with little question. We knew there was no room for error in our work, and those who surrounded us accepted the notion, true or false, that we rarely committed mistakes or misjudgments. People did what we told them, and we enjoyed the power and control that accompanied our status.

We were independent. We operated as small businessmen, running high-priced operations and hoping the door would open often for ready customers. Our offices worked like the corner grocery store, burdened by the costs of expensive equipment and personnel that had to be kept continuously busy to turn a profit. We charged patients and their insurers cost-plus, and they paid: our fees were rarely questioned. We cherished the power and control of being on our own, with no one to tell us what to do or how to do it.

We were mavericks. Like cowboys, we walked into the corrals of our offices and hospitals and hustled people into action. Our time was always of the essence. We knew what needed to be done and how to do it. Yes, we cared and we were concerned, though we were less interested in listening and more concerned with doing. We wanted to freely define our own style with little interference or control by others. We had the power to shape our universe into a comfortable domain that suited our self-image. We were loners in a sea of colleagues who wanted the same.

We were detached. Our linkages were primarily informal. We created our referral network through personal contact—the recommendations of satisfied patients along with the personal and professional events that brought physicians together. We made our reputations through these gatherings. It was through these meetings that we decided to whom we would entrust our patients. Reputations were built and destroyed within this informal network that bound us together.

And we were financially solvent. One of the most attractive features was the generous gap between our actual expenses and our charges. And with supporting personnel keeping us productively busy, we were able to yield plentiful and lucrative charges with enormous speed. We worked long and we worked hard. Our busy work schedule and the generous reimbursement system created a comfortable lifestyle to which we and our families became accustomed.

What could be bad? Medicine offered the allure of a respected profession, helping people at their time of greatest need, healing and saving lives. In our minds, we were bestowed our deserved lot, and society seemed to agree. We had power and control, wealth and prestige, security and comfort. Is it any wonder that physicians are clinging to what they once had? Is it any surprise that the profession now feels perplexed? And is it any shock that society, which has reshaped its view and expectations of health care, now demands something different?

There are those physicians who would hold on to the bygone era at any cost. I have heard colleagues vapidly threaten to leave medicine should it change. When they cloak their persistence for the status quo under the veil of better patient care, their resistance is seen for what it is: a desire to cling to what was relished in the old system. Having been there, I know well the allure of what was. I also know that the changes and the change process itself can be painful.

Having prospered in one system, it is hard for physicians to imagine a different balance among the many competing forces shaping health care and the practice of medicine. It is even harder to imagine an arrangement that could offer us ample, if not the same level of satisfaction.

Health care is changing, whether we as physicians like it or not. Our chances of fitting in depend on our effectively negotiating—now—the shape of medical practice in the future. That means we are part of the give-and-get of the negotiation process. And once this new system is in place, it means that negotiation will be part of what we do and how we go about doing it. That set of old assumptions and premises that worked well for a time are going to have to change.

◆   ◆   ◆   ◆   ◆   ◆

It was 6:00 P.M. Dr. Nick Norton was just sitting down to Sunday evening dinner. His wife had just placed a steaming bowl of green pasta in front of him when the beeper went off. His first instinct, to ignore it, was awakened by the fact that his family hated its noise, especially during dinner. "Just one minute," he apologized, his napkin dropping on the chair as he headed for the phone.

Dr. Norton is chief of orthopedics at the Oppidania Medical Center, and this Sunday evening is his turn to be on call. At the other end of the line was Lauren Lieber, chief resident for orthopedics. "Sorry to bother you, Dr. Norton. We just had a seventy-eight-year-old woman come in with a very serious, complex hip fracture. I'm in the emergency room and have been with her for about twenty minutes. She hasn't eaten all day, appears stable, and has been cleared by her internist. It probably would be best to do her now."

Norton knew what this meant. He would be going into the hospital for the surgery. It was only a matter of when. "Have you called the operating room? When can we get in?"

"They're talking eight o'clock. They have two rooms going, and it's been a pretty average night."

"OK, Lauren. You get everything set up, and I'll be there by seven-thirty." Norton returned to the table and a cold plate of pasta. His wife placed it in the microwave as he lamented his return to the hospital.

Norton pulled into his reserved space in the doctor's parking lot and was in the building and into his hospital greens by 7:25, ready to talk with Lauren, read the chart, and see the patient. Lauren walked up to him with a grimace on her face.

"I'm really sorry," she said. "You're going to kill me."

"Well, that depends. What's the problem?"

"There are only two operating rooms functioning tonight, and we've been bumped by the vascular team. We're set for nine o'clock. I tried to reach you, but you had already left home."

"Well, I'm not going to kill *you*, though that doesn't necessarily rule murder out entirely." Norton took a deep breath. "It doesn't pay to go home for the one hour. Anything else going on tonight?" Norton figured he would make the most of his presence in the hospital. He went up to check on the condition of several of his patients on the seventh floor. He went over the hip case with Lieber and was ready to roll at nine.

He got back to the operating room by 8:35 and was anxious to get going. Monday was what he called a killer day—OR cases starting at 7:30 A.M. and going all day—and he wanted to get home for a good night's rest. Just as he was heading into the OR, Diane Darling, the nurse in charge of scheduling the rooms, called him over. "Dr. Norton, I am so sorry. We just put an emergency C-section in your room. It shouldn't be more than an hour." Darling cringed to hear his reply.

Norton looked her straight in the eye and pointed his finger in her face. "Last delay. Do you understand? I don't want to hear one more delay. The end." Norton angrily turned around and steamed off to the surgeon's lounge. Why him, he wondered.

Two cups of coffee and one package of cookies later, he made his way back to the nurse's station in the OR. Diane Darling looked the other way when she saw him coming. Norton noticed the gesture and was ready for a fight. He liked to use a bit of humor and a firm tone when he was angry. It helped him keep in better control of himself, and it worked with other people.

He walked up to Darling's desk. "Diane, we are all ready to go, aren't we?"

Darling took a deep sigh and caught her breath. "Oh, Dr. Norton, I am *so* sorry. There's a bad auto accident coming into the ER and they need your room for a tracheostomy, chest tube, and repair of facial lacerations. I have no estimate of time at this point."

Norton decided to play it calm and firm. "No problem. Here's what I want you to do. Call up our favorite anesthesiologist, Dr. Walter, and have him get in here to open another room. End of story."

Darling had this sudden urge to run away. "Well, Dr. Norton, I thought you might want me to do that, so I already called Dr. Walter and explained the situation." She paused. "I told him about your patient and he said it wasn't an emergency. He said if you didn't want to wait for the room to clear, you would just have to postpone the surgery until the morning."

Norton was now seething. Walter, in his mind, was a typical young, lazy anesthesiologist, overimpressed with his own credentials. How could he make this decision without even the courtesy of a telephone call? It made Norton crazy!

"Until the morning? Who the hell does he think he is!" Norton's voice was loud enough for anyone within earshot of the station to hear it loud and clear. "Did you explain to him that this is an emergency?"

"Yes, I told him all about your case."

Norton demanded the phone and called Walter at home. There were no niceties. "Walter, what the hell is this? I've been waiting here, jerked around, since seven-thirty. What do you mean it's not an emergency?"

Will Walter had been through this before. "Just what I said, Nick, it's not an emergency. If you want, you can wait it out tonight. Otherwise, just do it in the morning. These things can wait."

Norton's voice grew tense. He enunciated one word at a time, so it would have maximum effect on Walter. "I have a full schedule tomorrow, hips and knees, and nothing can be changed. So tonight's surgery happens tonight. And I am not going to sit around here anymore waiting to be bumped. You get your ass in here, and then you have two choices. Either open a third room or put a note in the chart that this is not an emergency, and you and I will meet in Fisher's office in the A.M., before my cases!"

Walter knew what Norton's ravings would mean. He had been in this situation before. They complain to Fisher, who gets involved and then always takes the side of the surgeon. He did not want to hear another one of Fred's lectures about knowing when and when not to draw the line. He considered the choices and decided that it was still worth a bit of a try.

"Nick, is this really an emergency? Couldn't you get somebody else to do it tomorrow? It's not only a matter of inconvenience, it's big bucks to get that room up and going at this hour if it's not really necessary."

Norton was losing what little patience he had left. "Walter. It will really be big bucks when I stroke out. *Now.*" The telephone recoiled as Norton slammed down the receiver. He was not only tired, he was infuriated that he had to go through this ordeal. Not the best way to start a week.

Norton looked up at the clock in the OR as he was about to make his first incision. It was 11:42 P.M.

◆ ◆ ◆ ◆ ◆ ◆ ◆

The Travails of Transition

For a physician, many of the changes occurring in the health system today are undeniably tangible. They are easily measured: this year's decrease in income as managed care organizations restrict rates of reimbursement; an increased percentage of income eaten up by the insurance, rentals, and other costs of being in practice. These losses are distressing, especially when measured against the anticipated prospects for a maturing practice. For many physicians, one's self-worth is reflected in part by take-home pay, and as that income drops, so does one's self-confidence and self-esteem.

Many of the conflicts we experience now are generally presumed to result from the shift to capitated reimbursement systems and the new burdens and uncertainties they pose for our practice. It would be easy to explain all our conflicts as an outgrowth of these new organizational arrangements. In reality, this angle alone tells only part of the story. Conflict, after all, is experienced on the interpersonal level as well. Before we can appreciate the impact of these organizational shifts, we must understand our conflicts from the perspective of physicians as people.

These interpersonal conflicts arise over differing expectations of authority, collaboration, and control. They clash in the flurry of day-to-day decision making. When one person believes the call to be theirs and another believes it is negotiable, there is bound to be conflict, about the substance of the issue as well as the process by which it is decided. The bulk of these interpersonal conflicts swirl amid the complicating variables of age, gender, and turf. And they all result in a bottom line of money, power, and control.

This "age" dimension is illustrated by the conflict often seen between fifty-something and forty-something male physicians. How is this conflict manifested, and what does it tell us about changing expectations as they vary from one period of training to another?

The fifty-something physicians are beginning the home stretch of their careers, anticipating a decade of easy and lucrative practice to secure them for retirement. For years these physicians have submitted loyally to their superiors, mentors who dominated a rigidly hierarchical domain. They paid allegiance in the form of compliance and financial deference. Finally, the now sixty-something mentors are retiring, and it is time for those in their fifties to take over.

The fifty-something doctors now expect the same deference from their forty-something colleagues that they bestowed upon their own older counterparts. The physicians now in their forties, however, grew up in the period of Vietnam protest and the ferment of the sixties and seventies, which their older counterparts missed while in the ardors of residency training or while serving in Vietnam. The younger doctors, who cruised through the pop culture phases of "question authority," social mission, and the "me" generation, are unwilling to replicate a subservient relationship for their older counterparts. The dynamic manifests itself as conflict over money, with the older physicians expecting higher compensation and the younger ones expecting equal pay; obedience, with the fifty-something physicians expecting the younger ones to do as told; and prestige, with the older physicians demanding the recognition and status of senior statesmen. Neither group is wrong or right. They simply bring different expectations to the process of interprofessional relationships. When those differences are not clarified and resolved, there is certain to be conflict.

The conflicts between age groups arise from the different socialization these physicians experienced in their initial training and beyond. Budding doctors are exposed to the social mores, professional doctrines, and medical infrastructure that prevail during their time in medical school and as they move into residency and early practice. Those mores, doctrines, and structures shape their behaviors, relationships, and expectations. As these change over time, the profile of physicians changes as well. The physician trained in the early sixties differs markedly from his or her counterpart of the nineties, who is oriented toward gender equality, moderate gross earnings expectations, and practice in a managed care company. As these physicians of different eras work together, the distinctions can erupt into dysfunctional conflict, even though at the core there is more that binds than separates them.

Another source of interpersonal medical conflict is gender. This gender conflict is illustrated by Deborah Tannen (1990) in her distinction between how men negotiate and how women negotiate. Men tend to place primacy on hierarchical order in their dealings with others, as measured by various indicators of status, such as privilege, income, or reputation: "Am I higher or lower than the other person?" On the other hand, women tend to place more emphasis on relationships in their dealings with others: "Is this someone with whom I can relate?" Many of the associative shifts occurring in the health system now center on these very matters of status and relationship.

When you change the importance of status in a profession with a history of rigidly hierarchical ordering, you inflame conflict: between the resisters, who seek to maintain their position of dominance in a quickly crumbling system, and the reformers, who hope to change the nature and shape of that old order. And when you shift attitudes about relationships in an arena of close clinical contact, conflict becomes inevitable. The uniquely intimate nature of medical practice heightens the sensitivity to these matters of status and relationship. The potential for blunder and harm is heightened between people at different stages of change or resistance.

This gender conflict thrives at the cusp of frustrated expectations. At times it is men's presuming that all women are their subordinates, even female colleagues. As well, it is women's perceiving that all men are superficial, even those appropriately seeking to express themselves interpersonally. It gets meanest when men and women attempt to cross traditional lines. When a man seeks to interact relationally, men find him suspicious and women find him clumsy. And when a woman plays the hierarchical game, women see her as disloyal and men find her disingenuous.

At some point we are going to find some blended model in which people feel validated for who they are, not the script they play or defy. In the meantime, gender conflict is a presence for physicians. Though it's not a problem for medical practice alone, it is one we experience with particular poignancy, given the close interpersonal nature of our work.

Finally, turf battles. Who owns the patient, the primary care physician or the specialist? Who prescribes the medication, the nurse or the doctor? Who determines the necessity for a new piece of equipment, the manager or the medical director?

In medicine, turf is not an item of palpable space. Rather, turf is a metaphor for control. The greater one's turf, the greater one's influence or jurisdiction over decisions. And just as territorial battles generate fervent protection of property, so too is domination over clinical care zealously guarded by physicians and others who inhabit its domain. In recent years, traditional battle lines among specialists, between specialists and generalists, and between nurses and physicians have escalated. Some physicians are reticent to concede a meaningful role to patients in determining the course of their care.

Similarly, they are threatened by the encroachment of nurses and other nonphysicians into their domain. And many physicians are incensed by the expanded role of insurers in the determination of medical necessity. As an orthopedic surgeon, nothing infuriates me more than an inappropriate admonition from an unqualified insurance reviewer that I try aspirin to treat a patient who obviously requires a total knee arthroplasty.

"Who decides what?" is the common theme of these disagreements. Whether a matter of age, gender, or turf, decisional conflict arises when parties assume a different answer to this question.

Tasks and People

The frustrations that accompany conflict over decision making are greatest when the functional and relational aspects of our work do not augment one another. The functional aspects are the tasks we perform: repairing a femur, prescribing medication, performing an angioplasty. The relational aspects are the information exchanged, the time given, and the emotions understood.

Tasks and people are different. And tasks and people are the same. Incongruous statements? Perhaps. Though if these differences, similarities, and interdependencies remain incongruous in your medical mind, you will no doubt find yourself surrounded by conflict.

As physicians, it is imperative that our primary focus be on tasks. That is what we are entrusted to do. While other professions are allowed some reprieve for reasonable error, we, our patients, and our society permit little if any deficiency in our work. Our decisions, our actions, and the actions of others that we supervise have direct life-and-death as well as quality-of-life implications for patients. That vital association between what we do and people's lives is what makes medicine distinct. We cannot overlook a symptom, prescribe the wrong medication, or miscalculate a surgical procedure. Our work must be precise. It becomes an obsession for us, and that obsession could blind us to other essential aspects of medical practice.

In contrast to the importance of tasks, the relational aspects of our work seem secondary. Our time is precious. Our concentration is essential. And our status, necessary to ensure the adherence we require, must be enforced. This distance insulates us and makes us impervious to much that surrounds the practice of medicine. Some of this inaccessibility has been not only a function of distraction: for some it has been a tenet of practice.

As physicians, we have been schooled to erect a distance between ourselves and others: our colleagues, other health professionals, as well as the people we treat. In part this reticence is justified by the need for clinical detachment and professional independence. The separation offers emotional protection from the pain and hardship experienced by our patients. It allows us to move efficiently about our business without spending unnecessary time on social niceties. Unfortunately, in the process, we forge a chasm between tasks and people that can sometimes haunt our practice and reduce our effectiveness as physicians.

Do we want to integrate tasks and people to subdue decisional conflict and to yield a more balanced view of medical practice? If so, how can we ensure the benefits of this new profile for our practice now and into the future? And in what ways will negotiation fit into this emerging picture?

Crafting Cohesion

There is little about medical practice that is not changing. Computers are taking new command of information and robotics are performing more and more tasks. Our most important contributions, the extensive knowledge of our minds and the delicate maneuvers of our hands, are becoming inferior to the burgeoning intelligence and microscopic dexterity of machines. Managed care and emerging health policies are transforming how we conduct our business. Medicine is becoming more a cog in the health care network wheel than the hub around which a medical system revolves. Financial and societal readjustments are creating new expectations for the role we play in the lives of our patients and the welfare of our community.

Given these changes, can we generate and realize a new vision for the practice of medicine? Can that new role be one that satisfies the needs of our patients and the system, as well as our own professional objectives and financial expectations?

The answer is yes, *if* we are part of creating the change rather than the object of its agenda. As a physician I sometimes feel that health policy wonks, managed care utilization reviewers, and insurance company executives actively contemplate what they are going to do about us. Our perspective is ignored as a repetition of fading ideas rather than a voice for fresh and vital thinking. Our perspective is not part of the equation.

Being a part of the change means that we actively negotiate the contours of future medical practice. To negotiate rather than dominate means that it is not fully *our* process and not fully *our* solution. It means that we will give some things up in order to gain others. It means we listen and incorporate what others recommend. And it means that in the final analysis, we are a constructive part of the balance that represents new health care.

The negotiation to which I refer is not politicking that happens in Washington regarding rates of reimbursement, though it includes that as well. It is not merely negotiating a new arrangement with a managed care company, though it includes that too. And it does not merely mean changing our relationships with one another, with other health professionals, and with our patients, though it is that too.

To flourish in this new system, you must become a different kind of physician. The waning relative preeminence of your intellectual and mechanical prowess is replaced by something new and expansive. You assume a new profile as a caregiver. That new profile influences how you think, the manner in which you interact, and the process by which you come to decisions. Central to that new profile is negotiation.

This new profile means that as a physician, you negotiate all the time. You craft cohesion between what you do and the people with whom you do it. You are part of designing balanced policies to reduce the chances that you, and your patients, are not waiting all night for an operating room to open. You articulate, with others, what you hope to achieve in your practice.

As a negotiator, you become a catalyst for good patient care decision making, adjusting different clinical, financial, and social considerations in the process. Your purview, and that of others, is broadened. Negotiation is the manner by which you structure professional collaboration. And it is the way you resolve the day-to-day conflicts that emerge in your practice. Negotiation is fundamental to what you do and how you go about doing it.

As a mode of decision making, negotiation incorporates the appropriate contributions of those who effect or are affected by the choice. The decision is not made or dominated by one person. Rather, the frames of all the relevant parties are balanced to reap an outcome that is satisfactory to the complete range of their legitimate considerations. Those people who have the knowledge, understanding, or legal responsibility are involved and assume accountability for what they do and don't contribute. Your primary concern is for the effectiveness or efficiency of the decision, not necessarily your primacy in reaching it. As a physician, you are valued for actively enhancing this process; you are appreciated for knowing that you do not own it. I call it "mediating medical opinion."

As a process, negotiation binds the functional and the relational aspects of our work. Negotiation itself is task-oriented: it is directed toward the decisions and actions for which we are responsible. Negotiation defines the process by which we interact with people to reach those decisions and to effect those actions. As physicians, we do not act alone. Negotiation defines the two-way bridges that connect us to others.

To negotiate does not imply that everyone has equal say. I will continue to resist inappropriate admonitions from unqualified insurance reviewers that I try aspirin in place of necessary knee surgery. Rather, to negotiate means to actively engage in this process of give-and-take. Just as often, the call from an insurance company can raise and resolve legitimate interests. It can serve as an important check and balance for the system. My intention is to responsibly distinguish the extraneous from the legitimate concern. That is part of my negotiating profile as a physician.

To negotiate appropriately lifts a cumbersome burden from the shoulders of physicians. The reverse side of the paternalism that has characterized our relations with patients and the system is that it laid us open and responsible for all that went wrong. We fueled this illusion in the way we assumed decision control and in the false confidence we offered regarding our achievements. To change this outlook is not merely to add more legal forms on the way into surgery. Rather, to readjust this imbalance we must redefine people-to-people understanding: a give-and-take that clarifies what medicine reasonably can and cannot realize. This give-and-take, "negotiation," ultimately reduces a physician's burden because it explicitly requires others to assume legitimate responsibility for decisions in which they take part. It requires listening, explaining, and responding, and that is our job.

This shift is not only good medical practice, it is also downright pragmatic. The litigious nature of patient care today has caused many of us to retreat. Defending ourselves from legal repercussions, we have contrived a chasm between ourselves and our patients. Lawyers tell us what we should and should not divulge. While their counsel makes perfect legal sense, the perversions and repercussions of malpractice fright make little sense for patient care. In reality, our best defense against the dangers of the lawsuit is not silence. Rather, poor communication is the most common impetus for malpractice litigation. Even when a clinical mistake is made, good communication is the best antidote to legal action. Our medical integrity and personal honesty throughout the patient care process is the best avenue to avoid the potential lawsuit. When information, decisions, and actions are knowledgeably negotiated, whether with patients or colleagues, responsibility for known consequences must be shared by all at the table. In so doing, we are less on the defensive and more a proponent of productive coherence.

How do we initiate this shift to physician-as-negotiator? For as long as I have been in practice, physicians have been on a societally sanctioned pedestal. Because this exaltation has now become professionally problematic, it is time for the pedestal to be dismantled. To do so, we must truly integrate ourselves into the action. It is up to us to encourage integrative negotiation by the way we conduct themselves. We can transform what was our power and influence to enhance the quality of our decision making and collaboration.

Why would we want to do this? How could less power be more influence? Why would this shift to physician-as-negotiator be advantageous for us? The answer is simple. The changes we are negotiating are not a replication of the old power and control. Rather, we negotiate toward a new order and interdependence to enhance the health system's functioning. We are part of constructing a more even playing field on which we appropriately contribute and share decision making, accountability, and financial well-being. This is a more cohesive picture: one in which our role of coordinating technology and people and integrating decisions and actions is more valid and more indispensable. It is a table that fits what we can do and what we should be doing in the emerging health system.

◆ ◆ ◆ ◆ ◆ ◆ ◆

Fred Fisher maintains an active practice that occupies about half his busy schedule. He sees patients on an outpatient basis through the Oppidania Medical Clinic, located in the doctors' office building adjacent to the hospital. Although the shifts in reimbursement, the advent of managed care systems, and the efficiencies imposed by the clinic administration have changed the circumstances of his practice, the gentle attention and rapport he maintains with his patients have never altered.

He is on his way to a meeting in a private function room at a nearby Chinese restaurant frequented by the medical staff. The clinic's internal medicine physicians are gathering once again to discuss a reorganization of their practice: it seems like a never-ending topic. Fisher's agenda for the meeting is the same he has brought to every one in this series: he doesn't want anything imposed that will interfere with his practice. He does not want to change the relationship with his patients, his colleagues, or his support staff.

The announced purpose of the meeting is to discuss the transition of the clinic from a fee-for-service to a capitated independent practitioner association (IPA). As Fisher understands the distinction from his reading of medical newsletters, this means that the group will be going from charging for services rendered to receiving a set fee for a covered "life." Odd term. The less expensively they are able to serve that "life," the better off the organization will be financially. It all seems perverse to him.

Fisher takes a seat at the long table next to his old friend Rollins, "Dr. Ralph Rollins." Fisher and Rollins go back to college. They were together through medical school, residency, and on to Oppidania. Rollins is one of the few friends with whom Fisher is able to show his boyhood sense of mischief. He turns to Rollins and whispers, "You know, Ralph, they are trying to turn us here into an insurance company." Fisher hesitated for dramatic effect and then smiled. "Resist at any cost." Rollins considered the premise for a moment and a smile broke on his face as he went into his trademark low-decibel laugh.

Rollins and Fisher practiced the same kind of medicine, though Rollins tended to be much more low-key in his leadership and public activities. It was in keeping with their two different styles that Fisher was in a high-profile position while Rollins was primarily in his clinic seeing patients. It was also typical that Rollins was more willing to accept change than Fisher. In spite of their differences, Fisher depends on Rollins to give him an eye on what is happening within the medical staff.

"So what do you think of this whole capitation idea?" In Fisher's usual style, he asked a question and, before waiting for the answer, was off giving his own opinion. "I think this whole idea of doctors assuming risk is a lousy idea. It changes the fiduciary relationship with the hospital and makes us out to be competitors in our clinical relationship with them and other physicians. I think it's a mistake."

Rollins was not surprised at Fisher's attitude, nor at his compulsion to preach more than he listened. "It does change the fiduciary relationship, Fred, though it doesn't necessarily turn us into competitors. You could look at it another way, too." Rollins knew Fisher was ready to argue, even though he was listening closely. "We in fact do have a clear business relationship with the hospital. This arrangement merely brings it aboveboard, makes it explicit, and creates a different set of incentives. I wouldn't order this recipe if I had more of a choice, though in the long run I don't think it's as bad as everyone fears. And anyway, it's not a one-way street. We negotiate with them, and they negotiate with us. It's more balanced than you probably imagine."

"Oh, come on, Ralph. That's phony baloney. What are we going to do, take our business elsewhere? Or what is the hospital going to do, stop taking our patients? This is just giving work to a bunch of accountants and lawyers at our expense. Nothing is going to change, except our overhead costs."

"I am not going to defend the shift to a capitated system, Fred. I am also not going to resist it, because to do so would be lunacy. It's simply the way things are happening now, and we either go along or, you're right, Fred, the hospital could take its business elsewhere. Not explicitly, because we wouldn't let them get away with it. Implicitly, though, patients would just stop coming through our offices because insurance companies wouldn't send them our way. And the hospital would open up sources elsewhere, and we de facto would be out of the loop. Look, Fred, the hospital hasn't coddled us for all these years because they like us. It's because we send them our patients, and that means dollars and cents for them. The reason for looking at this new system is that it will ensure that we have patients. That is our leverage with the hospital, and that is our lifeblood. It's the same thing as it used to be, it's just different."

Fisher gave Rollins a look as if he said something that didn't make sense. Then he continued. "Right Ralph, and you know what the difference is. It used to be that we were paid for providing a service. That is what we do, what we were trained to do. Now we make money for not providing a service. We're like those farmers who get money for not growing corn. Except, Ralph, this is not corn, it's medical care, and the service we don't provide is not only wrong, it's dangerous. One of our patients gets sick and they can haul us into court. And you know where the insurance companies are going to be then? Running for cover. Don't you see, Ralph? We hold both the financial risk *and* the legal liability. The insurance companies have manipulated medicine into a corner, and here we sit eating Chinese food and going along."

"Fred, what's our job? Keeping people well, right? You have confidence we can do that, right?" Fisher nodded, though reluctantly because he was afraid he might be nodding about something with which he would ultimately disagree. "So that's what we are being paid to do: keep people well. And if we do a good job, we deserve the rewards. And if not, it's not doomsday, it's just not the automatic cash cow we have become used to. You know it yourself, Fred, all our financial incentives were for ordering tests, doing surgery, making referrals. The more we did, the better off we all were. Yes, much of what we did was justifiable. Though you know yourself that many of the tests were ordered routinely without considering the cost or benefit. Now, we must consider that cost-benefit ratio."

"Ralph, you are sounding like an ad for an insurance company."

That comment annoyed Rollins. It was tantamount to being called a traitor. "Fred, and you are sounding like you were born yesterday. What's the alternative? This is the marketplace, Dr. Fisher"—Rollins was trying to invoke his colleague's reservoir of professional common sense—"and you either play or call it quits. There are more of us out there than are needed, and the ones who are going to survive are those who are playing the game. And those who are ahead of it are going to thrive."

Fisher grunted a tone of acknowledgment and asked Rollins to pass the dim sum.

The waiters were clearing the plates and placing plastic-wrapped fortune cookies on the soiled tablecloth when Tim Thatcher rose to address the group. Thatcher has been the clinic's administrator for three years. A relatively young MBA, he had won the confidence of the medical staff by increasing efficiency while maintaining clinical practice intact. The management of the practice had been pretty sloppy before Thatcher arrived, and he was well liked by the physicians.

Just as he was about to begin, Dr. Gloria Green, president of the internal medicine group, put her hand on his arm as if to stop him. "Just a minute, everybody," she said, breaking into the many discussions around the table. "Before Tim starts up, I just want everyone to know that Tim and I have spoken about this issue of the capitated system, and I am pleased with the work he has done to put together this proposal. He has a good deal of material for us to think about, so I hope you will listen carefully."

Thatcher watched Dr. Green go through her unplanned speech with a sense of relief. Green realized that if this meeting turned into a doctor-administrator contest, it would be counterproductive. By introducing her strong endorsement of the idea, she deflected debate from divisive scoffing to serious consideration of some very complex issues.

Thatcher very briefly reviewed what everyone already knew about changing reimbursement patterns and what it meant for medical practice. He explained that in the current market, whether you are an insurer, hospital, or physician, you do what you need to do to ensure a steady supply of patients. The competition for patients is fierce, and they no longer come as individuals, they come in herds. The change is cost-driven, and Thatcher emphasized that this same factor affects everyone, though the implications are different for each. Patients and their employers want reasonably priced health care, and they recognize that they may have to sacrifice some though not all choice in order to get it. Given the high numbers involved, patients are likely to be more loyal to their pocketbooks than to their physicians. Insurers, Thatcher explained, are also under a great deal of financial pressure from their stockholders. They have to control the price of a service over which they have little direct control. They are essentially go-betweens, with expensive providers on one side and frugal buyers on the other.

Thatcher stopped to take his breath. "And here we sit in the middle of all this." A faint smile formed on his face, revealing the anxiety he felt about this meeting. He went on to explain that nothing is sacred in this new system. No one does anything because of tradition: you either are on the bandwagon or not. After much investigation, he is recommending that the group reorganize as a capitated IPA, negotiating competitive fees with a number of insurers to cover as many lives as possible. The future viability and size of the practice will depend on the number of patients they will be able to enroll and the overall "good health" of that group.

Thatcher most dreaded the question-and-answer period. He had prepared as best he could.

The first question was one he had hoped would come later, after people started getting used to the idea. "What about our relationship with the specialists to whom we refer in the hospital? Who pays for that?"

Thatcher opened slowly. "That's perhaps the biggest change for you in your practice. Now when you make a referral, the patient's insurance company pays your bill as well as that of the cardiologist. In this new system, you get one lump sum to care for all the needs of your patient. Essentially, if you must make a referral to a cardiologist, then you pay for it. So, the more you are able to handle on you own, and the less you use referrals, the better off all of us will be financially."

Someone piped in from the back of the room, "This is like a game of Russian roulette with all the chambers loaded. If we refer, we lose our money. And if we don't, and the patient has a heart attack, we lose our practice. If I were an insurance agent, it would make perfect sense to me." A subdued caustic laughter murmured through the room.

Rollins chimed in. "Look, it makes no sense to put Tim on the hot seat for this. He didn't invent the system. You're right, it puts us at some disadvantage. And I think after we are done venting some steam, we have to pay attention. I don't think the question is whether or not we do it, the question is how to make the most of it." Rollins's remarks silenced the room.

Thatcher picked up where he had left off. "There are two sides to this negotiation. We agree to a price with the insurers, and we budget accordingly. Then we go to the hospital and the specialty groups. We want to get as good a price as we can from them. If one of the cardiologist groups gives the same level of quality of care and a better price than the others, it's in our best interest to send business their way. Even more important, we'll want to send patients to specialists that get us the *most* for our money: good efficient care that is responsive to our continued involvement with the patient. The specialists need to be working with us, not wandering off in their own isolated world. If they are not with us, we don't send them patients, and soon enough the word gets out. We get a good level of service for our patients or we walk. We have some leverage in this system as well."

Gloria Green cued him with a question that she knew was on everyone's mind. "What about the financials, Tim? How might the books look after this?" Green knew the answer, though she wanted to give Thatcher the chance to answer it before too much dissent grew.

"Financially, we could do as well if not even better than where we are now. Our advantage in this whole new puzzle is that we have control. We decide where the patient goes, who they see, and ultimately what it costs. Though you do carry some risk, it's like any financial deal. The rewards go to whoever takes the risk and manages it well. We could even be talking 'lucrative.' It's just a matter of playing the game right."

Wil Wainwright raised his hand. Dr. Wainwright typifies the aggressive young forty-year-old physician who is working hard to establish a practice against all the challenges imposed by the system. His practice is not nearly as solid as he had expected it would be at this point in his career. "I recommend we go forward with Tim's proposal as fast as we can. A week doesn't go by without hearing of some new merger, alliance, or deal. I say every day we wait, we fall farther and farther behind. The fact is, if someone comes along and provides more cost effective care, in one day we could lose everything we have worked so hard to build. And it wouldn't crack in one day. It would just slowly fade away. And before we realized what hit us, it would all be gone. And all the lamenting in the world wouldn't bring it back. Personally, I'm not interested in being around to turn off the lights on this group. I say we move fast." Wainwright's comments turned the mood in the room.

The discussion period continued for another forty-five minutes. As the meeting was drawing to a close, Thatcher handed out some stapled sheets showing current and projected financials for the practice, arranged in three columns: best case, worst case, and reasonable case. Thatcher explained that the group's strategy would determine in which column they'd end up.

After the meeting, Fisher and Rollins were in the corner of the coat room getting ready to venture out into the evening chill. Fisher lamented, "You know, Ralph, the biggest buildings in this town belong to the insurance companies. In this litigious, risk-averse society, our greatest architectural temples are built in their honor. That is their business—collecting lots of money, assuming risk, and paying out when there is a claim. I just think it's wrong for doctors to start taking over their function. It changes the texture of medical practice, and don't tell me it's for the better."

"Fred, when you started off in your practice, weren't you concerned about cost?"

"Sure. It was different then. Many of my patients were paying out of pocket, and I had to be sure that I kept their costs in line. It was just a part of what I did."

"Well, Fred, think of it in those terms. You would still be providing the best medical care you can. You are just doing it with half an eye on the pocketbook. And just to make sure you don't forget, this time it's every patient's pocketbook, as well as your own."

With that, each man sent regards to the other's family, and they were off on their separate ways.

♦ ♦ ♦ ♦ ♦ ♦ ♦

The Evolving Doctor

Successful evolution is marked by continual readjustment between the parts and the whole. In the case of medical practice, this means shaping a compatible fit between changes in professional practice and shifts in the health care environment. How do we frame this adaptation so it works for both medicine and the system?

If the system is evolving, then so too must the physician evolve. There are two sides to this symmetry for us. On one side, our own changes in medical practice. On the other, our influence on the course of that evolution. These two dimensions exemplify negotiation: what we give, what we get, and the tone that guides the exchange. I term the physician who constructively engages in the process the "evolving doctor." This physician contrasts with the bygone model I described earlier in the chapter.

The bygone doctor was independent, a maverick, and detached: the evolving doctor is interdependent, managed, and connected. This physician is a partner, contributing to and deriving benefit through collaborative patient care networks, physician practice organizations, and medical services organizations. It is the surge in this type of interdependence that characterizes recent shifts in the health system. Historic rivalries have been forgotten as hospitals seek and achieve innovative alliances. To ensure a necessary flow of patients, community hospitals are linking to tertiary care centers, creating a spoke-and-hub referral partnership. To ensure a place for themselves and their patients amid the flow of patients, physicians are joining these networks. It is this affiliation that becomes the most important distinguishing characteristic of a physician. When prospective patients call my office, they are more concerned about my managed care affiliations than my medical school training.

This change is not new. It has been in progress since the early 1980s. What has evolved is the attitudes of physicians. The same doctors who once vowed they would never join now cannot imagine being outside the loop. They had resisted control: they did not want their practice nor their income dictated by someone else.

This apprehension is valid when the relationship between the managed care organization and medical staff is not considered a negotiation. When any interdependence is unilateral, it becomes imbalanced and even dangerous: there is no check-and-balance system to ensure that one side will not impose imprudent policy on the other.

To be an effective collaboration, the rules of policy and practice, as well as the exceptions to those rules, must be considered negotiable by all parties, including patients. The system works best when constituent interests are reasonably recognized and satisfied: when patients' concerns are fairly addressed, so they remain with the plan; when physicians' needs are fairly met, so they follow plan policies; and when management needs are observed, so the plan can efficiently go about its business. This sort of interdependence is what defines health care: for the system to function well, negotiating this balance is part of our medical responsibility.

And it is my premise that if the evolving doctor incorporates all of the above, one important characteristic will be shared with the bygone doctor: he or she will be financially solvent. Not all physicians will be able to succeed in the future. I do believe, however, that the success stories will be about those who collaboratively shape and actively negotiate the evolution.

Conclusion

Physicians can take a lesson from the dinosaur. When the earth's environment went through drastic changes, the dinosaurs' slowly changing physiology was unable to adapt to new climatic conditions and food supplies. I am not suggesting that the medical profession is facing extinction. Rather, I am warning that we have our dinosaurs among us: colleagues who refuse to adapt their practice and attitudes to a new type of health system. They will no doubt perish or languish in the system.

The evolving doctor, on the other hand, will find this an exciting time to be in practice. The contours of medicine are changing, and the present offers a unique opportunity to be part of shaping that change into the future. For those who are part of the action, medicine will remain a financially rewarding field of endeavor. It will no doubt be different than the previous "golden age," and so be it.

How does the lesson of the dinosaur fit the concept of whole image negotiation? As physicians, we are part of a bigger picture, the "whole." For years we ignored the rest of the system as we comfortably rested on its pinnacle. Now it is our turn to be part of the action. If we don't understand our place at the table, we will not be part of its deliberations.

I am not a prophet. I cannot predict what medical practice will look like in the future. It is the unknown quality of change that is the essence of evolution, the "image." The very purpose of negotiation is to incorporate and balance the many facets of change. What emerges from this process will not be any one purview. Rather, future medicine will be the creative product of the interplay itself.

To formulate that picture, we negotiate. We can no longer assume the preeminence of our interests alone. Rather, we play as one of many parties. Interest-based negotiation is the fitting way to frame this process, as it opens the door to mutual understanding, activity, and gain. It searches for compatibility. Conflict resolution, after all, is about turning incongruity into congruity: whole image negotiation serves the task and the time.

I often refer to health care as a Rubik's cube. There are many sides, colors, and twists and turns that describe the action. When you change one side, the move affects the alignment of the others.

This intricate cube is now changing. To be a part of the action, we must understand, articulate, and negotiate the intricate balance between the functional and relational aspects of our practice. Along with the rest of the system, we physicians need to engage in the evolution of a picture that functions well: one that has a place for those willing to be a part of the process.

♦ ♦ ♦ ♦ ♦ ♦ ♦

The conversation in the physician's lounge revolves in waves as new people come and go, different combinations gather, and topics flow from one to another. Someone walks in to make a call, grab a cup of coffee, take a snooze or just relax for a few minutes on the inviting chairs and couches. Every so often, a particular issue lingers in the room, moving from one group to the next. The Cummings affair quickly became one of those lingering topics. Four animated male physicians were alone in the corner debating the matter.

"Cummings got screwed." Dr. Steve Schilling, a second-year resident, was making the point while waving a half-eaten apple in the air. "What did he do? Look at some nurse's boobs? I mean, this place would turn into a convent if they knocked a guy every time he checked out the territory. Give me a break."

Another second-year resident, Dr. Cliff Clemens, chimed in his agreement. "The screwy thing is that they let it get so out of hand. They are talking about disciplining him. What the hell?"

Uncomfortable with the conversation, Dr. Charlie Collins watched the two of them and wondered if it was worth violating the macho code. Suggesting that maybe there may be a different view of the incident would definitely offend the dictums of male bonding. On the other hand, he couldn't live with himself if he didn't say something. "I disagree. I think Cummings deserves to be called on the carpet."

"Called on the carpet?" Schilling asked quizzically, as if he assumed Collins was joking. "You think Cummings should be penalized?" He was incredulous. "Pray tell, what did he do that any of us wouldn't? He touched her shoulders and arms. He maybe glanced at her breasts. You call that sexual harassment?"

"That wasn't the whole of the problem, and you know it, Schilling. The problem was that he was pushing morphine incorrectly for a patient and was trying to seduce her into going his way. I've seen Cummings operate before. It's his character. He was bound to eventually cross the line, and that nurse simply called him on it."

Ken Kavanaugh, chief of the ICU, occupied the fourth side of the box of couches. Kavanaugh likes to come into the lounge periodically, even though he has his own office, just to get a pace on the place. As the oldest of the foursome, Kavanaugh decided to listen before he chimed in. "Collins is right. What Cummings did was wrong. First, he crossed the line with Heather Harriford. Every woman sets her own line, and even if what he did is OK with one woman, it doesn't mean it's OK with another. Heather was doing her job, and coming on to her was wrong, no doubt about it." Kavanaugh paused to draw a distinction between his points. "The other thing, about the medication. He should have been more careful, and Heather was saving his ass. He was too proud to admit it, so he tried to change the topic by playing Mr. Tough. I'm sorry if this is not cool. There is social touching and there is sexual touching, and from what I heard of what went on, he pushed beyond mere friendly touching. I'm not saying that they take away his license. They should do something, though."

As the senior physician in the group, Kavanaugh carried a lot of weight. Schilling couldn't drop the topic, though. "OK, Ken, so where do *we* draw the line? What about the whole role of physicians here? If everyone is going around second-guessing doctors, then what's our use? I think we have to set an example with Chuck. If we are soft on this one, every nurse in this hospital is going to be filing a report every time we check out what's written on her T-shirt or complement her on nice earrings."

Clemens jumped in to support his friend. "It's not only harassment. We have to draw the line on nursing, Ken." Cliff was hoping to appeal to a common denominator and turn Kavanaugh around. "Everybody is trying to take a chunk out of medical practice, and I don't think we should give in. If we don't stick together, then they've got divide and conquer on us. We have to think about that, too."

Kavanaugh couldn't believe what he was hearing. He thought these young guys would be more aware. He decided to play the mentor role: he couldn't help it. "First off, women have a right to send a message and have it respected. That goes no matter where they are: in the hospital, on a date, or in public. Heather stepped away from him. That was his cue, and he ignored it. If the cue is clear and you ignore it, you're on thin ice and you open yourself up to legitimate accusation. Second, I think it's great for people to meet here and get together. Great. Just don't do it on company time, and don't mix it up with doing your job. Meet after your shift, go out, do whatever you want. Just don't mix your come-ons with your responsibilities. Finally, Heather was giving Chuck a clear message about a mistake he was about to make. Never, ever ignore a warning sign if someone is flashing it for you. It could be a nurse, a patient, a family member, or a colleague. That warning could save your life, to say nothing of your patient's life. Don't let your ego take control so that you feel some macho compulsion to ignore the warning. Check out what's being said, why, what you may have missed. Only after you are completely sure do you go ahead. It's like those warning lights on airplanes. The pilot doesn't ignore the light, even if it's only a problem with a broken bulb." Kavanaugh stopped to take a breath and suddenly heard someone behind him clapping. He turned around to find Dr. Beatrice Benson beaming.

"Good job, Ken. I liked it." She was smiling. Ken blushed.

"We were just debating this whole Cummings thing," Kavanaugh explained, somewhat embarrassed now about his passionate speech.

Beatrice plopped herself down next to Kavanaugh. "What's to debate? The guy's a jerk."

"Well, there's not a unanimous vote for that sentiment." Collins gestured to Schilling and Clemens.

Benson turned to them. "What?"

Schilling opened up somewhat cautiously. "I just don't think the guy should be fried. I think everybody is making too big a thing about what Chuck did. That's all."

Benson turned to Kavanaugh and gestured to the others. "Where were these guys when the women's movement was born?"

Clemens felt the steam blowing out of their argument. Nonetheless, he couldn't stand not defending himself. "I think it's unfair holding doctors to a different standard than everybody else. What Cummings did was not that terrible."

Kavanaugh lifted up out of his chair to make the point. "There, you've got it, Clemens. But you're wrong. It *is* fair to hold doctors to another standard. We are involved in the most intimate aspects of our patients' lives and bodies and emotions. That is a trust that society places in us. That is something you take with you everywhere you go, because now that you've got that M.D. behind your name, society always thinks of you as a doctor. Always, every minute. Yeah, that is a burden. And it's because you are carrying that burden that society is willing to pay you a decent salary and give you an extra measure of respect. Cummings is learning that lesson the hard way. Do yourself a favor, pick up the advice before you find yourself walking in his shoes."

With that someone noticed the clock, and everyone realized that they had to run off someplace else. Benson patted Kavanaugh on the back and glanced him a smile as he got up from the couch.

♦ ♦ ♦ ♦ ♦ ♦ ♦

Part IV

. . . .

Creating and Resolving Conflict

Part IV

Creating and Resolving Conflict

• •

11

Positional Bargaining

To this point we have raised whole image negotiation—collaborative problem solving, interest-based interaction, and integrative bargaining—as the preferred mode for reaching decisions and taking action. This method adapts best to the close, personal work that typifies health care. By enhancing constructive exchange, whole image negotiation synthesizes common purpose and generates opportunities for inventive outcomes.

Nonetheless, there are situations when aboveboard, interest-based negotiation is not your best strategy. The intent of this chapter is to help you identify those instances: what are the cues that alert you to the need for positional tactics? Once you have made the choice, what methods and maneuvers can improve your chances of success and reduce the risks of retribution? And how can you incorporate the wisdom of the negotiation chameleon, crafting a balance of interest-based and positional techniques to maximize your objectives?

This chapter comes with a cautionary note. In a training session, when we reach the section on positional bargaining, the mood of the room turns. There are some who rub the palms of their hands back and forth and mutter, "OK, now to the good stuff—this is how to *really* win." For others, the topic brings up negative associations: it reminds them of times when positional tactics were used on them, and they really *lost*. Others shy away, afraid of engaging in potentially contentious negotiation and concerned that their inadequacies in this area render them "negotiationally challenged."

Conflict and its negotiation is in effect a synthesis of heart, head, and gut. It involves a combination of emotion, intellect, and instinct.

Emotions and passions run high as people are compelled to confront difficult choices and consequences: it is the reality of these choices that sweeps them into the process or that drives them away from its commitments.

The intellect encourages the parties to conduct the transaction in a reasonable and civil manner, just as it can constrain them to distort and pigeonhole the problems into meaningless categories. Understanding can easily slip into intellectualizing.

Instinct refers to the innate impulse that can arouse a negotiation. Sometimes it is a defensiveness that drives the parties to self-protection. At other times, it is an affinity that compels them into compassion.

What combination of impulses guides our negotiations?

Adversarial methods derive from our instinctual drive for self-protection. Fearing our own demise, we ensure our survival by overcoming our enemies, real and perceived. Control becomes a matter of defense. In a physically violent situation, we protect our bodies. In a professionally dangerous circumstance, we guard our career. And in a personal predicament, we preserve our self-respect. Fearing brutality and defeat, whether physical, professional, or personal, we alleviate our anxiety by outdoing the destructiveness of the other side.

When parties believe their survival is at risk, they are likely to behave positionally. At times, there is an inclination to view even small matters as a gauge of survivability: "If we give on this issue, who knows what will hit us next!" That temperament is a reflection of professional insecurity. Such jeopardy has been exacerbated in recent years by health reform efforts. In reality, the increasingly competitive health care environment has spawned professional as well as organizational winners and losers. In such an environment, the question "How can I win?" assumes a vital importance for people who want to ensure their professional future. In fact, the true winners are learning that the best way to ensure their survival is by finding new ways to collaborate.

Unravelling Positional Bargaining

We humans invest great energy in cloaking our animal instincts into higher-order activities. I need to eat just as does my dog, though she doesn't adorn the activity with silverware, napkins, and classical music. Her romping in the park—pushing, biting, and chasing other dogs—resembles many health care organizations, though the dogs do not glamorize their activity as a struggle for professional dignity, "serving the patients," or departmental integrity.

To bring positional negotiation into its appropriate balance, you must see it for what it is. These defensive and offensive urges are many times real and warranted. To misjudge them, however, could be fatal. If you persist with interest-based negotiation when others irretrievably seek your professional ruin, you indeed will be destroyed. Likewise, when the other side holds out a hand and you perceive a fist, you not only erase their good intentions, you become self-destructive in the process. It is a matter of knowing yourself, understanding others, and then cleverly choosing from a set of viable options. The better your understanding and the wider your options, the greater are your chances of achieving satisfying outcomes from your negotiation.

When you are negotiating with reason and compassion and the other side is negotiating for conquest and control, you have two choices. First, you can try to move them toward your frame: appeal to their head and heart by reframing the problem into an interest-based negotiation. Emphasize your overlapping objectives, common purpose, and mutual desire to avoid negative consequences. By hearing as well as responding to their innate fears, you begin their move beyond those apprehensions. However, when you are convinced that appealing to their reason and compassion cannot work, then put your own guard into gear. Be clear about your objectives, the tactics likely to succeed, and the methods you will use to maintain self-control throughout the process.

As you read this chapter, the tone and tactics of contentious bargaining may ring familiar. So too should its costs and consequences. This chapter is not an endorsement of positional bargaining. Rather, it is a dose of reality. When adversarial negotiation defines the culture of your workplace, then the building itself feels more akin to the wilds of an untamed jungle than a place to attain the higher purposes of health care. You learn to judiciously play the game before you can change it.

Choosing a Positional Approach

There are three sides to the choice for positional bargaining: what you want, what they do, and your appraisal of the exchange. The key for you is relationship. As you assess the other side, the gauge is tactics. And the back-and-forth between you defines the exchange.

Plan your strategy to best accomplish your objectives. When the parties are part of a shared "whole," then a strategy that offers "gain-gain" potential works best. When the parties are unalterable adversaries, the only course is between a win or a lose. You want to expand your chances for the win that is clean: one that optimizes your objectives as it softens any harm to your own standing. What cues help you make your choice?

Positional Relationships

One of my colleagues aspires to an epitaph that reads "He left the world a better place." He is not a rocket scientist, brain surgeon, or philosopher; by his own description, he is just an ordinary person. Making the world a better place is something he works on every day: when he talks with the ticket agent at an airport, when he sees a patient in his clinic, and when he interacts with professional colleagues. "Relationship" for him is not just the long-standing personal connections he has with people he knows well. Even if for just a moment, relationship is that link with others for which he continually strives. He is ready to admit a selfish motive: "I figure that one day I'll help someone, they'll help someone else, and finally, maybe weeks later, it will come back to me."

In health service organizations, these sort of short yet intimate encounters are the norm. Patients enter a clinic sick and vulnerable, expose their symptoms and their bodies, and hopefully feel better on the other side of their stay. For patients, relationship refers to the care and confidence that maintains their identity and respect through the process.

There are times when this relationship is not important for you. Perhaps the circumstances are urgent and allow little time to attend to others. Perhaps you are distracted or involved with something more important than interpersonal matters. Perhaps the value of the tangible transaction—money, space, or status—supersedes the importance of your association. What others think of you is less important than what you tangibly receive from the exchange. You assume there to be little or no utility for the relationship, and you bargain accordingly.

Likewise, the other side may signal you that the relationship is unimportant for them. This message is conveyed by what they say and don't say, the dirty tricks they play, and their ostensible obsession to win. They are little concerned about your regard for them. Intimidation, coercion, and impudence characterize their attitude. Negotiation becomes a game of domination. According to the rules of their game of conquest, the victor is entitled to harass the loser. The preferences of the loser are immaterial. After all, if you are truly defeated and no longer around, what you think is irrelevant. The tenor of these sorts of battles is more akin to children in a sandbox fighting over who gets the shovel than it is to professions engaged in responsible debate.

Negotiation is a two-way street, and the mode of interaction, implicitly and explicitly, is determined by both sides. Just as you can bring the horse to water, if the other side does not want a rapport, you can't make them drink a conducive relationship. If they are determinedly antagonistic, you might decide to carefully adopt parallel tactics so you are not devoured by the process.

♦ ♦ ♦ ♦ ♦ ♦ ♦

"Dumb-ass fool. I hope she gets what she deserves. We've been putting up with that crap for years, and we don't fall apart every time some doctor gives us a look." Cathy Crow seemed to be oblivious to what she was saying as she unscrewed the top of her coffee thermos. Her eyes followed the steam from the coffee as she poured it into her cup. She was tired and eager for the caffeine that would return her pep.

Pauline Patrick glanced to her side as she unwrapped her sandwich. Five nurses on the Seven West general medical floor were taking their dinner break and discussing the latest gossip in the Harriford-Cummings "affair," as it had ironically become known. Pauline had not signed on to the disgust some nurses felt for Heather. She could see something in both sides.

Sylvia Sheffield looked over to Cathy with a wry, experienced smile. Sylvia was nearly sixty years old and had watched all manner of hullabaloo about nursing come and go. She gave it all little concern. She knew what the job required and had little patience for all the haggling that went on. "Actually, I think Cummings is a good-looking young man," she said. "I wouldn't mind it if he made something over me." Sylvia garnered the glances and smiles from Cathy and Pauline that she had been hoping for.

Judy Johnson stared at the three of them at the far end of the table. She could not believe what she was hearing. She froze in rage. Finally it blurted out. "You disgust me. How could you say such a thing?" She spoke directly to Cathy. She had written off Sylvia's comment.

Cathy was quick, almost as if she were expecting—even prodding—Judy. "Well, look who's getting hot under the collar. What's the problem, Judy? Rejected because he didn't go for you?" Cathy's ridiculing agitated Judy no end.

Judy gritted her teeth. She spoke slowly and deliberately. "Cathy, don't you have any respect for us and for what we do? When Cummings violated Heather, he violated all of us, personally and professionally. If we don't stand behind her on this, then"—she paused, not certain how grandiose to make her next statement—"then we are compromising ourselves. Then what Cummings did to Heather is nothing compared to what we are doing to ourselves."

Cathy relished the fact that Judy was so bothered. "Oh, come on, Judy. What are we doing to ourselves? Get off your soap box. Cummings made a pass at Heather, and she misinterpreted it. If I made such a fuss every time that happened to me"—she mimicked Judy's pause—"why, I wouldn't get any nursing done."

Cathy's sarcasm pressed every one of Judy's buttons. She pointed her finger straight at Cathy. "You call what *you* do nursing? You have an attitude problem, Crow, and that's not what nursing is all about."

Cathy's demeanor turned angry in an instant. "You puny little thing. Don't you question my attitude about nursing. My mom was a nurse, and my sister is a nurse, and you don't make fun of nursing around me. All I'm saying is that Heather made a stupid move, and it makes us all look bad."

Debby Donnelly sat quietly through the whole conversation. She agreed with Judy, though she was afraid to say anything. There was a heavy silence in the air after Cathy spoke. It felt like it lasted a long time. She finally spoke. "I think you guys missed the point. If Heather feels she was violated, she *was* violated. And I don't think any woman should have to put up with that—I don't care if she is a nurse, or a doctor, or a housewife. And it's all the worse because Heather was doing what we do all the time. She was sending out a warning cue to a doctor who wasn't paying attention. And his fixation on Heather instead of the patient was going to cost that patient a lot of suffering, if not worse. That, to my mind, is the crux of the issue, and I think it should be respected as that. No more and no less."

Cathy and Judy were both feeling rage mixed with a measure of foolishness. Again there was silence. This was a sensitive topic, and the incident with Heather was a tough issue. There was a blending of what each felt was right and wrong about sexual harassment and doctor-nurse relations combined with their own personal feelings for Heather.

Sylvia was always the "smoother-over." It had always been her role in her family, and it was the role she played at work. She tried to change the mood. "Look, it's no matter in the long run. Heather will come back just the way she used to, the doctor will probably get his wrist slapped publicly while the guys slap his back when we're not around. This has been going on since before you were born, dearies." She sighed a measure of weathered experience. "Just used to be that we had more of a sense of humor about the whole thing."

Judy was outraged. She liked Sylvia and realized she was of a different generation. Nonetheless, she could not let that remark go unchallenged. "There is nothing funny about what happened to Heather, Sylvia. And there is nothing funny about what happens to other women, women who work in this hospital and women that are brought into this hospital on a stretcher. We have to start drawing the line, and I respect Heather for having the courage to do it. She deserves at least our support, if not a whole lot more."

Cathy lifted her hands and started clapping. The clapping lasted for an endless moment. Everyone was silent and tense. "So what do we do, start giving out medals? Great. Heather made a big deal about something that goes on all the time. And it's not wife beating. That's the problem, Judy. You've got the whole thing confused. You don't know what real wife beating is. If you cry wolf over everything, then when the real stuff hits, nobody's going to be paying attention."

Debby jumped in before Judy could respond. "Cathy, you're not hearing what Judy is saying. Are you suggesting that all this pushing around we have to put up with is a good thing?"

Cathy was quick. Her voice was tense, and she raised her hand to point at Debby. "No, I never said it was a good thing—" She stopped as she glanced toward Heather approaching the room.

Mrs. Hayward's condition had deteriorated further. Her family was gathered in the hushed room down the hall. They needed a great deal of care and attention. They were very distressed. They asked Heather often if their mother was experiencing pain. There was a lot of crying. Because they had established a good relationship with Heather, the family found a great deal of comfort in her presence. Heather sensed that and decided she couldn't leave, postponing her dinner break.

Heather walked into the nurse's lounge briskly. She was emotionally drained, though invigorated. The time she spent with Mrs. Hayward's family helped her forget everything else that was going on at work. She plopped her bag of sandwiches and drinks on the table. The room was silent, and no one made eye contact. Her mood switched to sarcastic. "Let me guess. You were discussing the weather. I know, all these warm days we've been having. Could it be global warming?"

Debby sometimes had a way of getting carried away with the obvious. She hated silence. "Actually, we were discussing this whole mess with you and Dr. Cummings. I think it's fair to say that there is a good deal of arguing going on about the whole thing."

"Let me guess. Cathy, you think I should have gone to bed with him." Heather knew exactly what she was doing with that comment. She and Cathy came from very different backgrounds. Heather had had a middle-class upbringing, finished her nursing training at a major university, and was applying for entry to an advanced-practice master's program. Cathy came from a working-class background, and even her community college degree was a first for her family. The animosity between them ran deep, and this incident with Dr. Cummings was just another hook on which to hang their feuding.

Cathy was quick. "What are you saying?" She did not wait for an answer. "Let me tell you one thing, cutie pie. I was around here long before you could spell 'hospital,' and I'll be here long after you get your next fancy degree. And I have to survive in this place. And survival is not about complaining every time some Tom, Dick, or Harry looks you over. What you are doing is helping no one but yourself. I don't know what the hell you're hoping to accomplish, but you can get off your high horse about doing something for the rest of us. You are nothing but a pain in the ass, and don't you forget it."

As tough as it was to hear Cathy out, Heather was ready for this onslaught. She knew it was coming. She stared Cathy down and didn't say a thing. Sylvia spoke through her stare. "Now, now—enough, the two of you. It's a shame that this is dividing us so." Sylvia paused, as if what she had said was as revealing to herself as it may have been to others. She continued. "Actually, it is all too bad that it is dividing us up." Her afterthought lingered in the air as she packed away the remainder of her dinner. "Well, it's back to the mines. I've got to get to work."

Cathy echoed Sylvia and noisily packed away her bag, shoving back her chair and noisily marching out of the room. Pauline followed, offering Heather a sympathetic look as she raced after Cathy.

Heather placed her yogurt on the table and looked over at Judy and Debby's sympathetic looks. "Now, doesn't this do wonders for an appetite," she said. She looked down at her meal and let her hands go limp as she gave up on eating. Judy and Debby stayed a few minutes to lend comfort and support before they also had to return to their patients.

Finally, they too left, stranding Heather in the room, feeling alone and defeated. "What good does integrity do you at a time like this?" she thought to herself.

♦ ♦ ♦ ♦ ♦ ♦ ♦

Positional Tactics

How do you know whether the other side is leaning toward positional or interest-based negotiation? The tactics they use offer the most revealing clues. Attention to their moves helps you plan your own. At some point, the time comes to invoke the reciprocal rule of negotiation: if you play dirty with me, then I'll play dirty with you.

The inventory of positional tactics, of course, is endless. Several categories are commonly seen in health care settings.

Misinformation

The most common ploy of positional bargaining is bad information. In the work of health care, nothing is more harmful than misinformation: falsehood, deception, fabrication, fraud, deceit, pretext, exaggeration, and unfounded rumor. Why?

Information is the currency of decision making. Whether it is a matter of finances, administration, personnel, or patient care, the scientific proclivity of health care craves logical conclusion. Distortions foster a precarious atmosphere for clinical and managerial work. Misinformation detracts from both process and product: like a virus, bad information takes on a life of its own. Those trapped in the cycle of misinformation justify their misjudgments by defending their information. Soon, fantasy turns into fact as organizational myth is born and cultivated.

When you are convinced that rumors and innuendo about you are intentional and not the result of miscommunication or mistake, you are faced with a situation that warrants decisive action. By tolerating deception, you implicitly concede to it. This is your cue to adopt a more positional strategy.

Why would someone propagate misinformation? It is usually due to a combination of character and purpose. For some, such deceit is a tactic of fair play. Perhaps it was used on them by parents, supervisors, or colleagues, and by virtue of this experience it has become acceptable for them to use on others. It is their customary practice.

How else could duplicity be justified? For some, commitment to a higher purpose sanctions conduct that itself is disdainful: the ends justify the means. Misdeeds are cloaked in the sanctity of the cause, and the harm inflicted upon victims is rationalized as just punishment for their obstructions. Though venal in nature, this breed of arrogance is not uncommon in health care, given the vital importance of the work. The challenge is to avoid stooping to this level while somehow toppling it.

"Gotchya"

The gotchya game is one of the most insidious of the signals warning you to shift into positional gear. How is the game played? Your overall record is exemplary. When weighed against your accomplishments, your mistakes are insignificant. You notice your reputation dissolve as minor missteps are converted into major problems. When you commit a legitimate though trivial error, you hear a loud "Gotchya" resound from your opponent. Every slip becomes an explosive complication, and you feel like you are walking through a minefield of humiliation.

What is happening? Your antagonists are building an illusory case against you. The specific points are vacuous. The issues themselves are petty. The real problem is not the poorly completed travel report, the miscommunication with a secretary, or the file that was temporarily misplaced. The real message is that they are out to undermine you by documenting your every mistake. Your challenge is to understand their motives and methods and then mount your own campaign to put your purpose back into perspective.

Achieving that perspective is no easy matter. Your vulnerabilities and insecurities have been revealed. You feel in jeopardy. The very pettiness of the affair is insulting in and of itself. If you permit yourself to believe that the poorly written travel report is evidence of your incompetence as a clinician, that the unhappy secretary reveals your inadequacy as a manager, or that the misplaced file displays your ineptitude as a planner, then you are in real trouble. You have fallen into the gotchya trap. That is their ruse. You begin doubting yourself. You become frustrated.

Your challenge is to distinguish the allegations from the message. The greatest danger is your own self-doubt. If you merely respond to the allegations, you become caught in their very trivial pursuit.

What should you do? Recognize the game, document the insignificance of their allegations, and then mount your own campaign. And remember, you must be doing pretty well if they have to plunge so low to assail you.

Other Toxic Tactics

The list of troublesome tactics is endless. You may find blackmail, extortion, threats, and coercion at your professional door. Even more painful than the hostility aimed directly at you is the cross fire directed at others with whom you work: colleagues, associates, and employees who are harassed simply because of their allegiance to you. Everyone around you has taken sides. Your work becomes embroiled in conflict tangential to your principal purposes. When those principal purposes begin to take a backseat to the conflict at hand, it is time to mount decisive action.

Mere acquiescence is neither preferable nor prudent. There is too much at stake, and you know that you are unwilling to bear the humiliation and the tangible losses of a positional defeat. You also know that you want to avoid tumbling to the level of your opponents. To do so would put you at even greater risk. Both professionally and personally, there is one attribute you best be unwilling to sacrifice at any cost: your integrity. Why?

The cornerstone of negotiation is trust, that intangible trait not to be bought, borrowed, or manufactured. It is a quality that you carry into every negotiation, be it interest-based or positional. Should you employ toxic tactics yourself, you will demean your stature in the eyes of those at the table as well as in the minds of others who are watching. Your opponents can take much from you: they can even score some victories. The one distinction they can't seize is your integrity. Your best chance of rebounding, whether from victory or defeat, is by safeguarding the foundation of your future negotiations: your integrity and the trust people have in you.

The positional game itself is not particularly difficult to pick up. We each carry preprogrammed, instinctual instructions that guide us to some pretty nasty tactics (and as a male, I acknowledge that my half of the species seems to have acquired a particular abundance of these genes, though certainly not a monopoly). In fact, the real challenge of the positional game is playing as a contender while maintaining your professional credibility. That quandary is the focus of the next section: How do you prepare yourself? What is your strategy? How can you ensure that you will achieve a clean win?

Preparing for Positional Negotiation

You have already made the most important decision of positional negotiation: you have decided to use it. Let us assume your choice to be a wise one.

As with any form of negotiation, you are always preparing. You prepare for the first round. When the first round is over, you prepare for the next. Preparation requires you to collect and mobilize three essential ingredients: information, options, and choices. At each point in the process, what you acquire accumulates, and what you deduce fluctuates.

Information

You want to know whatever you can about the other side. What is their strategy, and how might you outmaneuver it? What have they done in the past, and might their patterns be repeated? What motivates them, and can you appeal to those incentives? Where are their alliances, and how strong are they? What are their sources of power and influence, and can you muster enough strength to prevail? What are their options, and which are they likely to choose? The more you know, the more extensive your options and the more judicious your choices.

How do you acquire this information? There are the usual sources: documents, colleagues, and others who are familiar with your opponents. It is a matter of tracking them down, asking the right questions, and accurately assembling and interpreting what you have learned. These third-party sources do offer useful data. Oddly enough, though, I have found that with a bit of clever enticement, the most valuable disclosures come from the other side itself.

It is astounding what people are willing to reveal about themselves, either overtly or indirectly. Every meeting with the other side offers opportunities to collect such information. For example, at the opening of a discussion, I must decide whether to speak first or second. When involved in an interest-based negotiation, I usually prefer to speak early in order to set or reinforce the tone of the exchange. However, when I am involved in a positional negotiation, I choose to go second. I am more interested in what the other side has to say than in divulging my own strategy. People hate silence and are all too willing to blurt into the void with an unrehearsed remark. Catching them off guard, learning their concerns, and allowing them to make statements they will later regret not only gives me information, it also makes them feel more vulnerable.

To assess what they are divulging, I listen to more than just their literal words. My focus is on what they mean: their intentions. This message is reflected through body language. It is communicated just as much by what they don't say as it is by what they do say. Their tone and intonations reveal much about what lies inside.

And what do I do with this information? I let it sift through both my intellect and my intuition. I know that learning about someone else requires me to know a lot about myself. What and whom can I trust? What is real and what is a ruse? What distortions do my own filters create? This combined information and insight helps me craft my options.

Options

Chapter Five highlighted the utility of generating a wide range of options from which to cultivate negotiated solutions. Option building is an essential exercise in all negotiation, though there are marked differences between interest-based and positional negotiation. In the former, option building is a collaborative endeavor. As the parties develop options and find mutually compatible solutions, they learn about one another, share needs, and voice concerns, all while building a constructive relationship. The outcome meets the tangible, short-term objectives as well as the long-term, integrative purposes of the parties: they reap immediate gains in the current negotiation and they anticipate continued fruitful exchange.

By contrast, in positional negotiation option building is not a mutual effort: it is a private matter. You do it on your own or with your own constituency. Your purpose is to construct a list of viable possibilities and preferences. While you might feign joint option building as a ruse, you are really developing your own roster of options to meet your own needs, objectives, and concerns. To strengthen your position, some of your options you will reveal, others you will exaggerate, and some you will conceal. Certainly you are calculating in your disclosures, being careful not to weaken your stance. For example, in a job dispute you might broach your willingness to break with the organization because you have other offers, without indicating the source of those offers or your distaste for most. You hide what will weaken your position; you reveal what will strengthen it.

Another significant distinction between interest-based and positional option building is the mine fields you find in the latter. Your options in an interest-based negotiation usually range from fair to good to fabulous: "Just imagine what the synergy of our combined efforts could accomplish!" By its very nature, interest-based negotiation tends to be hopeful and optimistic. On the other hand, positional bargaining has a dangerous edge which must be calculated into the assessment of your options. It is a win-lose game, and you must appreciate the likelihood and consequences of a loss. If you lose, you could end up forfeiting your job, reputation, money, or whatever else might be on the line. To ignore the real potential for losing not only limits your strategy, it could also be the source of your defeat: "I never really considered the possibility that I wasn't going to win." It is that confidence that keeps you fighting, and it is that fallacy that could distract you from gauging grave professional and personal setbacks.

In a positional negotiation, the wider your range of options—the more viable and realistic, the more pragmatic and strong they are—the greater are your prospects. Imagine yourself a mouse in a maze: the more routes to the cheese, the better are your chances of getting the prize; and the finer your reading of the traps, the better are your chances of avoiding and escaping them.

Choices

When you are at the juncture between preparing and doing, it is time to exercise your options and make your leap. How do you craft your preliminary choices?

Most important, you want to be clear with yourself about what it is you want to accomplish. This is the most vital yet difficult tenet of successful positional negotiation. Know and live your objectives. For many positional bargainers, the problem is a preoccupation with revenge. Rather than focusing on their manifest objectives, those caught in the revenge trap become obsessed with seeing the other side writhe in pain. They want to inflict upon their opponents as much if not more suffering than they have experienced themselves. Punishment is inflicted through professional renunciation, financial devastation, or outright personal ruin. This punishment not only provides personal satisfaction, it also vindicates and validates the rightness of the hangman's cause: "Ding dong, the witch is dead! Which old witch? The wicked witch!"

There are two problems. One, while you are dismantling the other side, you are distracted from your own objectives. When the mouse in the maze forgets the cheese, it is unlikely that he will get the prize. Your energies, thinking, and resources are uncontrollably diverted, and you lose your aim and momentum. If the other side is wise, they will pick up on your obsession and use it against you: "You see, he is not really interested in improving services. His campaign is no more than a personal vendetta in disguise." Second, you and those who watch you are left with a lingering doubt about whether the punishment fits the crime. Only the rare positional battle is fought in a court of law. Has justice truly been served by your sentence, and if not, how might its severity come back to haunt you? Your colleagues, concerned that they may be your next victim, might congratulate you on the outside, while inside they have lost respect for your professional judgement and balance. Revenge in professional circles is a high-cost proposition. Is that how you want to invest the limited resources of your war chest?

The distinction between objectives and revenge sets up a wrenching inner battle. It is the dilemma between reason and instinct. When your revengeful instinct is in control, you go for punishment. When your reason is in control, you are clear on your journey and destination. Your focus is on what you want to accomplish and how to make it happen. You build your strategy and make your choices accordingly.

Positional Strategy

Having placed your impulse for revenge into a contained box (allowing retaliation fantasies to run wild in the private dens of your imagination is a healthy way to satisfy these urges), you can turn to step one in developing your positional strategy: focus on what you want to accomplish. The more coherent your list of objectives, the more reasoned your choices, the more vigorous the support from your allies, and the more explicit your target, the better will be your chances of winning. Again, this is a win-lose game, and you want to do what you can to enhance your chances of winning.

Your professional negotiations will likely revolve around two types of concerns. The first involves exchanges of tangibles and intangibles: salary, space, and equipment as well as recognition and information. The second involves professional behavior and status: from career advancement and promotion to censure and accusations of wrongdoing.

Both exchange and behavior negotiation and conflict may call for you to employ a positional strategy. In each case, your task is to find and establish a standard measure, preferably one favorable to you. This standard allows you to compare your position against a commonly acceptable and reasonable gauge. Your game plan is to employ that standard to advocate your position. For example, in a contract fee negotiation, establish the usual range for professionals with your qualifications, and then demonstrate how your unique added value and experience justifies a higher amount.

There are three benchmarks to calibrate as you plan your positional strategy. Your target range is what you reasonably hope to accomplish. Your high range is the inflated stipulations you open with and are willing to concede in order to make the deal. And your low range defines the point at which you leave the negotiation to pursue other offensive or defensive alternatives.

The Target Range

Start with your target range. Consider that you want to sell your car for $2,000. You have researched the book value of the auto, the market demand for the vehicle, and the time of year: it is May, and students are looking for summer transportation. The amount you want is reasonable, and you are confident that you can find a buyer willing to pay the price.

As you formulate your target range, assess what is negotiable and what is not. Be clear on the scope of issues and their ramifications. Know that what you have staked out is achievable.

In American culture, cars are on the list of negotiable items. Each culture and organization has its own list of negotiable and nonnegotiable items. Spaghetti in a grocery store, salary in a government agency, emergency medical care in a hospital—all are nonnegotiable items in this country. Cashiers are not authorized to haggle over the price of groceries. Public agencies offer salaries established by a grading system, with little flexibility for individual circumstances. And it would be unethical to discuss billing during a life-and-death situation in a hospital. On the other hand, items such as cars, houses, and salaries in private organizations are permissible items to negotiate. Similarly, department budgets, office space, and institutional policies and procedures are legitimate negotiable items. You do not want to bargain or advocate for matters that are inalterably nonnegotiable, because it is a waste of time and effort and it makes you appear uninformed.

What distinguishes the negotiable from the nonnegotiable, the definitive from the disputable? An object or service without an absolute, recognized value is open for deal making, as is an issue without a conclusive, agreed-upon outcome. The purpose of bargaining is to establish an acceptable value or outcome. Placing an object into a category with a set of standard values—for example, the book value of cars—is the essence of negotiation. Likewise, the cost of medical services can be set on the basis of generally accepted community billing rates. And a public health issue can be debated based on the experience of successfully or unsuccessfully addressing it elsewhere. The question is whether the standard value or agreed-upon outcome is convincing or applicable. Do car buyers endorse the recommendation of book value, or are they perceived as tilted in favor of sellers? Are community billing rates seen as reasonable, or are they seen as inflated by providers? And is the public health experience elsewhere comparable to the conditions seen locally?

Similarly, when you have been accused of a personal or professional transgression, what standard is used to determine whether you have committed the offense? What is the accusation, and by what standard is your act considered wrongful? Is there valid evidence against you, and does it prove your culpability? Is there a congruence between the accusation of negligence, liability, or mismanagement and the acts committed? Furthermore, were there mitigating circumstances that must be taken into account as the charges are assessed? How will the problem be judged, and what are the implications for all involved?

The distinction between what is and is not negotiable likewise applies to questions of professional behavior. Sexual misconduct, gross financial embezzlement, and actions intentionally harmful to patients each call for disciplinary action against the offender: the question is only what that action will be. Continued patient contact is likely out of the question. However, minor infractions taken as major offenses can also fall within the purview of positional negotiation. You must clarify that a simple miscommunication, misunderstanding, or miscalculation does not belong in that category of condemnable violations.

While the courts may subscribe to the precept "innocent until proven guilty," in the councils of professional practice, such equanimity is rare. Once branded by the arbiters of public opinion and gossip, your sentence will have devastating implications for your career. Just as you must establish your target range for a car sale, you must be deliberate about what you hope to accomplish in response to a professional vendetta. What is your win?

Likewise, if you are advocating for professional promotion, a salary increase, or other advancement, what is the basis of your position? What standards have you chosen to gauge your requests: are they reasonable and recognized? Do others value your accomplishments as much as you do? What tangible benefits have you delivered, and how might your continued success benefit the organization?

Whether a purchase and sale, a professional dispute, or an organizational negotiation, test your target range on the scale of reasonableness. If your target range is not tenable, you set your own trap of greed, disappointment, and miscalculation, invoking your own defeat before you even begin the fight. Assess the necessary considerations and take aim for an objective that is both feasible and satisfying. Your objectives should be clever, resourceful, and street-smart: one win can lead to your next victory.

The High Range

Your target range is private: you keep it to yourself or share it only with trusted compatriots. Your high range, however, is public. It is what you say you want in your opening bid. Incorporated into this initial proposition is room to move, a cushion. Why and how do you create this latitude?

Positional negotiation is a game. Unlike organized sports, in which explicit rules determine winner and loser, in positional negotiation you determine your own criteria for winning. Thus it is possible for the other side to think you have lost when you know that you have won. How can this be?

Between your target range and your opening bid, you place a set of requests that you would love to have and which you are willing to concede. In the give-and-get of negotiation, you give up what you did not care about getting in the first place. In the face of your "concessions," the other side is motivated to come to an agreement. With this ruse, the other side may feel that you caved in, when in fact you got everything you wanted.

There is an art to setting your high range. If it is too high you will appear unreasonable, and the other side will score points against you. For example, if I advertise my $2,000 car for $4,000, I leave plenty of room to move down; the problem, of course, is that the people who come to view the car will be in the market for a car of much higher value than my junk heap. They want a car worth about $4,000 to $5,000 in caliber and quality. I will have attracted the wrong buyers, and my advertising investment and time will have been for naught. No concession on the price will convince these buyers to purchase my car. Similarly, if you are negotiating for building space to house your department, insisting upon a whole floor when you are likely to get little more than a wing makes you appear unreasonable and ridiculous. Your request will appear outrageous, and your competitors will flamboyantly tout the folly of your miscalculation. And finally, if you claim zero responsibility for a professional misdeed in which you did have some culpability, you set yourself up to have the book thrown at you. If your opening bid is beyond reason, you sacrifice your credibility and give the other side command of the shots—not a desirable situation.

On the other hand, if your opening bid is too close to your target range, you afford yourself little room to move and meager leverage. Even if the other side receives a generous bargain, they will feel cheated if they anticipate some concessions and you offer none. This is the enigma of the interest-based negotiator who does not comprehend the game: the other side always wants to think they got a good deal. It is the logic of retail salesmanship: inflate the original price, and then give the consumer the satisfaction of a 25 percent "reduction." If the same slacks have the identical price in two different stores, the consumer is more likely to buy the pants marked with a discount. Furthermore, if your opening bid is too close to your target range, the concessions you are forced to give may take you below what you hoped to achieve. You needlessly negotiate from a deficit position.

Someplace between too high and too low is the right spot for your opening bid. How do you set it? Short of common sense, there is no universal rule of thumb. Much of the calculation relies upon context, such as the generally accepted and unwritten rules of the organizational culture in which you work. At budget time, it might be generally known that in anticipation of a cut, everyone inflates their proposal by 10 percent. It is part of the ritual of the apportionment process. To request only the budget you really need will leave you with a shortfall. To request 30 percent over your target makes you appear greedy and may raise questions about your managerial competence.

The difference between the good negotiator and the conqueror is that the latter wants it all. He is not willing to concede anything. That stance tends to drag the negotiation process out endlessly. It is the difference between the win, which you can achieve through negotiation, and the conquest, which might sow the seeds of your own defeat.

Choosing the right opening bid is a matter of strategy. And who knows? Perhaps savvy and luck, resourcefully combined, will yield you some of the surplus.

The Low Range

On one end, you calculate an opening bid that gives you room to move. On the other end, you establish a point beyond which you are unwilling to concede: your low range. In the case of the auto, for example, the low range is the price below which you are unwilling to sell. If your target is $2,000 and your opening price is $2,500, you might set $1,500 as your bottom price. You presume there must be someone out there willing to spend at least that much for the car. If your first customer offers not a penny over $1,200, you decline the offer, confident that someone else will bring a better price. In health care negotiations, the low range could be defined by staff working conditions, patient care decisions, or service reimbursement rates beyond which you are unwilling to concede. For example, you might be unwilling to accept more than six patients to one nurse in your hospital unit, unwilling to allow restraints imposed upon nursing home patients who are usually competent, or unwilling to accept rates of reimbursement that are below your real cost of providing care.

Your low range defines what Fisher, Ury, and Patton (1991) describe as your BATNA, the "best alternative to a negotiated agreement." Your BATNA determines the point at which you walk from the negotiation table. Given the meager and unacceptable offers proposed by the other side, the better alternative may be resignation, a strike, going to the press, or a lawsuit. Exercising your BATNA means disengaging, at least for the time being, from constructive, solution-oriented discussion. Your BATNA could be passive: you simply leave the scene. If you are a valued staff member or colleague, your departure inflicts a high personal and professional price upon the other side. Ideally when you invoke your BATNA you have a better option than sticking around for the punishment, such as a terrific or at least acceptable job elsewhere. Your BATNA could be aggressive: you seek the total destruction or partial impairment of the other side. In the case of international conflict, for example, the better alternative could be an armed invasion if the other side is unwilling to accept specified bottom-line concessions.

There are two important reasons for appraising your bottom line and setting your low range early in the process. First, you do not want to remain at the table when the other side has transgressed into what you consider professionally, morally, or pragmatically repugnant tactics or demands. Many negotiators stay too long, hoping they can somehow convince the other side to change their position. Wake up! Their position is clear: you just don't get it! For you to endure conditions that the other side knows you find unacceptable is a strategic mistake. You weaken your own position when the other side finds you are willing to graciously suffer their taunts. You will have issued an invitation for punishment, and if the other side is evil enough, they will have a good time with you. When you stake out your bottom line before you get there, you are less likely to get snagged in the spiral of an escalating assault.

Second, by anticipating your low range, you strategically are best able to cope with the pressures of bargaining. Some negotiators panic at the mere thought of making a concession, even a minor one. In their mind, it is a sign of weakness to give up anything, no matter how paltry. Because they have not clarified for themselves what is important and what is not, they are more likely to get trigger-happy and immediately reach for their BATNA. They stomp out of the room before giving negotiation a fair try. This is a strategic mistake.

If you are altogether inflexible and immediately threaten to pull out your BATNA, you cue the other side into pushing your panic button. If you appear too desperate to leave, the other side might just call your bluff and then flaunt the rigidity and unreasonableness of your position. Leaving the table prematurely creates the impression that you are interested only in domination. It is not sportsmanlike. You render yourself too easy to dismiss.

As you contemplate your low range, you also discover your own bottom line of process preferences and substantive principles. Your process preferences constitute your own code of negotiation. There are some who are ready, with proper warning, to walk from the table when the time is right. There are others who, having given the other side proper warning, maintain that persistence at the negotiation table is the only way to settle differences. These people will continue collaborating, talking, or conceding, no matter the cost. They view walking, striking, attacking, or suing as a violation of their philosophy. They are opposed to exercising any BATNA. This unwillingness ultimately (and unfortunately) could impair their negotiation effectiveness. If the other side detects this attitude, they just might boost their goading, knowing that there is no limit to what they can pull off. By ruling out any BATNA, you weaken your negotiation effectiveness.

Your substantive principles refer to your own code of professional ethics. What are you unwilling to tolerate, and are you willing to pay the price for exercising your BATNA when faced with wrenching moral dilemmas, professional improprieties, or personal misbehavior? At what point are conditions so deplorable that you are willing to accept the financial uncertainty of unemployment, the professional risks of a public scandal, or the high costs of a court battle? Ample experience has proven that not every dispute can be resolved through negotiation. Where do you draw your line?

When it comes to identifying and exercising your negotiation BATNA, there are two primary types: the perseverers and the bolters. A perseverer might say, "If only we can improve our relationship, we could find a solution to this problem." There is a reluctance to declare a BATNA, no matter the cost. On the other hand, bolters might conclude, "I'll leave right now and show them that I can't be pushed around." There is an enthusiasm among bolters to jump at the BATNA, no matter the situation. Whatever your own tendency, combining self-awareness with strategic decision making improves the chances that you will neither stay too long nor leave too fast.

Remember, there are a range of options to consider as you plan your BATNA; time and energy devoted to planning those better alternatives is a worthy investment, if nothing else, for your sense of negotiation security. To do so requires both courage and creative thinking. Mahatma Gandhi, Martin Luther King, Jr., and other leaders have advocated nonviolence at times when followers were all too eager to adopt more destructive tactics. A work slowdown is less severe than a strike, as are a deluge of letters of support, a sympathetic news article, and a run to the board of directors. Whatever strategic method you choose, it is essential that you do not in the process lose your most important asset: the supporters and allies who legitimize the actions you are taking.

Balancing High, Low, and Target Ranges

How are these three strategic ranges used in practice? In positional bargaining, you open the bargaining by associating the item in question with a value that is slightly outside your desired end point. The car seller might point to the pristine appearance of the car to justify its slightly above-book-value price. The buyer might counter that the unusually high odometer reading in fact places it slightly below book value. As there is no absolute value for the used car, they go back and forth over the relative merit of appearance versus performance. Each emphasizes his own claim while privately considering the merits of the other's arguments: yes, the buyer lusts at the thought of driving that red convertible, top down, on a sunny day; and true, the seller reckons he did get a lot of use from this now well-worn vehicle. Whether they come to an agreement depends on whether, amid all the objective and subjective information, they can find a value that falls into the acceptable range for each. What tactics do they use to get there?

◆ ◆ ◆ ◆ ◆ ◆ ◆

Public opinion has a funny way of turning complex issues into simple dichotomies. That was the nightmare for the Community Health Plan (CHP). When news spread of their withdrawal from the Oppidania Medical Center (OMC) in favor of Urbania Medical Center (UMC), a well-intentioned effort to trim health

costs and save money for their subscribers turned sour. Rather
than being heralded for their bold leadership in curbing health
inflation, they were castigated for threatening the viability of a
venerable institution, and in the process cheating their customers
with bargain-basement health care. Newspaper editorials gave
the issue reasoned though critical consideration. Radio talk show
hosts were not as generous. And public opinion, being what it is,
greatly disfavored CHP and all associated with it, especially the
Urbania Medical Center.

UMC, caught in the cross fire, was cast, somewhat unfairly,
as the cheaper and clearly inferior alternative to the Oppidania
Medical Center. Though Urbania had never shared Oppidania's
stellar reputation, no one had ever before gone to the trouble of
pointing out UMC's mediocrity. Now it seemed that everyone in
town had their favorite Urbania slur story, which ranged from
major gaffes to everyday inefficiencies. And while Oppidania
may have suffered its own shortcomings, in the polarized, bad-
guys-versus-good-guys mood that had overcome the city, no one
was ripe to tell unfavorable stories about Oppidania (except, of
course, the people at CHP). There was no doubt that the antagonism had become vindictive when CHP released Oppidania's
price list, detailing exorbitant costs for everything from an
aspirin to a triple-bypass procedure.

The question at Oppidania was how to handle the situation,
both from a public relations perspective and from a strategic
perspective. The general consensus among the leadership was
that there was no need to enter the fray directly: everyone else
in town was doing it for them. OMC could take the high
ground, emphasizing their historic and continued commitment
to high-quality patient care and community service. There was a
growing consensus in town that while OMC may be slightly
more expensive, their life-giving accomplishments made their
costs worthwhile. Amid the controversy, the conventional wisdom was that people were willing and should be able to make
the choice for themselves and their families. Oppidania, in its
news releases on the matter, outlined aggressive measures it had

taken to reduce costs whenever possible, though never to the detriment of quality patient care.

While Oppidania kept a low profile during the controversy, the Arena Health Plan (AHP), CHP's major competitor, did not. Much to the chagrin of the OMC leadership, AHP launched an aggressive marketing campaign featuring full-page newspaper ads touting their continued commitment to high-quality care and patient choice. With upcoming open enrollment periods for a number of major employers, the insurer wanted to implant the impression that anyone who did not choose AHP was risking their health and cheating their family. The people at Oppidania, hoping to keep their options open, were afraid that the AHP strategy could backfire on them, just as the CHP strategy had inadvertently damaged Urbania.

After much discussion, Oppidania's executive leadership agreed that the best strategy was not to make calls about the matter to any of the key players. They had considered contacting Urbania to diminish any possible rifts between the two. It was decided that little good could emerge from such a conversation, and it might be interpreted as an apology when none was warranted. They likewise rejected the idea of asking Arena Health Plan to moderate its aggressive ad campaign. As long as their were no overt inaccuracies, it was not up to Oppidania to instruct a major client on how to manage their marketing campaign. And finally, they decided not to call CHP, as they already had the upper hand in any potential negotiations. It was CHP who had walked away, and it would have to be up to CHP to walk back. The senior staff recognized this as a risky strategy, as it offered only precarious control and limited maneuverability. On the other hand, it was one that kept the options open, even though the options themselves were not all that attractive. The decision was to wait, anxiously, and see.

For the next few days, the phone did not ring, and the attention of the media did not subside. The reports went from facts and figures to sappy human interest stories. Finally, newspaper editorials began to question why the health care community was allowing this mess to get so out of hand. The local health department commissioner, Manuel Mendez, said that it was really up to these private companies to settle the matter on their own. On the advice of the mayor's office he decided not to get involved, concluding that to do so at this point could lead into a political quagmire.

The telephone finally rang at Oppidania. It was Nathaniel Norquist, chief financial officer for CHP. He wanted to meet with Iris Inkwater. The meeting was arranged for the next day. Iris spent the afternoon with her senior staff, developing a strategy for the session. They concluded that it was in the best interest of the hospital to resume their relationship with CHP, and if they played it cool, they would probably end up with a favorable financial arrangement.

It was just Norquist and Inkwater; as usual, they met on neutral turf, the same restaurant that had seen so many of their lunchtime discussions. The customary opening niceties were tense and cold. Iris waited for Nathaniel to make the first move.

"Iris, what can I tell you? We took a beating over this deal with Urbania. We want to reconsider an arrangement with you."

"We are willing to consider what you have to offer." Iris tried to sound as noncommittal as possible.

"Iris, what we have to offer is very simple. We'll bring you on at the same rates we gave Urbania."

"We looked at those figures after our last round. They are fantasy numbers. We don't know how they are going to survive with those dollars. They have to be cutting their staff to dangerous levels. We're not willing to have our candy stripers perform nursing functions. The figures are impossible." Iris knew what she was doing. Norquist needed her now more than she needed him, on the one hand. On the other hand, she could not afford to lose this contract.

"Well, Iris, *that* is a fantasy. Urbania is not using candy stripers in the surgical suites. They did, however, cut where it is appropriate to cut. You know yourself that they are getting a bad rap in the papers. Don't let yourself get caught up in the propaganda." Norquist wanted to demean Iris's comment to divert this level of discussion. It did not work.

"I find that offensive, Nathaniel. We are talking dollars and cents here, and I have a commitment to keeping Oppidania viable as a high-quality institution. I am not willing to compromise on that quality." Iris wanted to paint Norquist into a corner. It did not work.

"So what will you get for it, Iris? An expensive funeral? Oppidania has simply been unwilling to go through the belt-tightening that everyone else in this country has accepted. That is the reason for this mess. We have our responsibilities as well, Iris."

The discussion was descending to finger-pointing. "Nathaniel, you will get nowhere personalizing this issue. You have created your own mess, and now you want me to bail you out. We are not willing to do that for you." Iris caught herself. What was she saying? The strategy was to play hard to get and then to ultimately play ball with CHP, since the hospital really did need the contract. She had allowed the conversation to turn into a divisive confrontation.

The echoes of their interchange punctuated the silence that followed. Norquist was beginning to panic. He had strict instructions to bring back a verbal agreement to continue discussions leading toward reinstating the contract. It had to be done quickly, before enrollees made their decisions about possibly switching plans during the upcoming open-enrollment period. He could not jeopardize the company's financial viability.

Norquist broke first. "Well, Iris, if you can't meet the Urbania numbers, what are you talking about?" Norquist knew he could be creating an impossible situation for himself. Urbania would protest being pressed financially if Oppidania got a better deal. This controversy had been too much in the open to hide anything. And since CHP had already negotiated several contracts with large employers, any increase in costs would hit the plan hard. He had little, if any, room to maneuver.

Iris came back slowly. She knew if she said 10 percent,

Norquist would balk. In reality she needed 5 percent. She decided to play the numbers a bit high to leave herself room to come down. "Seven and a half percent, Nathaniel. My numbers people said that the difference between your figures and what is scarcely livable for us is seven point five. If you want us, that is what you will have to pay."

Norquist was getting worried. "Iris, I will tell you point blank. That number will kill us." Actually, Norquist had some room to move. He wanted to panic Iris before giving in.

Iris knew he was calling her bluff. She was not going to be tricked. "Nathaniel, the numbers are not going to kill you. You've done it to yourself. You are making impossible promises. You've squeezed yourself in two directions. You got carried away with your own ability to control this market. It's not that simple, Nathaniel. No one did it to you but yourself."

Norquist was here for a negotiation, not a scolding. He resented Iris's lecturing, and he was overcome with a sudden urge to leave the table. He caught himself, and spoke slowly. "Iris, you need us much as we need you. If you are left with AHP alone in this town, they will squeeze you dead, and there will be no one left to bail you out."

"Squeeze us the way you are squeezing, Nathaniel? We are getting nowhere, my friend. I suggest you go back to your shop and think hard about what you are proposing to us. Begin to sound reasonable, and we will be willing to talk."

The meeting ended abruptly. Neither Iris nor Nathaniel walked home with what they had hoped to achieve.

The headline in the next day's morning newspaper summarized the predicament: "OMC and CHP suspend talks." The headline did not play well at OMC. Nor did it play well at CHP.

◆　◆　◆　◆　◆　◆　◆

Combining Tactics and Strategy

Negotiation is the art of persuasion. In the case of interest-based negotiation, the carrot of mutual benefit and the potential for future gain motivates both parties to make rational choices. In the case of positional negotiation, it is the stick of leverage that prods other parties toward the direction you desire. You pose a convincing argument by imposing your power, influence, and clout upon the other side's deliberations. Your positional tactics define how you do this.

Basic to the development of your positional tactics are perceptions. It is the perceptions you foster, embellish, and sway that convince the other side. Just as there is no absolute value for an item in a positional negotiation, there is also no absolute distinction between what is real and what is merely perceived. You may believe that you have great power within your organization. However, if the other side perceives you to be a weakling, then you have little power during your negotiation. Likewise, your real organizational influence may be marginal. However, if the other side believes you hold the key to their future success or failure, then your bargaining power is greatly enhanced.

The use of perception to fortify one's position is a common ploy of positional bargaining. In military conflicts, for example, an army magnifies the apparent size of its force; in legal disputes, one side exaggerates the size and legitimacy of its claim; and in professional negotiations, one party magnifies the consequences of a budget reduction. The key is not the actual size of the army, amount of the suit, or consequence of the cutback. The key is what the other side believes and what action they take as a result. Positional tactics are used to create the perceptions necessary to stimulate the hoped-for reaction from the other side.

This tenet of positional bargaining raises an awkward ethical question: do the ends always justify the means? The answer is no. It depends on the context. A tactic that is morally correct in one instance may be immoral in another. Having exhausted other avenues to address the problem, going to an investigative reporter with a story about patient abuse would be appropriate as you balance ends and means. To use the same tactic for an internal professional dispute would be improper. The responsible alignment of ends and means must be assessed for every negotiation. One can be a successful positional negotiator while remaining within the bounds of what is considered appropriate professional and personal conduct. The credo of the British diplomatic corps offers a guide: "Never lie, and never tell the whole truth."

How does one create the necessary perceptions and desired reactions in one's opponent? Following is a sampling of positional tactics to inspire your thinking. Again, use the reservoir of your imagination to construct a scheme appropriate to your situation.

Learn Their Strategy

International negotiation is marked by the intrigue of intelligence agencies which spy on the workings of their opponents. Apart from the romance associated with these operations, they illustrate a fundamental premise of positional bargaining. The more you know about the other side, the more effective your own strategy will be. What are their target, high, and low ranges? To maximize your gains, you want your opening bid to be as close to their low range as possible. What perceptions are they trying to manufacture, and how concerned should you be about them? You do not want to misread what could be a real threat. And how do they perceive the signals you are sending them? If they do not take you seriously, you may have to raise the stakes.

You only abet their cause if you violate the law or organizational policy to uncover their strategy. Nonetheless, there is a range of perfectly legal and proper ways to learn what the other side is thinking. Going out to lunch with the right people, tracing public memos, getting the inside scoop from trusted colleagues, reviewing your opponents' past behavior to predict future patterns—such tactics can provide useful information to help you discern what they are doing and to anticipate what they will do next.

The Boomerang Effect

Having assessed your opponents' strategy, you have the opportunity to get one step ahead of them. Once you know their options and choices, defeat them by gently closing those choices so that they are adversely painted into their own corner. If you learn that they are on their way to the director to blast you, get there first with your own version of the story. By the time they get to the boss to launch their offensive, the boss will have already set them on the defensive. If someone plans to embarrass you at a meeting with a malicious accusation, privately warn the other participants beforehand about the regrettable performance they are about to witness: your opponent will look like a fool. If another department is about to steal some of your office space, contract for customized renovations and then let them hold the bill. Like a bullfighter, you want to outsmart the opposition by fostering illusions to invoke their own collisions.

These calculated, proactive moves must be taken with great caution. If your opponent does not show up at the director's door, does not make the impassioned speech, or does not go for a territorial grab, you are left looking an even greater fool. Remember, they are playing the same game.

Diversionary Tactics

Imagine that you are confronted with two issues: issue A and issue B. Issue A is of vital importance to you. Issue B is of secondary importance. Upon which one do you focus initial public attention?

Many people respond "issue A—you fight for your priorities." In fact, the better choice is issue B. To achieve a win on matter A you formulate an inconsequential issue B. During your negotiation, you ostentatiously concede on that issue. You appear to be magnanimous. In return, and for what is a paltry price, you gain success on what is really important. Issue B is usually the increment that separates your target range from your high range. As you retreat from your initial proposition, you will create the perception of having made a compromise, though all along you have adhered to what is essential for you.

Say, for example, that your organization acquires a new office building. As space in the building is being apportioned, your concern is more for location than for square footage. You want to be close to other departments, to patients, and to amenities for your staff. The primary point of contention among the various departments is square footage: everyone argues that they have unique requirements and require a lot of space. You too sing these blues—and then offer a concession. You will accept a smaller space than you would prefer in exchange for a better location. If the administration is having headaches over excessive demands for space, your concession could win you points and the location you desire.

Create Leverage

There are issues about which the other side cares and those about which they do not. Focus on the former. What motivates them? What incentives would prompt them to shift? Once you understand what can induce them, create and demonstrate your capacity to influence those very outcomes. In so doing, you raise the stakes for not complying with your wishes. You have created real choices, with the potential for uncomfortable consequences. In the process, you have devised leverage: the power of persuasion.

For example, in the course of a budgetary dispute at a public hospital, you learn that a significant sum of money recently has been diverted into an unusually generous administrative line item. These funds have, in fact, been generated by your department and are necessary for the continuation of services to vulnerable populations. The bargaining has become positional. You know that the commissioner of the local public health agency, a relative neophyte, is particularly sensitive to bad publicity because of his tenuous political appointment. Your reputation is long-standing and solid. At some point during your negotiations, you gently comment on the interest which the mayor might have in this gross misappropriation of funds. Later in the conversation, while on a different topic, you let it drop that an advisor to the mayor, a close personal friend, is coming to your home for dinner. You have pinpointed one of the commissioner's primary anxieties, and you have demonstrated your capacity to influence that motivator. Chances are that your budget will be restored before the advisor arrives for dinner.

Sow Info Bits

There is an old army trick that might inspire some useful positional maneuvering on your part. Consider the dilemma of a small group of soldiers facing a full battalion on the other side of a wide valley. There is little hope that reinforcements will arrive before dawn. They want neither to surrender their position nor to fight the battle, which they would surely lose. What can they do?

Once darkness falls, they drive their few trucks quietly and without lights down from their position on the hill. At the bottom of the hill, the drivers turn the trucks around and illuminate their lights. They ascend the hill noisily, only to turn off their lights and drive back down once they get to the top. This continues and is watched by the other side all night. The opposing army, convinced that they now face a full legion, decides not to attack.

Whether you create a perception of power by walking through the corridors with someone of great stature, having your name appear frequently in the press, or touting your professional accomplishments, the impressions you create and employ will be carefully watched by the other side. What they do will be influenced greatly by what they perceive. Carefully orchestrating those perceptions to your advantage is a potent ploy of positional negotiation.

Reasonable Mischief

There are endless possibilities for making the other side uncomfortable. Cultivate fear by having others plant incendiary comments. Negate your opponents' actions by convincing others of the insignificance of what they are doing. Undermine them by appealing to superiors, subordinates, and colleagues. Foster the general impression that even associating with the other side casts someone in an unfavorable light. Surround them with tactics until they give in. If you must, undermine the very ground upon which they stand.

Threats and the Duel

The tactics listed above are devious by their very nature. Your aim is to manipulate the professional and personal habitat in which the other side functions: all that surrounds them turns hostile. The advantage of this strategy is that it is not you who carries the smoking gun. Altering perceptions with reasonable mischief is a sublime way to force the issue. The general consensus turns against the other side as their professional assets slip away.

At some point, however, these circuitous maneuvers may not be enough. You may have to mount your own scheme to destroy your opponents outright, by whatever means necessary.

The customary rules of warfare, be it military or professional, require fair warning before launching an attack. If the warning is taken seriously, you may be able to attain your objectives without engaging in the messy business of open conflict. In most cases, you are better off if you can win without going to battle.

Make your threat known to the other side: explicitly outline the choices and consequences they face. There are three necessary ingredients for an effective threat. First, your opponents must be convinced that you have the will to go through with your scheme. If not, they will call your bluff, hoping to make you appear the wimp. Second, they must be convinced that you have the means to implement your plot. If not, they will allow you to attack, confident that they will defeat you in battle. And third, when they do not conform to your demands, you must carry through with your threat. If not, they may try to stall or deplete you into defeat.

A successful threat affords you a win without encumbering the costs of a legal contest, the time required for a full conflagration, or the public scorn of a war. A threat, when successful, is less dangerous than exposing yourself to the perils of battle. And if your threat does not succeed and you must proceed to a duel, do what you must to win.

* * * * * * *

Dr. Ted Tuckerman had seen it all in his thirty years of internal medicine practice: the aches, the pains, the discomforts. He had a good reputation as a careful doctor, which he carefully guarded. The day that changed his practice happened slightly over one year ago.

Mrs. Betty Brown had been a patient of his for nearly ten years. A grocery store clerk, she seemed to live for her ailments. She was a complainer, and Dr. Tuckerman imagined that she spent her time with her friends recounting, in great detail, the minutiae of each of her visits with him. Nonetheless, Tuckerman grew a fondness for Mrs. Brown, who brought a poppy seed cake into the office every holiday.

It was three years ago when the trouble began, just after a very cold and inclement spell of winter. Mrs. Brown complained of dizziness and colds. She was enrolled in a managed care plan, which she had joined through the supermarket chain where she worked. It was a frugal plan, and they were particularly careful about limiting what they considered unnecessary tests and referrals. At the time, Tuckerman had assumed that her complaints were just another of her cold bouts. He encouraged Mrs. Brown to put them into perspective and not be too worried. He was reluctant to go through the hassle of sending her for another full workup for naught.

It was three months later, in the middle of May, when the complaints had not abated, that Tuckerman finally became concerned. Her condition had deteriorated, and she was having trouble breathing. She had never been a smoker, though on questioning, Tuckerman learned that her husband had been a pack-a-day smoker throughout their marriage.

The X rays came back with what Tuckerman had most dreaded. Mrs. Brown was suffering from a progressed case of lung cancer. At this point, even aggressive treatment would give her only a few more weeks. Against the wishes of her family, Mrs. Brown decided to forego chemotherapy. She returned to her home with hospice support and died two weeks later.

It was thirteen months until the letter arrived from the state board of medical registration. Mrs. Brown's daughter, Leslie Long, had filed a complaint against him with the board. The complaint alleged that because of his negligence, her mother had suffered a cruel death that could have been averted had he conducted tests earlier. Ms. Long had written the board a long letter detailing Mrs. Brown's medical history, her illness prior to the diagnosis, and her painful death. It described her centrality to the family and the deep loss they had experienced since her passing. There was nothing positive in the letter: it neglected to mention anything about the many years of exemplary care Dr. Tuckerman had given Mrs. Brown. It was a stinging attack. It ended with a plea for the board to remove his license to practice medicine. The family could not endure the possibility that someone else might have to suffer as had their mother.

For Tuckerman, the letter was a nightmare. He sat moribund in the office of his attorney, Larry Levine. Levine was matter-of-fact about the situation. He had successfully walked other physicians through similar problems many times.

"So, tell me everything you can about this Mrs. Brown," Levine asked. "Was she a whiner?"

Tuckerman spoke glumly. "She was difficult. Whenever she came in, she had an endless list of aches and pains for me. I listened patiently to each, though I couldn't take every one seriously: I would have spent her whole plan's yearly budget on senseless procedures. The trouble, of course, was that there was the danger that I would miss something. And as it turned out, I did. Nothing much more to it than that."

"Ted, Ted, you've got an attitude problem." Levine paused to consider what could bring Tuckerman to his senses. He got up from behind his massive mahogany desk to sit closer to his client. "I have a question for you, Dr. Tuckerman. Are you still planning to continue your practice of medicine?"

Tuckerman looked up as if Levine had just asked an absurd question. "What kind of a thing is that to say? Of course I want to continue my practice. That's what I hired you to guarantee me."

Larry smiled as if he had just won a small victory. "OK, Ted, I'll do that. But I'll need your help. You see, we're fighting a good-guys-versus-the-bad-guys battle here. Right now, you're the bad guy. We've got to turn you back into the good guy who made a reasonable miscalculation—if that—all in the name of good yet prudent medicine. Do you understand?"

Ted felt like a small boy who had just been reprimanded by a teacher. His reply was reluctant: "Yes, I understand."

The problem for Tuckerman was that in fact he did feel a bit like the bad guy. This incident had shattered his confidence and his faith in his own medical judgment. Just as Ms. Long's letter had neglected the many achievements of his career, so too did his own current perspective erase those achievements. He did feel guilty. Not guilty enough to abandon his career. He did feel guilty enough to believe that he had somehow contributed to Mrs. Brown's demise, or at least deprived her of a chance for prolonging her life.

On the other hand, he had another mix of feelings that too were part of the confusion. His wife, his kids in college, his mortgage, his career, his future. He certainly did not want to sacrifice all he had worked so hard to build. When he looked at this mess from that perspective, he reminded himself that in the overall scheme of things, this was a legitimate oversight. His wife reminded him of that too, as did the few close friends in whom he confided this catastrophe.

So here he sat in his attorney's office, preparing a reply to the board's request for a response to Leslie Long's complaint. He had brought a sequential description of the medical facts, the necessary records, and his own draft of a letter. Levine assured him that he would look over the file and prepare an appropriate retort for submission to the board.

As the meeting came to a close, Levine jumped up and confidently put out his hand to Tuckerman for a good-bye handshake.

"Remember, Ted, you are a great doctor. When we are done with this, I am certain that you'll be looking here at little more than a blip in your career, not its demise. You hear me?"

Tuckerman, staring at the ground, nodded glumly. "That was a pretty rough letter, Larry." He looked up at his attorney. "Yeah, Larry, I hear you."

Dr. Tuckerman's reply to the board outlined his actions and justifications. It asserted that over the years he had seen her, Mrs. Brown had been given excellent care. It concluded that lung cancer, a devastating and swift disease, would have claimed her even if it had been detected somewhat earlier. He expressed his regard for Ms. Long's mother and his own sense of loss upon her death.

As he signed, sealed, and sent off the letter, his fears grew. He had seen what had happened to friends. He knew that the competitive marketplace for doctors, being what it was, could turn this black mark on his record, as minor as it was, into a fatal flaw.

It was now just a matter of waiting.

* * * * * * *

What If You Can't Win?

There is a popular misconception that if you cannot score a win, you are doomed to enduring a loss. Among those who hold this view, a lamentable lack of imagination presumes that the opposite of triumph is defeat. Is there another option?

Of course! If you absolutely cannot win at the game you are playing, change the game. There are a number of ways to do this. One method is to start playing football while your opponents are still playing baseball. If the fans in the stands show up to see football, your opponents will look quite silly. Turn a losing budget battle into a race for public recognition and deposit the accolades into the bank for later withdrawal. Another method is simply to leave the field with your ball. If your opponents continue to compete even without the ball, they will appear to be motivated more by the fight than by the real issues at hand. If you are locked into a losing battle for control of your organization's overall operations, preserve your professional autonomy and demonstrate a greater interest in achievement than in domination. You can simply start playing on a different field altogether. If your opponents seek your defeat within the organization, find a better job elsewhere and convey your talents and resources to a more hospitable arena. Your departure and subsequent accomplishments in that more attractive setting will offer the other side little more than a hollow win. After all, theirs is not much of a win if you elude the game and find more rewarding endeavors.

Finally, if there is no way to salvage the situation, know when to accept a loss and move on. There is no need to allow your opponents the vicious pleasure of watching you writhe in defeat.

A Clean Win

Just as there is a proper way to lose, there is a proper way to win. Earlier in this chapter, the notion of achieving a "clean win" was introduced. Many people are startled when their win reverses, turning into a loss. Their tactics and strategies may have won them the battle. However, in the long run the damage they did to their reputation, their resources, and their own self-esteem made them casualties of their own war.

The clean win is based on clean tactics and clean outcomes. It is a win that is fair, just, equitable, and honest. It is an outcome that mixes wisdom and compassion with triumph and good fortune. It is a victory that preserves ethical principles and virtue.

Certainly there is a temptation to gloat over the loser. Just as you allowed yourself private fantasies in order to contain your urges to destroy them, so too should you check these impulses to torment the other side after your win. Know when to let go. To attain your objectives, you need not annihilate your adversaries. You have outsmarted them—that is enough.

Mixed Models

In order to clarify the difference between them, this chapter has treated interest-based negotiation and positional negotiation as two distinct models. In reality, you are likely to combine and intersperse the two in your negotiations. For example, the tone of a discussion with representatives of another organization is likely to be collaborative for the most part. However, if you were to detect their playing games or being needlessly reticent, you might employ a few rounds of positional bargaining. In so doing, you demonstrate your capability and willingness to play hardball when you must. Curiously enough, a temporary positional stance is sometimes the most potent way to persuade the negotiation back to a tone that is interest-based.

As you shape your mix of strategies, strive for a suitable fit. Connect persuasive strategies to the specific circumstances of your negotiation. Mold that pathway by clarifying your own objectives, understanding those of the other side, and recognizing the general context in which you are negotiating: assess your picture, their picture, and the big picture. The process itself is pliable. Each frame evolves as the negotiation unfolds. With each step and each shift, test the waters, guiding your statements and tactics to assess reactions and explore alternatives. Proceed in small steps. If something works, move with it. When you are tripped up, attend to the cues your opponents are sending out and readjust your tactics accordingly.

Like tools, negotiation is about options. If you have only a hammer, you will pound at every occasion. If you have a toolbox full of options and strategies, and if you know how and when to use each, then you will be able to create the best fit between task and tactics. Use the right strategy at the right time and you will fly; use the same strategy at the wrong time and you will crash. Molding the right fit requires insight, courage, and perseverance. You must be willing to take risks. You must be aware that you will sometimes make mistakes, and you must have the common sense to learn from them when you do. Your insights will derive not only from your professional experience; more importantly, they will derive from your wisdom and your willingness to learn from both failure and success.

Conclusion

More than any other, this chapter has been incongruous with the general tone of the book. It was a challenge to write. And for you, the reader, some of the passages likely evoked visceral reactions. Why include this perspective?

To be an all-around effective negotiator, it is vital to know and understand positional bargaining: its design, methods, and consequences. First, you will be better able to spot its use against you. This is particularly important when you work with those who talk interests and play positional.

Second, you will know when to use it and when not to—perhaps the most difficult puzzle to balance in negotiations. It is the "do-gooder" trap of health care that makes this choice so complex. Some advocates, self-righteous in their cause, are too swift to adopt positional negotiation. Their mission becomes lost in the fray of battle as they create enemies and lose allies. Others are too reluctant to use positional strategies, eschewing these contemptible maneuvers which their goals demand. Their purpose becomes sacrificed to their unwillingness to fight for it.

Finally, in reading this chapter you may have discovered parts of yourself that you, in fact, do not relish. Are there times when you are instinctively positional when the battle is not necessary? Are there times when you give up on what you know to be right because you cannot face a positional struggle? To enhance your negotiating effectiveness, you may want to transform both your style and your strategy. Recognizing yourself is step one in making that shift.

12

· ·

Mediation, Arbitration, and Dispute Resolution

Disagreements and differences are common in the frenetic work of health care. The preponderance of these disagreements are routinely resolved by the parties involved through direct negotiation: they talk it out and eventually find a solution. Nonetheless, the disputes you most likely recall are those that were not so easily settled. Those are the disputes that painfully escalated so that others became involved in waging or resolving the issues: colleagues who took sides, supervisors who entered the fray, attorneys retained to represent the contenders. By the time these others were recruited, the fighting surged to vicious, passionate, and vindictive battle. What are the options in such a situation?

Escalating conflict ignites a storehouse of weapons: litigation, full-scale confrontation, and even violence, to name a few. Many such conflicts soar seemingly out of control into these high-stakes contests. The parties become so distant and combative that their only signals to one another are bombshells: a subpoena, a defamatory article in the press, a devastating threat, a shattering blow to one's reputation. Fearing defeat, the parties take cues from one another: "get them before they get you." Each new signal provokes the next assault, causing the conflict to surge into its next hostile offensive.

There are alternatives. "Alternative dispute resolution," or ADR, refers to a range of interventions intended to replace these tactics of escalation. Arbitration and mediation are the most common forms of ADR. Their purpose is to interrupt the escalation by offering the parties a structured, monitored framework to air and possibly resolve their dispute.

ADR has roots in a number of arenas. Legal reformers, seeking alternatives to the long waits, high costs, and contentious framework of the judicial system, created the "multidoor courthouse," which offers mediation and arbitration as alternatives to litigation (Goldberg, Green, and Sander, 1985). Labor organizers began using mediation years ago to resolve bitter labor disputes, and the federal government's mediation service is now regularly called upon before and during strikes. Out of the 1960s community justice movement, neighborhood dispute-resolution centers were established to resolve tenant-landlord disputes, fights between high school gangs, and disagreements over land use. Divorce mediation has become a popular avenue for settling potentially divisive family conflicts, and in the international arena, mediation and citizen diplomacy are used to ease tensions between nations (U.S. Department of State, Foreign Service Institute, 1987; Kelman, 1995).

ADR methods are now being explored for their application to health care–related dispute resolution (see Slaikeu, 1989; Dauer, 1993). ADR is used to handle disputes ranging from classic legal disputes to complex organizational, patient care, and family relations conflicts. A growing number of managed care organizations and hospitals require patients to sign an ADR clause so that disputes arising in the course of their treatment will be less likely to result in litigation. Similar provisions are being incorporated into staff contracts and interorganizational agreements. In Massachusetts, the state medical board has instituted a voluntary mediation program that offers patients who file a complaint against a physician the opportunity to seek resolution through mediation. At the Montefiore Medical Center in New York, a mediation model was developed and tested for its effectiveness in resolving bioethical disputes (Dubler and Marcus, 1994). This and similar models are being incorporated nationwide to resolve complex patient care disputes. In Washington, D.C., the American Bar Association is experimenting with a program to build mediation into nursing home dispute resolution.

What is the value in making a dispute resolution alternative available, especially in the high stakes and emotionally charged arena of health care? What are the options for interrupting the escalation and resolving the dispute before it spirals further into mutually destructive conflict? How do you encourage the disputants to begin talking?

Guiding the Parties to the Table

Parties involved in a boiling, high-stakes dispute often become focused on one objective: "the complete and virtual annihilation of the other side" captures the sentiments often heard. Whether it is a malpractice issue, a conflict between departments in a medical center, or an internal staff dispute in a health clinic, each side gauges their survival and their satisfaction by this somewhat vicious criterion. Conflict becomes obsession as time, costs, and distractions accumulate for each side.

This accumulation of burden affects more than the primary parties to the dispute. In a nursing strike, for example, the costs are borne not only by the nurses themselves—the conflict is likewise felt directly by the secondary parties: those people left behind to do the necessary work. It is also endured by the tertiary parties: the unserviced patients and the members of the general community, who wonder if the hospital will be there for them should they need it.

What shifts the battling parties' attention toward a possible settlement? At times it is the secondary and tertiary players who pressure the sides to talk. A weary hospital staff member walks out to the picket line and compassionately explains the dire consequences of the strike for the patients in the hospital, questioning whether the strike is really worth it. The media rebukes the hospital's administration for imposing the working conditions that led to the strike, admonishing them for neglecting their public responsibility by placing the community at risk. The hospital's trustees turn to the CEO, just as nurses on the picket line turn to their union representatives, each imploring the primary players to negotiate in earnest.

Similarly, an outside impetus to settle might come from a supervisor, judge, colleague, or spouse. Such pleas represent a wake-up call, a perspective from someone not invested in the battle who can therefore see its boundless costs and its finite benefits. In a very heated dispute, only rarely do the parties reach this realization on their own. There is a reluctance to acknowledge the desire to settle, as it creates the appearance of capitulation. Or it might be interpreted as a concession of waning energy, a signal of vulnerability. By contrast, if the inducement comes from an outside source, a third party such as a mutual friend or an impartial authority, the disputants are relieved of the illusion of surrender. In the process of being eased to the negotiation table, each side, either implicitly or explicitly, begins to reconsider their objectives and tactics.

This third party must be able to win the confidence of both sides in order to ease them, one step at a time, from battle toward conciliation. Without this attention, one inflammatory remark by either side can propel the parties back into their hostilities.

Talking is a tenuous process. It is fraught with danger: you could say too much; you could give the wrong impression; the other side could pummel you when you are vulnerable; your regrets about the meeting could overwhelm you; you could be provoked into lashing out, verbally or physically, toward the other side. An outsider can help keep these passions in check and retain the disputants' willingness to talk.

In the process of allowing themselves to be eased to the negotiation table, each side, either implicitly or explicitly, begins to reconsider their objectives and tactics. The turning point emerges when both sides, separately though somewhat simultaneously, honestly assess the costs, risks, and potential benefits associated with the dispute. It is a sobering moment. It has built within it some mix of humiliation, defeat, fear, bravado, and vulnerability. The mounting downsides of the dispute are no longer tolerable, and the drive to escalate evaporates. The delusion of reaping substantial benefits wanes as the realization of the dispute's real costs looms. It is time to call off the cannons. It is time to talk. How can this negotiation be initiated?

This willingness to talk is a mutual signal for both sides. There are some who resist the shift: they regard talking as an expression of surrender. It is and it is not. The distinction is important. It certainly is a suspension of the escalation. It surely need not be a surrender of the concerns, principles, or objectives that brought the parties to dispute. After all, resolution emerges only if a way can be found to honor and reasonably satisfy these desires. Talking this out, rather than fighting through combat, can offer a different form of persuasion. Guiding the disputants through this distinction between suspension of hostilities and surrender and on to negotiation is crucial.

For some, it is hard to accept negotiation. In their mind, the only legitimate form of persuasion is intimidation: it is what they understand and what they know how to do. Their worldview is one of winners and losers. They can only "win" by fighting hard and significantly harming or destroying the other side. They believe the adversarial method is the best, if not the only, means of true justice. However, life (like health care) is not a game of football: barreling toward a single all-important objective, pummeling others along the way, does not enhance necessary collaboration. Even members of one's own team may be aghast at such offensive maneuvers. Those who would use this method must be convinced that resolution usually emerges from a balance between the sides. A third party can help accomplish this transformation, legitimizing an alternative that is better than a fight to the bitter end.

Whether the negotiation is voluntary or mandatory, such as when the parties are contractually bound to first use ADR or when they are ordered by a judge to an ADR procedure, the decision to attempt the ADR option does not foretell the settlement itself. It simply demonstrates a willingness to explore the options. ADR reveals the prospect that differences do not have to be waged as a destructive contest. It exposes the high financial and social costs of the adversarial method. It reframes the dispute and offers a process for bringing it to conclusion.

Getting the parties to the negotiation table is one hurdle: getting them to settle is something else, as in: you can lead the horse to water, and you can't make it drink. The purpose of this chapter is to introduce you briefly to alternative dispute resolution methods. The focus is on mediation, since mediation will be most immediately useful to you in resolving the everyday issues that you find in your workplace. Since the intent of mediation is, in part, to bring interest-based negotiation to the fore, the methods discussed here are also instructive for your own general negotiation and dispute resolution endeavors.

Negotiation, Arbitration, and Mediation

ADR involves the use of a neutral third party to help the disputants reach a resolution (see Crowley 1994; Singer, 1994). By definition this nonpartisan individual has no stake in the substance of the settlement. The impartial's prime focus is on helping the parties resolve their conflict and reach agreement. The detachment and lack of bias of the third party allows the disputants to ascribe the necessary trust and confidence and to move toward legitimate settlement. The task of the neutral is to introduce a process that can help the parties reach that settlement. As such, the neutral forms an understanding of the issues and a strategy for resolving the dispute.

The most important distinction between negotiation, arbitration, and mediation is the matter of partisanship. As negotiator, you are naturally partisan. You advocate your own interests or those of your constituency. Since you have a stake in the outcome, it is presumed that you are biased on your own behalf. You are predisposed to assess the scenario from your own subjective lens, as are other negotiators, and you are naturally partial to solutions that benefit you. Even as you ponder and acknowledge the issues from other perspectives, you are predisposed to meeting your own objectives. A measure of selfishness is presumed.

By contrast, a neutral third party is introduced into a dispute precisely for his or her lack of partisanship. When the parties are locked in battle, the neutral is able to offer an objective analysis of the issues, a new set of eyes to consider options and a process for resolution that all parties could consider just and fair. The process works best when all the parties want settlement and when they believe the neutral third party to be honorable and objective in handling the dispute. That confidence is fundamental to approval of both the process and the person.

The negotiator begins as a partisan and is partisan throughout. The arbitrator begins a case as a nonpartisan. When pronouncing a ruling, the arbitrator becomes partisan. The mediator begins as a nonpartisan and remains nonpartisan throughout.

In arbitration, the neutral third party hears the arguments of both parties and then issues a determination. The parties advocate their position to the arbitrator, each hoping the case will be judged in their favor. When the parties choose binding arbitration, they are contractually obligated to abide by the ruling. If they violate the terms of the settlement, they face the consequences delineated beforehand in the arbitration contract. In nonbinding arbitration, the arbitrator's ruling is offered only as an opinion. It remains for the parties to negotiate a mutually acceptable settlement, using the arbitrator's opinion as a benchmark. The advantage of binding over nonbinding arbitration is that the case usually ends with the ruling, thus limiting the expense and time invested in the dispute. The disadvantage is that the parties lose control of the end result, which is why some disputants prefer nonbinding arbitration.

Disputants choose arbitration over litigation because it is private, it avoids courtroom backlogs, and it does not impose formal rules of evidence. Many workplace grievance procedures operate on an arbitration model. A grievance is submitted by an employee and appraised through a hearing process. An individual reviewer or a representative panel hears the case and issues a judgment. Depending on the grievance procedures in place, that determination could be final or it could be open to appeal based upon specified criteria.

Mediation is the use of a neutral third party to help disputants find and agree to an acceptable resolution of their conflict by way of a private and confidential process. A mediator does not issue a ruling. The purpose of mediation is to assist the parties by offering a process for reaching a settlement (see Folberg and Taylor, 1984). The mediator does not act as a judge and has no power to impose an outcome upon the parties. Rather, the mediator facilitates the process of negotiation between the parties, helping them to better understand their options, choices, and consequences. The mediator is a catalyst for settlement, not an advocate for one party over another. The outcome of mediation is determined by the parties: they each have the authority to reject or accept the offers presented to them.

Disputants choose arbitration over litigation when they want to settle their dispute without the complications of a courtroom battle. They confer to the arbitrator control of both process and outcome. Disputants choose mediation over arbitration when they want to maintain greater control over the settlement itself. They confer to the mediator control of the process, and they maintain control of the outcome. The parties remain with negotiation over mediation when they want to settle on their own, without an outside intervener. They control both process and outcome.

Mediation: Setting a Frame to Resolve Health Care Disputes

This chapter highlights mediation. (For a further discussion of mediation method and practice, see Moore, 1986; Laue, 1987; Kressel,

Pruitt, and Associates, 1989; and Folger and Jones, 1994.) The process offers a readily useful, constructive framework for resolving health care disputes. Its methods can be adapted to facilitate the complex process of convening involved parties in a meaningful, defined, and pragmatic manner. Because control of the outcome remains with the parties to the dispute, the process attends to their varying roles, stakes, interests, authority, purposes, and expectations in reaching a mutually acceptable outcome. Given the need to balance these many considerations, the adaptability and inclusiveness of mediation is key to its success.

Dispute resolution is in fact a routine aspect of health care work. On a regular basis, health care professionals facilitate agreement among a complex web of issues and people. In most cases this reconciliation is accomplished without particular attention to the process by which it is performed. The mediation framework offers a set of systematic methods to assess and settle existing and anticipated conflicts. Mediation can be incorporated within a health care organization so that it is easily accessible, offering parties a safe meeting ground to fairly discuss and resolve their differences.

Mediation is most beneficial when applied flexibly and creatively. Two models of mediation, with their different settlement venues, apply to health care situations: formal and informal mediation.

In the process of formal mediation, the impartial facilitator makes it clear that the parties are being brought together for the purpose of mediation. The neutral is an outsider and is clearly known and accepted as mediator for the case. He or she establishes the process at the outset, describing the roles, rules, and steps necessary to find settlement. The parties recognize their involvement in a mediated dispute-resolution process. This formal set of procedures is particularly helpful when the dispute has advanced into combative sides with inflamed emotions and adversarial interactions. The structure itself calms the tensions and creates a venue for constructive negotiation.

Familiarity with the professional context of the dispute, be it a commercial, environmental, or health care disagreement, can be an advantage for the mediator, though it is not an absolute require-ment and sometimes can even be an obstacle. A fundamental knowledge of the subject at hand allows the mediator to legitimately and knowledgeably focus on primary issues and advance the parties to a feasible resolution. Nonpartisan health care professionals, for example, can successfully serve as mediators, as long as they are per-ceived and behave as neutrals. That perception is critical to the effectiveness of the process. For example, in patient-physician dis-putes, a physician as mediator or co-mediator is a boon to under-standing the issues, involving the parties, and forging resolution. Just as often, a patient feels that the presence of a physician as medi-ator tilts the process in favor of the doctor. In this scenario, a health care manager, a lawyer that specializes in medical cases, or a nurse may be agreeable to both parties.

How can one secure an outside mediator to help resolve a dis-pute? Mediation and arbitration services, some specializing in health care, are sprouting up around the country. In addition, courts are offering ADR services, as are law firms. Federal agen-cies offer mediators to help resolve major labor disputes. One should confirm the credentials of the proposed mediator. Among the more important criteria for recruiting a mediator are the accept-ability, neutrality, and legitimacy of the impartial for each of the disputants.

Disputes most likely to call upon mediation are those in which there is a clear and tangible cost to nonresolution, such as when the anticipated extravagant expenses of a protracted legal dispute pro-pel the parties to a more low-cost, private process. These could include malpractice disputes, conflicts regarding physician-hospital privileges, labor disputes, or disputes over institutional jurisdiction, to name a few.

By contrast, informal mediation incorporates the methods of mediation, applying them liberally to meet the particular circum-stances of the dispute at hand. Informal mediation is useful to resolve immediate issues as they arise in the course of health care. Bioethical conflicts, staff disagreements, interprofessional disputes, policy issues, and matters that arise between family members, patients, and staff are typical of the types of day-to-day disputes that can benefit from the flexible application of mediation methods. In these types of issues, there is usually neither the time, the resources, nor the willingness to call upon an outside neutral to intervene in the case. In these instances, an individual with the training and recognition to mediate from within can be an invaluable resource for the institution and those associated with it.

What is the difference between formal and informal mediation? Formal mediation is a structured process, with clearly defined roles and expectations. The mediator sets and maintains this framework, directing the parties from exploration of the issues to option-building and settlement. For example, during formal mediation, the mediator opens the session with an introduction about the process, the voluntary nature of the parties' involvement, and the meaning of the neutral role. However, in the type of circumstances facing the bioethicist, a formal discourse about mediation likely will detract from the matter needing resolution. For example, an ethicist entering an intensive care unit to help resolve a disagreement regarding a do-not-resuscitate order best not lecture the parties about the methods and processes of mediation. Yet, these very methods of mediation can offer a useful framework for resolving such matters. Using mediation methods as a guide, the bioethicist adapts the process to the circumstances of the dispute.

There are legitimate problems and pitfalls in the use of informal mediation, and they are best acknowledged if they form an obstacle to resolution. Foremost is the problem of neutrality. For example, someone employed by an institution does not pass the test of pure neutrality in a dispute between a family and hospital regarding an unwanted discharge to a nursing home, especially if administration is pressing the action to relieve itself of a costly financial burden. It would be disingenuous to present yourself as impartial if your boss dispatches you to mediate a resolution of the problem with the proviso "And just make sure the patient is out of here pronto when you're done!" You can help resolve the problem using your mediation skills, *and* you are not a neutral in this case, especially if you want to keep your job.

Other problems with informal mediation are the loyalties and biases that may get in the way of neutrality. If you are asked to informally mediate a dispute between a nurse supervisor and a physician on a medical floor, you may be too familiar with the physician's boisterous behavior to enter the fray unbiased. Similarly, the disputants may know too much about you to trust your objectivity. If your reputation is one of favoring one side or the other, or if your allegiance to the agenda of your boss is mistrusted, your influence as an informal mediator could be compromised.

In spite of these problems with informal mediation, it does offer a practical and systematic avenue for resolving the myriad of disputes common to health care organizations. The best way to describe and understand the mediation process itself is from the perspective of formal mediation. Following is a description of mediation as a formal process, with recommendations for adapting the process to the realities of health care decision making.

◆ ◆ ◆ ◆ ◆ ◆ ◆

The Long-Tuckerman case was reviewed by the state medical board. A staff member investigated the complaint, looking into the care given Mrs. Brown and Dr. Tuckerman's overall medical record. While it was felt that the doctor had made a miscalculation in this case, the board decided not to take disciplinary action against him. Such action could have included temporary suspension or full confiscation of his license to practice medicine. The board generally restricts such unilateral action for more serious cases, of which there are a significant number in the state. This case did not meet the criteria for such action, especially in light of the physician's general record.

Nonetheless, the board did not want to fully dismiss the case.

It decided to refer the parties to the board's voluntary mediation program. The chief investigative officer for the case called both Leslie Long and Ted Tuckerman to describe the program and to inquire of their interest in meeting to see if a resolution might be possible. The investigator explained that if a mutually agreeable solution could be reached, and with the consent of both parties, the case could be removed from the public files of the board. The board would keep a record that the case had been settled. If the case was not settled, it would remain an open case on file with the board. This system offers some leverage to the complainant to even the table, and it offers incentive to the physician to participate and be amenable to settlement. If the complainant's demands are unreasonable, the physician is under no obligation to accept them.

They both agreed to meet with a mediator. Tuckerman asked about bringing his attorney. The board staff member said he could do so if he insisted. She recommended against it, as the presence of an attorney tends to turn the discussion slightly more adversarial than if only the direct parties are present. Tuckerman discussed the question with his attorney, who recommended to give mediation a try without the presence of counsel.

The case was referred to a local mediation agency with a state contract to provide the service. The agency's independence from the state medical board enhances the neutrality and confidentiality of the process. The agency was able to schedule the mediation without a long delay.

On the day of the mediation, Bob Bennett, an experienced mediator with the agency, invited Leslie Long and Ted Tuckerman into the mediation room. He introduced himself, shook their hands, and checked whether they knew one another. Bennett took his place at the end of the conference table. Long and Tuckerman sat on either side, facing each other.

Bennett opened the session. "First, I want to thank you each for coming here to discuss the complaint brought through the board of medical registration. I have spoken with each of you about the issue, and you each said that you would be willing to meet through mediation to explore the possibility of coming to some sort of settlement. Because you were both positive about sitting down and talking this out, it was decided to go ahead and schedule the mediation.

"Let me explain a bit about mediation and my role as a mediator. Unlike litigation or arbitration, in which a judge, jury, or arbitrator decides the outcome of a dispute, in mediation the development and acceptance of the settlement is up to you. We explore the issues together, considering the options for reaching a resolution you both can accept. Then *you* decide whether you are going to accept the outcome. That outcome is not imposed upon you. You create it, and you decide whether to accept it.

"That, of course, does not mean that you will each get everything you want. If the settlement is one that both parties can accept, it usually means that there has been a good deal of listening and understanding, along with some give-and-take in order to reach agreement. That is, the settlement has to be acceptable to you as well as to the person sitting across the table.

"My role as the mediator is to help you move through the steps of listening, understanding, developing options, and coming to an agreement. My role is not to tell you how to settle your differences. At times, I will help you better understand your choices. The acceptance of the choices and the consequences, though, is totally up to you. I am not here as a judge: creating and accepting the settlement is your task.

"Both of you will get a chance to tell your story as you see it and to air your feelings about what happened. At times we will meet together, here in this room. There may be a need for me to speak privately with one or both of you. Then I will ask one of you to wait in the waiting room while I caucus with the other. There may be things you want to share with me in confidence.

"As I mentioned on the phone, the process itself is confidential. Obviously, the three of us sitting here are not in the public glare of a courtroom. We are also not operating under the direct rubric of the board. I am obligated only to report back whether or not we reached settlement: yes or no. I must also remind you that under the laws of this state, whatever is said here cannot be entered into a courtroom hearing. As a mediator, I cannot be called into court to testify should this conflict get to that point. These protections have been enacted in the hope that they will encourage people to resolve their disputes honestly and directly with one another, well before they get to the courtroom. Therefore, I hope you will each use this opportunity to genuinely express what is on your mind, to hear what the other person is saying, and to sincerely explore this opportunity for settlement.

"You are both here on a voluntary basis. If you feel we are not making progress, either of you can call off the talks. If you are satisfied with the results of this mediation, we will conclude the process with the preparation of a written agreement that responds to the needs and interests of both of you.

"One important ground rule: I ask that one person speak at a time. It is vital that we hear and heed what is being said. Are there any questions?"

Both Long and Tuckerman shook their heads.

Bennett continued. "Oh, I have one. Do you prefer first or last names?" He hoped they would be comfortable with the greater informality of first names. He looked to Long, who said, "Leslie is fine with me." Tuckerman too agreed to be called Ted.

"Fine," Bennett continued. "First, I would like some background. Leslie, you initiated the complaint. Could you please tell me what led to the filing?"

Leslie went through her story. Her emphasis was not on the medical facts, though she made reference to the fact that Tuckerman had missed the beginnings of the cancer. She spoke more of what her mother meant to her. The implication was that Tuckerman was guilty of murder. Bennett listened carefully, nodding to indicate his active concern for Long and periodically looking over to Tuckerman to assess his reaction.

When she finished, Bennett synthesized her comments. "Leslie, if I understand what you are saying, you feel that Ted missed some important diagnostic indicators which, had they been found earlier, could have saved your mother's life. Is that correct?"

"Yes, that captures how I feel."

Bennett next turned to Tuckerman. "Ted, tell me your view of what happened."

Tuckerman talked directly to Long. "Leslie, first I want you to know how much I cared for your mother and that I too felt a sense of loss at her passing. As I'm sure you know, I was her physician for ten years. Not a holiday passed without her bringing in a poppy seed cake."

Leslie turned to the mediator to explain. "Mom made the best poppy seed cake in the world."

Tuckerman continued. "Now, being a doctor, you have to make a lot of tough judgment calls. I don't think I would be telling you anything new to say that your mom was very concerned about her health."

There was a moment of silence. Finally, Leslie spoke. "Actually, Dr. Tuckerman, you're being kind with that. Mom was obsessed with her health. Whenever she had a visit with you, she would call me up to tell me every gory detail: the pills, the aches, the pains, the tests. There were times, love her, that I felt like putting down the phone and then coming back twenty minutes later when she was done. She was a little bit of the sufferer in that way."

Tuckerman listened intently and then continued. "Well, I won't disagree with you on that. Now, as a physician, I am sometimes in a tight situation. I have to weigh very carefully the tests I order for each patient. I always want to be as careful as possible, on the one hand. On the other hand, there is a lot of pressure to be prudent about health costs. So I have to balance out what I do. If you didn't put down the telephone"—Leslie shook her head to indicate that she had only thought of not paying attention, she never did it—"then you know that your mother got a lot of attention and a lot of tests and whatever medications we thought could cure her, whatever the ailment."

"I'm not saying, Dr. Tuckerman, that you didn't give her good care for all those years. All I'm saying is that in the crunch, when it really counted, you weren't there. You didn't come through, and it killed mom."

Bennett watched Tuckerman tense up. He decided to jump in

to cool down the situation. He turned to Long. "Leslie, to say to a doctor that he killed his patient is a pretty hard accusation. Are you sure that is what you mean?"

"She's dead, isn't she? And Dr. Tuckerman was her doctor, wasn't he? What do you call it?"

Bennett turned to Tuckerman. "Ted, I'm not an expert on cancer, though I know a bit from personal experience about lung cancer. Could you explain the disease to us?" Bennett was hoping that the pointed question would help calm down Tuckerman. The mediator could see that the physician was seething from the implication that he had somehow murdered his patient.

Tuckerman took a deep breath. "Lung cancer is in fact an insidious disease. In some forms it comes on very quickly, and it is deadly. It is still among the most difficult, if not impossible, forms of cancer to treat. Your mother had a particularly bad case. Even if we had caught it slightly earlier, it is unlikely that the outcome would have varied by much. She had been exposed to a lot of secondary smoke, even though she wasn't a smoker herself. The problem was that the symptoms that would have alerted us to the lung cancer, in some ways, were masquerading as a common cold. Those colds were a pretty usual winter occurrence for your mom."

Bennett allowed Tuckerman's comment to sink in for a few moments. He watched Leslie carefully. "What do Ted's comments mean for you, Leslie?"

Long took a deep breath. "I don't know. I guess it was inevitable that she was going to die eventually. I mean of the lung cancer, given that it was in her system. I just can't buy that Dr. Tuckerman, I mean Ted, wasn't negligent for not being more careful about checking for it."

Bennett looked at Tuckerman. The doctor looked like he was about to explode. "I think this would be a good time for a private session," Bennett said. "I would like to speak to each of you privately. Ted, I would like to start with you. Leslie, could you go out to the waiting room for a few minutes?" Leslie nodded and left the room.

Once the door was closed, Tuckerman let loose. "Look, Bob,

you're a real nice guy and all, but this simply is not going to work. She has it stuck in her mind that I killed her mom, and no amount of gibberish is going to change that. You're siding with her by legitimizing all this bullshit she's throwing on the table."

"Ted, I can understand why you are frustrated. She seems to be contradicting herself. On one hand, she agrees that her mother was obsessed with anxiety about her health. That admission was an important insight for her about you as her mother's physician. I also get the sense that something else might be going on with her. Any clues as to what that might be?"

"No clues. I'm not a mind reader." Tuckerman was fuming.

"She is grieving the loss of her mother, and she wants to blame it on someone. You, Ted, are a safe pick. She is having a hard time accepting the loss, and she is putting all that energy into blaming you. Your statement that you too felt a sense of loss was heartfelt, and I could see that she heard you. She is going through a change, from seeing you as a murderer to someone who cared for and cared about her mother. That shift is not going to happen instantaneously. You might have to be a bit patient with her."

"It's hard being patient with someone who is so stubborn."

"I understand. What's your choice?"

"You said it yourself. I can walk out of here whenever I want."

"What good would that do you at this point? Wouldn't it just reinforce her impression of you?"

"Yeah, it probably would."

Bennett stayed with Tuckerman until he calmed down. Next, he asked Long into the room for a private session.

"Leslie, what are you feeling about where we are so far?"

"I don't think Dr. Tuckerman gets it. He doesn't understand what I am feeling."

Bennett wasn't sure that Long herself knew what she was feeling. "Leslie, what are you hoping to get out of this?"

"I went to a lawyer about this whole thing. He said maybe we could get some money for this. Insurance companies like to settle sometimes. But it wouldn't be for big bucks, nothing in the millions, because mom was old and the medical facts weren't big-time wrong. Anyway, after I was done talking with the lawyer I realized that money is not what I was after. I wanted something more."

"What more?"

"I want to make sure this doesn't happen to anybody else. That's the main thing. That's why I wanted his license removed. So that he wouldn't do this to somebody else."

"What could satisfy that?"

"I heard that sometimes in these settlements, the doctor agrees to go to a medical education class about the subject. At least if he took a class on the warning signs for lung cancer, then he would know what to look for."

"That does not sound unreasonable."

"And one more thing, he should have to make a contribution to the American Cancer Society. That also will help make sure this is not repeated."

"And those two things would satisfy you?"

"Just one more thing. I want to know that he is sorry. What happened hurts us forever. I need to know that he understands that."

"When we come back together, can I present those three items to him?"

"Yes, I would like you to do that."

Bennett walked out to the waiting room and invited Tucker-man back to the room. He reopened the discussion once they were both settled. "My private sessions with both of you were very helpful. I have a better understanding now of what is going on for each of you, and thanks to your comments, there are some ideas for possible settlement."

"Ted, Leslie has mentioned three things that would make it easier for her to settle. The most important thing for her is knowing that this will not happen to another patient and family. She wanted to know if you would be willing to take a medical education course on lung cancer?"

"I too want to make as certain as possible that this doesn't happen to another patient. I have to take medical education courses often, and if it would help settle this matter, I would be happy to make one of them on the topic of lung cancer."

Bennett was encouraged. He hoped the next concession would come as easily. "The second is a little tougher. Leslie would like to see you make a contribution to the American Cancer Society. There is something significant about this request. The family is not interested in getting any financial gain for themselves from what happened. They sincerely are more interested in making sure this does not reoccur for others."

"What kind of a contribution are you talking about?" Tuckerman asked.

Leslie was quick. "Three thousand dollars."

"Three thousand dollars? That's a lot of money."

Bennett put up both hands as if to call a time out. "Hold on. Can we first talk about the concept before we get to an exact dollar amount? Ted, in concept would you be willing to make a contribution?"

"Sure, in concept that would be fine. It just depends on how much."

"What would you propose?" Bennett asked.

"One thousand would be fine. I think that would be a fair amount."

Bennett turned to Leslie. "What do you think?"

"How about we split the difference? Two thousand. It's a good cause."

Tuckerman took a deep breath. "OK, if that's what it'll take to settle this thing, I'll make the contribution."

Bennett continued. "Finally, Leslie wants an apology."

Tuckerman turned directly to Leslie. "That's easy. Leslie, I don't know if you can imagine how hard it is for a doctor to lose a patient. I felt a tremendous sense of loss when your mother passed away. It's hard to accept this, but lung cancer is a terrible disease. There is a limit to what we doctors can do, and that is frustrating for us. I wish I had caught your mother's condition earlier. Maybe if there had been a better prognosis she would have been more willing to try treatment. I was surprised and frustrated that she didn't want to attempt chemotherapy. It was her decision, though, and we all had to respect it. Yes, Leslie, I feel terrible about what happened. I lost my father to cancer, so I have some feeling for how devastating it can be. I truly am sorry."

Tuckerman's words lingered in the air. Long broke the silence. "That helps. That helps a lot."

Bennett had a sense of what Tuckerman was thinking. Bennett wanted to raise it before Tuckerman fumbled with how to put it on the table.

"Leslie, given what Ted has agreed to and said, would you be willing to settle and allow the complaint to be removed from the board's public files?"

Long hesitated. Tuckerman was beginning to fume. He had a sudden impulse to push away from the table and run for the door. Who was she to determine such an important question for his medical career? She didn't say a thing. The anxiety was driving him crazy. Bennett sensed Tuckerman's frustration from the corner of his eye.

Leslie spoke slowly. "Yes, this settles the complaint. The case can be removed from the board's public files."

Tuckerman was overwhelmed with relief. He looked at Bennett and then to Long. "I'm glad we were able to settle this."

Bennett summarized what had been agreed to, jotted down the points, and had each sign an impromptu document. The settlement was reported back to the board of medical registration. A letter of acknowledgment for the donation was sent by the charity to both Long and Tuckerman. Tuckerman took the course on lung cancer within three months of the mediation, and the case was removed from the board's public files.

◆ ◆ ◆ ◆ ◆ ◆ ◆

The Role of the Mediator

Fundamental to the process of mediation is the impartiality and perceived neutrality of the mediator. (For a comprehensive overview of mediation processes and techniques, see Moore, 1986.)

Impartiality refers to the mediator's attitude. Neutrality defines the relationship between the mediator and the disputants: the mediator is a neutral if he or she is so perceived by the disputants. What is the significance of neutrality for the success of mediation?

The mediator serves as a fulcrum—balancing, connecting, and resolving the differences between the disputants. By not leaning to one side over the other, the mediator establishes the importance of finding a settlement that fairly accounts for the legitimate needs and interests of all sides. If a proposed settlement unfairly favors one party, it will likely be rejected by the other. Since agreement itself is voluntary, such a rejection represents a breakdown of the mediation process. The mediator personifies the common ground toward which the parties are encouraged to move.

The generative importance of mediation is the discovery of solutions that will simultaneously satisfy the interests of both sides. As they develop trust in the neutrality of the mediator, the parties reveal their underlying concerns, and in the process, the mediator helps them derive and combine workable solutions. Finding those options and gaining that consensus is the key to bringing the parties to a settlement.

Of course, maintaining the impartiality of perspective and the neutrality of perception is a monumental challenge. At times, the mediator does form an opinion about the people or issues involved in a case. However, if the mediation process is to succeed, the mediator must not reveal those biases in what is said or done in the mediation process. To undermine that nonpartisanship would be to damage the very legitimacy of the intervention. The ultimate test of neutrality, however, does not lie simply with what the mediator says or does. Rather, the most significant measures of neutrality are the perceptions and beliefs held by the parties.

How does their perception of neutrality affect the disputants? Parties involved in a dispute often fear that outsiders will align with their opponent, thereby weakening their own position. Similarly, one's position is bolstered by the outsiders who endorse it: disputants crave allies. In a highly polarized dispute, the mediator represents a unique value-added dimension to the process. In most cases, attempts by the opposing sides to gain favor with the mediator do not succeed, as the mediator maintains his or her impartiality. If the mediator were to take sides, the parties would reinforce their positions, thereby reducing their willingness to offer concessions. The fairness of the process is not upheld if it is biased.

The mediator's impartiality offers a unique perspective on the dispute. (For a useful discussion of perspective in the negotiation process, see Ury, 1991.) Invariably, by the time the parties call upon a neutral for help in settling their differences, the conflict has become obstinately polarized. The mediator is able to offer a fresh perspective: a new set of questions to reframe the parties' differences, an opportunity to reflect on real choices and consequences, and new options that the parties have not previously considered. The mediator moves each party away from the conviction, or perhaps even obsession, that theirs is the correct resolution. In its place, the mediator offers new thinking and new options for considering the dispute. There is less emphasis on one perspective's being right or wrong. Rather, the mediator opens perspectives that offer multiple options and opportunities for resolution.

In mediation, the parties create the settlement: it is not created by the mediator. Their participation in the process is voluntary, as is their acceptance of the settlement. To maximize the chances for settlement, the agreement must be mutually beneficial, producing a "gain-gain" outcome. In such a scenario, the parties recognize that they achieve more by accepting the agreement than by continuing the dispute.

The Process of Mediation

When it comes to mediation, negotiation, arbitration, or communication, the word "process" is regularly bandied about. There is good process, bad process, no process, ironic process, and far too much process. What is process?

If substance is the ends, then process is the means. It is not the decision; it is how the decision is reached. At times, process defines an established sequence of steps, clear roles, definitive authority, and specific criteria for reaching decisions. The parties follow a predetermined script. At other times, the assumed steps, roles, authority, or criteria do not work; or there is no predetermined method for reaching a decision; or the parties do not accept their part in the script. In these cases, another process must be developed if the parties are to reach their objectives.

Good process is not defined by a specific formula. The most appropriate vehicle delivers parties efficiently and effectively to a mutually acceptable agreement. The right people are involved in the decision, the criteria are fair and sensible, the information used is valid and objective, and the outcome is reasonable and legitimate. Sometimes the process is established beforehand. Sometimes it evolves naturally between the parties. The key is whether it takes people where they hope to be.

Bad process excludes people who feel they should be a part of the decision, does not use objective information or criteria, or reaches an outcome that is infeasible or unlawful. Bad process is inefficient: it keeps people on the train and never advances them toward their destination. The greatest process conflicts are between people who like train rides and those who simply want to get someplace, as well as with those who want to dictate the destination and cancel the train ride that others feel is necessary.

Ironic process is that unfortunate predicament in which the parties actually agree on most substantive points, and yet are unable to communicate constructively to take themselves beyond their own obstinacy. The absence of process hides the presence of concurrence. Even when they agree on specific points, their polarization has them repudiating statements that ultimately are reasonable. Paradoxically, they are simply unable to get themselves unstuck.

In order for the parties to reach an agreement on the substance of their heated dispute, there must be some broad consensus and acceptance on the means for getting there. This is often a stumbling block, since it may appear secondary to the conflict: everyone is so focused on the ends that little attention is placed on the means.

In fact, process may be central to the dispute. One party complains, "If you had asked my opinion in the first place, maybe we wouldn't have gotten to this impasse." Another retorts, "It is not my intention to talk endlessly. We have a job to get done here, and in the long run, that's all that counts."

Certainly if the parties are overwhelmed by hostility on substantive matters, there will be little attentiveness left to focus on process. That is the contribution of mediation. The mediator structures and guides a procedure, first to prove that it is possible to get the parties talking, and then to turn their discussion into a constructive outcome: the resolution of their dispute based upon overlapping yet different objectives. It is this methodological balance of process toward outcome that is the essence of mediation.

In this way, the mediator reframes the tenor of the disputants' negotiation. At the point when the mediator is brought into the conflict, the parties are most often locked into a positional and distributional negotiation posture. The mediator hopes to transform the negotiation into an interest-based, integrative process. The task is to assess whether an appropriate reframing is possible given the history and attitudes of the disputants. If there is a reasonable chance that a settlement can be achieved, the mediator must construct a process to move the parties from confrontation toward cooperation and ultimately to resolution. As mediation is voluntary, at any point either of the parties or the mediator himself or herself can suspend or postpone the mediation. (For a discussion of ethical questions in dispute resolution, see Laue and Cormick, 1978.)

The Sequence of Mediation

There are eight steps in formal mediation process: premediation appropriateness, premeeting investigation and party buy-in, party meeting, issue clarification, option building, option assessment, movement toward mutually acceptable solutions, and resolution and implementation. Each step is discussed briefly.

1. Premediation appropriateness. There are many avenues by which a dispute can reach mediation. At times, one of the disputants brings an inquiry to the mediator. Often, it is someone who knows or is associated with the party who suggests and contacts the mediator. Rarely, the disputants request mediation together. The initial task of the mediator is to assess whether the matter is appropriate for mediation (see Potapchuk and Carlson, 1987). The mediator describes the process and then poses a critical question: "Are you interested in finding a settlement?" If the answer is yes from all parties, then the mediator has established the basis for continuing to the next step. If, on the other hand, all or one of the parties prefers merely to defeat the other side, then the mediation effort most likely will be fruitless. An affirmative response need not specify the conditions of the settlement. It needs merely to express a general desire to move beyond the dispute and a willingness to accept mediation as a reasonable process by which to attempt a resolution. It is a signal from each party to the other that there is a willingness to put aside the weapons and negotiate a settlement. Having brought the parties to this point, the mediator informs each about the general approach and process of mediation.

2. Premeeting investigation and party buy-in. Having completed a cursory analysis of the issues and parties to the case, the mediator delves deeper into the background, objectives, and obstacles facing settlement. The mediator's most important tool is a good question: the mediator uses his or her inquisitiveness to discern options and opportunities for settlement and encourage the parties themselves to see the dispute from multiple perspectives. In the process of this investigation, the parties develop trust in the mediator. By the end of this stage, the mediator has developed a strategy

for building the mediation process, which is shared with the parties. The mediator plans the format for the meetings and establishes a time line for moving forward. These proposals are shared with the parties for their approval, with the cautionary note that each should be reasonable about expectations for the outcome: there can be no promises about what will or will not be achieved. The mediator has now gained support for the process and objectives of mediation.

3. Party meeting. There is often a good deal of tension between the parties. In most cases, the parties are well known to one another and are accustomed to adversarial discourse. It is the very inclusion of the neutral third party that makes this first meeting with the mediator unique. The mediator uses this opportunity to create a clear change in tone from the parties' previous encounters. At the opening session, the mediator sets the table, controls the course of discussion, and ensures that everyone has a fair chance to speak and be heard. The mediator opens the forum with a brief discussion of mediation, the purpose of the meeting, and the processes that will be used in the hope of reaching a settlement. Importantly, the mediator reminds all parties that everyone at the table has agreed that they are ready to find a settlement and that each has agreed to participate in this process in an effort to find it. Particularly during this initial session, the parties vent their anger and frustration toward one another. Some opportunity must be allowed for them to let off steam, though it is up to the mediator to decide when to move on toward the search for a settlement.

4. Issue clarification. The mediator arranges the parties' issues into two broad categories: points of agreement and points of disagreement. The disputants are often surprised to discover that there are items upon which they agree: they both want a settlement, they both have found the dispute to be painful, and they both hope that the agreement will be consonant with their values. Beyond these general points of agreement, the mediator may find specific points of agreement on substantive issues related to the conflict. Next, the

mediator points to matters of disagreement. These points are arrayed from the easiest to settle to the most difficult to settle. The mediator suggests that the parties begin with the least complex matters of dispute. In the process of gaining agreement on several easy issues, the parties build a constructive dialogue, move toward trust, and assume a less adversarial stance with one another. As agreement builds on specific points, the parties shape the momentum and confidence needed to address the most difficult matters facing them. Once they are confident of their ability to agree on the bulk of their disagreements, finding consensus on the final difficult issues is more likely.

5. Option building. The mediation process helps the parties find settlement options they could not find on their own. Often the mediator finds two incompatible proposals advanced by the disputants. The challenge is to generate a new set of choices that creatively combines the essential ingredients of each party's interests. In the process, the mediator helps to prompt a new set of options, some combination of which will be acceptable to all sides. To do this, the mediator brings his or her imagination to the process and likewise sparks that of the disputants. The task is to create a set of ideas that were not readily apparent to the parties prior to mediation. The mediator uses brainstorming and laundry list techniques to formulate a list of plausible ideas. Brainstorming asks the parties to quickly express a range of ideas without editing or comment: it is intended as an unobstructed, creative exercise. The laundry list exercise has the parties categorize the brainstorming ideas into lists, such as good options, bad options, feasible options, and unrealistic options.

6. Option assessment. In the course of their option building, the parties classify their choices: from mutually rejectable to mutually acceptable. It is wise to begin with what is unacceptable to both, as it is easier for the parties to reject than to accept. The mediator walks the parties through an appraisal of each option, stressing that

it is a choice and it has a consequence. Each party must be willing to address their own preferences and the associated consequences, as well as the impact of that choice on other parties and the likelihood that the other party would voluntarily accept such an outcome. In so doing, they move from their "fantasy win" to a more realistic goal: they begin to realize that each party must leave the table with some substantive gain if the process is to end in settlement. The parties are asked to assess the options in light of their own interests and in light of the recognized interests of the other parties. The mediator encourages the parties to use interest-based negotiation to reframe their relationship (see Fisher and Ury, 1991; Fisher and Brown, 1988). During this process, some of the parties' options rise to the fore and others fade. Attention focuses on a set of proposals that is agreeable to each party.

7. Movement toward mutually acceptable solutions. By this point the mediator has built an incremental process that has the parties converging on a range of specific settlement options. This agreement outlines a substantive exchange, the process by which the exchange will occur, and the protections to ensure its implementation. At this point, the mediator notes on paper the key points of agreement and requests buy-in from each of the parties. The mediator repeats each point so that the parties can voice concerns, changes, and consent. This acceptance is focused on the note pad of the mediator while it is being clearly heard and understood by both parties. It is at this point when the "fantasy moment" is likely to occur: the parties hear what they are getting and giving and compare this real outcome with their original fantasy solution of "I win, you lose." The difference between the actual settlement and the fantasy solution is disappointing, and the parties begin to retreat from the agreement. Bringing them back to the table tests the mediator's patience. As one party gets cold feet, the other says, "You see, I told you he can't be trusted." The mediator must once again remind them of choices, consequences, and reasonable outcomes. By

the end of this stage, the mediator reiterates the agreement and gains final acceptance.

8. Resolution and implementation. Moving from resolution to actual consummation of the deal is a delicate stage in the mediation. The parties have progressed from their initial adversarial stance and anger to a feasible proposal that offers them some degree of satisfaction and closure. The mediator hopes for more than a mere handshake: the outcome must be one that will endure, an agreement to which the parties will abide. Therefore the agreement should include incentives and a means of enforcement to ensure that each party adheres to its provisions. Often there is limited trust between the parties, so such assurances help build mutual confidence in the agreement. At times it is wise to build in a formal implementation process, to be monitored and executed by an outsider. This outsider could be the mediator or, more likely, some other third party trusted by both sides.

Mediator Activities

There are six streams of activity interwoven throughout the mediation process. (For a further discussion on mediation actions and technique, see Honeyman, 1990, and Honoroff, Matz, and O'Connor, 1990.) In each phase, the mediator simultaneously engages in investigation, empathy, neutrality, managing the interaction, inventiveness, and persuasion.

1. Investigation. The mediator is much like a detective, searching to understand the problem, its history, and the interests and objectives of each side. The mediation process is like piecing together a puzzle, exploring the pieces' different shapes and trying various arrangements in search of the right fit. What could one side offer the other to spur settlement? Were there any key moments or points of misunderstanding that escalated the dispute? What

are each party's interests, and how might they complement one another? In the course of this investigation, the mediator distinguishes truth from exaggeration and falsehood. The better the mediator's insight and understanding, the more likely will he or she be able to move the parties toward a mutually acceptable agreement. Mediation requires a good deal of information gathering, and the mediator searches for and encourages the use of high-quality data: objective information that is verifiable and accepted by both sides.

2. Empathy. In order for the parties to accept the process, they must build a trusting relationship with the mediator. That relationship with the neutral is antecedent to their developing a more trusting relationship with the other parties to the dispute. Key to this building process is confidence that their concerns are acknowledged and understood. The mediator employs active listening to offer tangible assurance, voicing and demonstrating his or her own concern and understanding for the disputants' feelings and emotions. At moments when the parties are overwhelmed by emotions that could derail the process, the empathic listening and assurance of the mediator can keep the negotiations on track. The problem for the mediator is balancing empathy with overidentification, which could compromise perceived impartiality.

3. Neutrality. As discussed above, the parties bring an understandable suspicion of the mediator's neutrality into the mediation process. It is natural for them to test the mediator, closely watching what is said as well as what is implied by body language and voice intonation. The mediator is alert to these tests and slips of confidence in his or her neutrality. Similarly, the mediator is conscious of the fact that pure neutrality is a mix of myth and professional credo: people bring their own biases and history into any dispute. Mediators competently distinguish what they think from what they say and do. The proof is in the outcome.

4. Managing the interaction. The mediator is in charge of what occurs at the mediation table. He or she establishes the rules of

interaction—one person speaks at a time, no one person dominates the discussion, everyone arrives at the session on time—and then enforces compliance by each of the parties. The key to this process is creating an equitable balance of time, concern, and attention. In so doing, the mediator fosters a somewhat level playing field, in which the parties accept that their interests are being fairly represented at the table. Even when the parties are engaging in constructive negotiation on their own, the mediator periodically interjects a comment into the discussion—perhaps to note progress, contribute an observation, or pose a question. Why? The mediator is aware that at any moment, friendly discourse can turn confrontational with one hostile comment. He or she wants to maintain a presence in order to protect the mediation from potentially stumbling down the slippery slope toward dissolution.

5. Inventiveness. Not only must the mediator help the parties develop resolution options which they had not previously considered, he or she must also fashion the process so that the parties feel they are part of the creative endeavor. The mediator wants the parties to own the discovery of ideas and solutions. Rather than merely announce an option, the mediator may lead the parties through a series of questions so that they find solutions on their own. In so doing, the mediator not only takes the party through a new line of thinking, he or she likewise learns a great deal about the background of the dispute and the possibilities for resolution. The mediator is attempting to build compatibility of ideas, proposals, and people in a scenario of significant discord. To do so requires an abundance of creative and imaginative thinking and maneuvers—and patience.

6. Persuasion. The mediator seeks to create movement toward agreement. To do so, the mediator must convince the parties to recognize their predicament. In so doing, they begin to change their attitudes about the other parties and the settlement proposals facing them. The parties, of course, ultimately shape their own choices. The mediator, by definition, is without authority to impose a reso-

lution upon them. He or she encourages the parties to reframe their understanding of the problem and potential common-ground solutions. This is accomplished by clarifying the choices and the consequences that face the parties. There are costs to conflict, measured in wasted time, lost opportunities, and expended resources. The parties are encouraged to honestly weigh these costs against the benefits of settlement. It is this contrast that is the mediator's most effective tool of persuasion. In this process, the mediator persuades by questioning rather than by prescribing. The temptation to advocate an obvious solution—apparent to the mediator and stubbornly refused by the disputants—is a desire that the mediator must constantly resist.

Mediation Forums

The mediator employs a variety of meeting arrangements to conduct the discussions between the parties. The classic image is of the mediator sitting at a table with the disputants evenly distributed on either side. Indeed, the shape of the table, the closed-door atmosphere, the arrangement of the parties, and the placement of the mediator are all carefully orchestrated to illustrate and enhance the principles of mediation: neutrality, a level playing field, confidentiality, privacy, and voluntary participation.

In addition to meetings with all the disputants, the mediator may conduct private sessions with each of the parties. Before mediation begins, the mediator contacts each party to gather information necessary to assess whether mediation is appropriate for the case. During a joint mediation session, the mediator or one of the parties may call for a private caucus. In most cases this refers to a meeting between the mediator and one of the parties. The disputants may also hold private meetings among themselves. Finally, the mediator may engage in shuttle diplomacy, in which he or she separates the parties and then carries information and proposals between their private locations.

Mediators are often flexible with form and format in order to enhance the parties' inclination toward settlement. In most cases the mediator meets with the parties to work together, face-to-face. However, in some cases it is prudent not to bring the parties into the same room: the meeting would so inflame emotions that progress would become impossible. The mediation then becomes a process of shuttle diplomacy. In other cases, the antecedent to an actual meeting is a long procedure that ignores substance in favor of process: the shape of the table, who will be there, the rules of order, and the manner for concluding a settlement. Progress on these matters then prepares the parties for their meetings on substantive matters. Whatever it takes, mediation itself is an adaptive process, molded to facilitate progress toward resolution.

◆　◆　◆　◆　◆　◆　◆

Two years ago, Iris Inkwater established a dispute-resolution committee to handle the range of issues not dealt with by existing hospital procedures. The grievance process for employee complaints had tended to become adversarial, especially when unionized staff were involved. The bioethics committee dealt well with difficult patient-related conflicts; however, it was sometimes approached to resolve other kinds of disagreements simply because no other mechanism existed to address them. Standard management procedures handled most issues smoothly, except, of course, the most difficult. And more disputes than necessary were going to court, including malpractice, medical privileges, and even building contractor disputes.

The dispute-resolution committee was designed to temper the adversarial nature of conflicts, with the hope of helping parties find mutually acceptable solutions. It was composed of seven members: a representative from the medical staff, a representative from the nursing staff, the chief operating officer, the hospital's general counsel, the social work director, a pastoral counselor, and a representative of the unionized staff.

The committee saw its role as that of providing a reasonable forum for people to talk out their differences. Such discussion ideally came at a specific moment in the course of a conflict: at the crossroads just between the vociferous venting of rage and the onset of full-scale war. The committee did not replace existing hospital governance procedures. Rather, it stood alongside them, clarifying the issues and often offering solutions that were much preferred to a reprimand, censure, or dismissal. The key to the process was the active participation of the disputants in expressing, understanding, exploring, and resolving the issues. The role of the committee members was to informally aid this process. Since its inception it had been used for physician privilege disputes, interstaff conflicts, and several management squabbles, to name just a few.

The committee was flexible in how it went about its work. Each of its members had training in dispute resolution. The group met monthly, with special meetings called for specific problems. Its role was not to act as judge. Rather, its purpose was to facilitate and encourage the adoption of a negotiation process acceptable to both sides. At times members met with disputants as informal mediators. At other times the committee would recommend the parties to an outside, formal mediator or arbitrator. Finally, the committee served a counseling function, hearing the particulars of a case and recommending a process for resolving the dispute (though not an outcome). The hospital found that the very presence of such a committee facilitated earlier and more amicable settlements.

Any member could be approached about a dispute, and periodically they each received calls about various issues. Because there was so much general discussion about the Harriford-Cummings case, however, the committee learned about the issue through the grapevine first. It seemed like a natural for the committee's dispute-resolution process.

After a few calls among members of the committee, it was concluded that this issue was quickly growing out of proportion to the initial incident. It had brought to the fore a number of underlying controversies that had been waiting to explode: gender conflict, nurse-physician antagonism, nurse practice divisions, physician practice apprehensions, and the way the hospital does or does not deal with these problems.

The committee decided to attempt to bring Cummings and Harriford together for mediation. The physician on the committee, Larry Lumberg, called Chuck Cummings; Katherine Knight, the nursing staff representative, called Heather Harriford. After a volley of calls between them, it was determined that Lumberg and Knight would meet with Harriford and Cummings to informally mediate a discussion. Both parties were reluctant to accept such a meeting at first. They each agreed after they had taken some time to consider both the offer and the realistic options facing them. They accepted that it would be better to try for a settlement than to allow the matter to escalate further.

They met in one of the small hospital conference rooms not far from the cafeteria. Lumberg and Knight arrived well before Harriford and Cummings. They agreed that it would be best for Katherine to open the session and introduce the process. Larry would discuss the possible outcomes that might emerge.

Cummings arrived first, a few minutes before Harriford quietly walked in and took her seat. Knight and Lumberg greeted them both. Cummings and Harriford shared only icy glances with each other.

Katherine opened the meeting. "First, I want to thank you both for agreeing to meet with us today. As you know, Larry and I spoke with both of you, and you both agreed that it would be best to sit down and discuss this matter privately, together.

"As mediators, Larry and I hope to facilitate a discussion about what happened, what it meant for each of you, and how it might be resolved. Our purpose is not to judge whether one of you is right or wrong. It is up to you to assess what happened and how it might be resolved. Also, what goes on here will remain confidential. Larry and I will discuss your dispute only with each other, and we will report to the dispute-resolution committee only whether or not your dispute was resolved, nothing more. The purpose of this confidentiality is to try to get us away from all the hype, rumors, and gossip that have spread around the hospital regarding this matter." Katherine turned to Larry so he could continue.

"Whether you can come up with a mutually acceptable resolution is up to you," Larry began. "One part of this process is going over what happened, to see if there are any misunderstandings. Another part is exploring what each of you needs in order to move beyond the problem, what you need for yourselves and what you need from each other. Our purpose here is not to smooth over matters that should be addressed. Rather, we hope to encourage an open discussion of issues that are of concern to both of you. Before we begin, do either of you have any questions?"

Chuck shook his head. Heather spoke slowly. "Let's say we can't reach anything through this process. Then what happens?"

"Then the complaint you filed will be reviewed through the normal administrative review procedure. The complaint will be assessed through the medical staff governance process. Your charges will be considered; though, as you know, you will not necessarily find that what they decide meets with your approval. The disposition of the complaint will be their decision, not yours, so you are no longer in the loop at that point. By contrast, if we can come up with something here, you are obviously a part of developing and accepting the solution." Larry finished, and Heather nodded in acknowledgment.

Katherine spoke next. "We like to begin by getting a sense of what happened." She turned to Heather. "Heather, you filed the complaint. Could you tell us what happened and what led you to take this action?"

Heather went through a very matter-of-fact description of the story, describing Mrs. Hayward's condition, her reaction to the morphine, and the touching and pressure she got from Cummings. "It was inappropriate. It was terrible, and I felt violated. He was making an advance while I was trying to ensure that the patient would not get the wrong medication. There is no reason why I should have to put up with that. Actually, there is no reason why anyone here should have to put up with it. He and all his buddies who think this is cool deserve to learn a lesson. This is a hospital, not a bar. We all share responsibility for our patients, and it is not a responsibility that should be taken lightly." She looked straight at Cummings. "This whole thing has been a nightmare for me. I did what I thought was right, and I am being punished for it. It's not fair, it's just not fair."

Kathy turned to Cummings. "Chuck, what is your view of what happened?"

Cummings described a busy and tense evening that had capped a twelve-hour shift. He said the tension was finally beginning to ease when he went into Mrs. Hayward's room. Her family was very upset, though they couldn't stop talking about how much they appreciated Heather. He explained that his intention was to pass along to Heather what they had said. He also wanted to relieve Mrs. Hayward's pain, because it was not only troubling to the patient, it also was very unnerving for the family to see her so uncomfortable. He explained that he only wanted to do well by everyone.

He said he really didn't know about Mrs. Hayward's previous reaction to morphine. There had just been too much going on, and he hadn't had a chance to study her chart. He admitted that he had been wrong, and he said he appreciated Heather's warning him about it.

"The more difficult issue for me," he continued, "is the misunderstanding between Heather and myself. I just meant to be friendly, that's all. I didn't want her to feel uncomfortable about a come-on, or anything. It's not what I intended, and I am afraid that under the fatigue and stress I was feeling, I got carried away."

Heather jumped. "Carried away? I would call that a bit more than carried away!"

Chuck jumped right back. "Look, I didn't feel you up or anything. I was touching your shoulders, that's all. I'm trying to be reasonable here, OK? If you want to rile things up, then this whole thing isn't going to work."

Larry jumped in. "Time out. Let's go back to the facts. Heather, what exactly did Chuck do that you found offensive?"

"Several things. He was rubbing my shoulders as if he were giving me a massage. He was playing with my bra straps. Then he blatantly stared down at my breasts. It was all very suggestive—all while he was ordering me to give the patient inappropriate medication."

Larry waited for Heather to finish. "So, Heather, if I understand correctly, it was the combination of touching, staring, and making suggestive remarks in a context that was very inappropriate. Is that correct?" Heather nodded.

Larry turned to Chuck. "Is that what happened?"

Chuck was quick. "Yes, that's what happened. I think it's fair, though, to consider what didn't happen, especially given all the fuss being made over this. I did not fondle her, rape her, or touch what is not ordinarily considered OK to touch between people who know one another. We're talking shoulders here, nothing more."

Katherine jumped in. "You're right, Chuck, there is a distinction. Nonetheless, even though it was just a shoulder, what makes the difference is how long you touch it, the movement you make while touching, and the context of that touching. Can you see that?"

This time his response was slower. "Yes, I can see that. I just think the punishment should fit the crime."

Heather reacted quickly. "What punishment? You haven't been punished. What's happened to you anyway?"

Chuck looked straight at Heather. "What are you talking about? A physician lives by his reputation. It is as essential as breathing. Whatever happened, and whatever might happen, this whole thing has put an indelible black mark on my reputation. You couldn't think of a worse punishment than that."

"Oh, give me a break." Heather's voice dripped with sarcasm. "What the hell is a reputation? And are you so dense that you didn't know about your reputation among the nursing staff long before the incident between us? Your reputation stinks, Cummings, and you might as well face up to it."

"I'm not talking about my personal reputation, which I can sense is what you are probably referring to. I'm talking about my professional reputation."

Katherine asked the next question. "Chuck, you are making a distinction. What's the difference?"

Chuck turned to Katherine. His voice calmed. "One thing has to do with who I am as a person. Yeah, I've had a reputation since high school of being something of a lady's man. And Heather, you are not the first woman to tell me that I'm a bit too fast. What I'm talking about is my reputation as a doctor. That's what is at stake here for me."

Heather's irritation grew. "How can you see those as separate? You *are* a doctor. That is the responsibility you took upon yourself. Every minute you are in this building, you are a doctor. You can't turn it on and off at your convenience, especially in the middle of talking about a sensitive patient-care issue."

Chuck was quiet. Larry noticed a change in his expression. He spoke into the silence. "Chuck, what's going on for you?"

Chuck looked perplexed. He hesitated. "This whole thing is getting mixed up for me. It seems that we're talking about two separate things, and when they get mixed up is when it gets so complicated."

Heather sensed that he was genuinely struggling. She was feeling a speck of empathy for him. "Do you understand why this upset me so, why what you did was wrong?"

"I think so."

Katherine interrupted. "Chuck, I sense that Heather would find it helpful to hear why you think it was wrong."

He spoke slowly, working to craft each word. "I think I crossed a boundary that is important to her, a boundary I may not have understood." He paused.

Larry coaxed him. "What was that boundary, Chuck?"

"I think Heather felt I was making a sexual overture, and I felt I was just being friendly."

"Just being friendly?" Larry asked.

"Well, maybe more than being friendly. I guess it's important to me that women find me appealing, especially women I find attractive. I was sort of checking out whether there was a spark there. You know, just being innocently flirtatious."

Heather was listening intently. "Maybe if the setting had been different, what you did could have been considered 'innocently flirtatious.' If we were at a party, or at a dance, and you did what you did, I would have turned around and gone for the punch—I mean the drinking kind—if I wasn't interested. Or if I was interested, I would have responded differently, and we might have danced. The problem is, our discussion about Mrs. Hayward was not the prom. We were in the middle of a discussion about a patient and about giving her medication that would have been dangerous for her. You were taking advantage of your position of power as a physician to intimidate me. That's not simple flirtation."

Chuck was looking at the floor, considering and clearly working with what Heather was saying. Heather's words hung in the room, resonating. Katherine and Larry looked at both of them and then glanced at each other, nodding slightly: they would let Heather and Chuck work this next exchange on their own. They did not interrupt.

Finally, Chuck looked up. His expression had turned from docile to hostile. "Fine. So you didn't like what I did. You told me that just when it happened. You could have left it at that and it would have been done with. But you couldn't do that. You had to turn this whole thing into a capital crime. You blew it out of proportion."

"You jerk. And I thought you were beginning to get it!" Heather was biting mad.

Katherine's voice leaped into the middle of the fray. She sensed they were about to go down the slippery slope. She knew it was important for Chuck to express what was on his mind and that Heather's quick attack would cause him to recoil. Because he seemed to have been working on understanding the issues, and because deep down he seemed to be conflicted himself, she wanted to keep him in the process. "One second, Heather. Chuck, what are you saying?"

Chuck took a deep breath. "All I'm saying is that this thing has grown so out of proportion that it's making me sick, OK? I don't think my whole career should be shot down because of this one complaint."

Larry picked up the discussion. "Who said your whole career is being shot down?"

"Well, it's obvious. Because of this complaint, I'm branded. You think that's fair?"

Larry intentionally did not answer his question directly. "Let me tell you what I see. Both of you have a line that can't be crossed, on a matter of great concern to you. Heather, for you the line is on someone making inappropriate sexual overtones at a time when there is a serious patient-care issue being discussed. To do that is unforgivable. Right?"

Heather nodded.

"And Chuck," Larry continued, "having someone threaten your career goes over your line. You feel that if someone has a problem with you, they should let you know about it, not threaten your career with their problem. Does that capture your sentiment?"

"Precisely."

"So, given that, it's hard to respond to what Heather is saying?"

"Yeah, that could be."

Larry turned to Heather. "Heather, is there anything Chuck can do that would satisfy you and, at the same time, assure him that it would not ruin his career?"

There was nearly a minute of silence as Heather thought. "Yes, if he sincerely apologized, and did something, such as taking a class, then I would be willing to drop my complaint. And he would have to convince me that it wouldn't happen again."

"Chuck, is that something you could do?"

He was quick. "Yeah, I'll do anything."

Heather was annoyed with his response. It was too quick. It sounded like he was willing to say anything just to get this matter off his back. Then he could go back to his old ways. "No, it's not 'I'll do anything,'" she said. "I want to know what you'll do specifically."

Chuck was beginning to realize that he wasn't getting it. Heather was looking for something deeper. He knew that he would have to respond on her level, sincerely respond on her level, if there was going to be any movement. He thought to himself that he would have to try harder. "Heather, I am sorry for what I did. Truly sorry. I'm not sure what more to say."

"Actually, there is something more to say. The Multicultural Institute is running a three-evening seminar on gender issues. Would you go?"

"What's involved?"

"Three two-hour sessions. People speak on just the type of issues we've been talking about here. And there is discussion time after the sessions. Would you go?"

"Yeah, I would go. Actually, I think it might help me out. Maybe that, plus I can tone down my libido some." He offered an apologetic smile. Heather nodded back.

"If I do this, there is something I would like in return," Chuck said.

Katherine responded. "What do you want in return?"

"My apology, Heather, is genuine. If I take this class, and if I assure you that I truly have learned a lesson, will you drop the complaint?"

Heather was slow to respond. "Yes, I would drop the complaint."

Larry summarized what had been discussed during the session. Katherine made it very clear what was agreed. She asked Chuck to contact her after he'd attended the class. She would let Heather know that he had complied, and only then would the complaint be formally withdrawn.

That evening, Heather spoke with one of her closest friends about the session. Her friend asked if she felt he had gotten off easy. Heather responded, "On the one hand, yes. On the other hand, if I had pressed the complaint, any mark on his record would have been relatively insignificant in the long run. He wouldn't have learned anything from it. It probably would've just ignited his anger without helping him get beyond it, and that anger would have been more of an obstacle to his changing than anything else. This way, I think the guy really learned something. If I wasn't convinced of that—if I hadn't seen the change in him even in the course of that short meeting—I wouldn't have agreed. He realized something about himself and others that he will carry for the rest of his career. On the chance that he will learn a positive lesson, it was worth the risk to withdraw the complaint."

Heather wasn't absolutely sure she had done the right thing. Nonetheless, both the process and the outcome had left her with a sense of satisfaction. She hadn't destroyed him with her anger. She had done something far more profound.

* * * * * *

Adapting ADR to Health Care Practice

Ideally, differences and disagreements between people involved in the work of health care are resolved before they reach the point where mediation or arbitration is necessary. The premise of this book is to advance resolution of health care disagreements by combining prevention and cure. In this integrated model, interest-based negotiation resolves most matters; mediation and arbitration are used to resolve only those that have escalated. Disputes arising from routine decision making and staff interaction are then seen on a spectrum from low-level matters that can be resolved on the spot to full-scale conflagrations that can benefit from ADR. Disagreements are identified and resolved at the least adversarial and most constructive level possible: the earlier we incorporate constructive resolution, the less likely that disagreements will escalate into costly and unnecessary distraction. Like surgery, ADR should be avoided if less intrusive and less costly options are available. (For a discussion of dispute system design, see Ury, Brett, and Goldberg, 1988, and Slaikeu, 1989.)

Nonetheless, when heated disputes do arise, an easily accessible and pragmatic mediation procedure is a useful and efficient way to bring parties to the negotiation table. These methods can be molded and adapted to fit the particulars of any case. Formal mediators are settlement-oriented, and they naturally adapt their methods to the situation at hand. Health care professionals can likewise adapt informal mediation methods to the unforeseen circumstances that regularly confront them in their practice. Perhaps the greatest attraction of mediation is the consistent inclusion of relevant parties in the dispute-resolution process. By definition, the parties have a voice in the final decision that is reached. The mediator upholds that perspective to ensure that it is reflected in the settlement.

Bioethical disputes offer an illustration (see Dubler and Nimmons, 1992). Bioethicists are caught in somewhat of a professional dilemma. On the one hand, they want to effectively help the parties reach a resolution. On the other hand, they maintain a responsibility to uphold the laws of their jurisdiction as well as general moral principles. What if the parties are considering options that would breach either the law or those principles? Using these laws and principles as the boundaries of what is acceptable, the bioethicist guides the parties through the mediation process. As a result, the parties are often able to find a number of options they hadn't previously considered, all falling within the range of what is legally and morally acceptable. Sometimes *when* a decision is made is at the crux of the issue, and a short delay facilitates agreement. Sometimes *who is involved* in making the decision is the primary point of contention—family members want to know that their concerns are heard. Sometimes the *criteria* used to determine an action are disputed: the bioethicist can help ensure that clinical measures are sensitively used to assess conditions and determine outcomes. The mediation process allows bioethicists to balance their organizational and societal roles while helping the participants resolve what are some of the most wrenching dilemmas faced in health care. The outcome of such efforts is termed "principled settlement"; it defines both the process (mediation) and the outcome—a mutually acceptable and ethically responsible agreement that conforms to both legal requirements and moral principles.

Mediation certainly is not appropriate for the resolution of every dispute. When a fair determination has been made that a decision will be imposed upon one or all of the parties as a function of legal, moral, organizational, or clinical considerations, and when there is no room for negotiation, then mediation is improper. It is fraudulent to even suggest that there is room for discussion when a given decision is foreordained.

A word of caution regarding the use of ADR procedures in

health care: at times the process itself can become unnecessarily ritualized. Since the ADR field has its origins in formal legal settings, the process sometimes assumes an aura of formality, despite its proponents' eschewing the use of restrictive procedural impediments. For the most part, these protocols make perfect pragmatic sense. For example, in order to disclose his or her role and to offer protection from subsequent legal ricochet (when the disputant takes legal action against the neutral), third parties engage a formalized contractual process to inform and protect all parties to the dispute. Certainly, during formal mediation these procedures are necessary and wise. However, as mediation methods are adapted to the unique, informal circumstances of health care disputing, these techniques too must be applied with flexibility.

One important adaptation of ADR to health care is in the matter of organizational or professional learning. Pure ADR is not always instructive or corrective in its orientation. Dispute resolvers measure their success on the basis of a concluded settlement. However, for those involved in the ongoing work of health care, our conflicts are a vital source of invaluable information. Especially when former disputants resume a close working relationship or when someone must return to the circumstances that generated the dispute in the first place, the lessons learned must be incorporated into a reformed practice style and system design. When a practitioner returns to routine patient care following a malpractice case with one patient, when nurses resume collaborative work following a dispute with the medical staff, or when administrators reestablish business ties following a disputed billing issue with a vendor, what follows resolution must be different from what happened before. It is essential to ask, "How can we improve the probability that the same dispute will not recur?" This question becomes a routine aspect of the settlement process, so that systemic learning is one more outcome of resolution. In this way, mediation can be helpful well beyond the culmination of a single dispute.

The term "alternative" in ADR is somewhat of a misnomer, left over from the field's origins in labor relations and law. Mediation and arbitration initially were promoted by reformers as an alternative to litigation, violent altercation, or further escalation. There are those who anticipate that one day, mediation and arbitration will be so widely accepted and practiced that litigation itself becomes the last-resort alternative, used only after all else has been tried and failed. Preferring to preserve the catchy three letters that have become a trademark for the field, some practitioners have renamed the process "appropriate" dispute resolution.

Conclusion

Mediation and arbitration are adaptive processes. They have been used to advance resolution of a wide range of complex issues. (For a critical overview of the applications of mediation, see Kressel and Pruitt, 1989). In each of these applications, ADR has been formed and reformed to fit the circumstances of its new arena. Its entry into the health care field is a relatively recent phenomenon. It is a two-way learning opportunity. Health care has much to learn from dispute resolution, just as DR has much to learn from health care about unique decision-making criteria, conflicts, and implications. In this way, new concepts, techniques, and methods emerge as the processes of dispute resolution adapt to the requirements of the health care field.

As we launch a new forum of utilization, we should continually question the fit of process to problem and outcome. How might we adapt the procedures to better respond to typical health care disputes? What parameters define situations inappropriate for mediation or arbitration? And in what ways can the lessons learned from the disputes we resolve inform us about what we are doing and how we might do it better?

Part V

Whole Image Negotiation

13

• •

Crafting the Essentials

Two fundamental considerations resonate much of the congruity and incongruity of our work in health care: what we do and how we go about doing it (Charns and Tewksbury, 1993). Betwixt them coalesces much of the fact and much of the myth that foment our conflict and build our resolution. What are we trying to accomplish? Are our efforts and investments compatible with those goals? Do our actions and decisions enhance those objectives? Do the answers to these questions fit one another? Do our results and outcomes resonate with what it is we are trying to accomplish? If not, why not?

Generating compatibility amid these dimensions is a vital and compelling process. That compatibility, or the lack thereof, is reflected by the intersecting pieces of the puzzle that comprise our health system. The better-tuned the fit, the better will be our shared objectives and our capacity to achieve them. When purpose and action mesh, we optimize our aggregate capacity. That is what good collaboration is all about (see Susskind and Cruikshank, 1987; Carpenter and Kennedy, 1988; Gray, 1989).

The problem is that for a long time, our health system has been out of balance. What we have been doing—our purpose—has not been clear. How we have gone about doing it—the process—has not been working as well as it could. And there has been only mixed satisfaction with the outcomes we achieve. As a whole, society certainly is clear that they are unhappy with what we cost. The priorities have not been right. And while we are able to dazzle with our new technologies and capabilities, overall health status and statistics do not reflect well upon our accomplishments.

The problem is that the very people responsible for fixing the balance are the same who would benefit or loose by the adjustment of the scale. That is why the imbalance for so long has been tolerated and transfixed. Things, however, are changing. Why? Because it has become generally accepted that those who can create and offer a well-aligned balance are those who will prosper in the emerging health care environment. The people who pay for, receive, monitor, and regulate health care, the "market," are demanding the change. There are tangible choices and clear consequences.

Amid this emerging new balance, negotiation and conflict resolution method offers you a vital toolbox: a reservoir of skills, techniques, and behaviors. Your task is to contribute to this process of defining, redefining, and refining the balance. In so doing, you foster fundamental understanding, cultivate pragmatic concurrence, and generate the necessary collaboration to make the system work. You understand others better. You are able to help them better understand you. And you are able to engage one another in a manner that is mutually beneficial.

Negotiation and conflict resolution method, however, is only method if practiced without purpose. Like the adept aircraft pilot, you may be able to fly the plane; however, if you don't know where you are going, chances are you are not going to get there. Or even worse, you might take the passengers to a destination where they don't want to be. The human and financial stakes are too high in health care to tolerate mindless wandering.

Some might presume this process of grappling with purpose is merely in the domain of legislative policymakers, corporate leaders, and major purchasers of health services. Not so in health care. Because of the close interpersonal nature of our work, this theme implicitly is manifest in every interaction between coworkers, patients, and providers, and the many organizations and departments whose work must be orchestrated. Defining purpose is an interactive process that spans all levels, from you as an individual to the web of countless individuals who comprise the system.

How do we understand and align our different perspectives, expertise, and values? How do we synthesize motives, incentives, and actions? How do we make for good health and for good health care?

What We Do

The work of health care embodies circumstances, choices, decisions, and consequences.

Those *circumstances* blend the needs of patients and populations, the considerations of professionals and policymakers, along with the ambiguous mystery that defines what is wellness and illness. It is this changing context in which we practice: the macrocosm never remains the same. Emerging discoveries, new diseases, innovative treatments, changing political winds, and redefined business calculations shape the shifting domains of our work.

Though health care rests upon the world of science, its endeavors dwell in the realm of the human. It is from this intersection that our range of *choices* emanates. Those choices derive not only from what is fact. Perception, preference, and philosophy too infuse what is acceptable to one person and what is reprehensible to another: a surgical or nonsurgical treatment? the purchase of equipment or the provision of vaccines? the appropriateness of a physician or the substitution of a physician assistant? As long as we respect that right to exercise choice, a range of expectation will always be with us. That range of choices must be assessed, weighed, balanced, and counterbalanced until the parties are ready to decide.

Decisions and *actions* are the substance of what health care does and does not do. They are the programs we implement, the people we hire, the treatments we administer, the administrative moves we make, and the human attentiveness we render. It is that to which we commit and for which we are responsible and accountable. What we do is a measure of our compassion, tenacity, values, and vision.

Consequences are what we produce. Because we work in the most vital and intimate of human endeavors, that achievement is measured for each individual patient as well as for society as a whole. Our challenge is to correctly balance the needs of each individual, whether as patient or staff, with the needs of the whole, whether professional group, organization, or populace. If we have successfully treated the few at the expense of the many, have we accomplished our purpose? And yet, if we abandon the few in favor of the many, have we justly allocated our capacity for producing well-being? Have we used our know-how and resources to best achieve healthy people and a healthy society?

Circumstance, choices, decisions, and consequences hang in a fluctuating balance. They each shift and then shift one another. When circumstances change, so too do the range of choices available to parties charged with reaching decisions: when patterns of service reimbursement are adjusted, so too must the inventory of service options be altered to ensure a workable flow of patients. If certain outcomes are no longer deemed acceptable, then choices must be reassessed to chart a course that reaches the desired objectives: mortality rates outside the range of acceptable for a treatment protocol, for a particular provider, or for an entire institution are the cue for corrective action. As each of these factors resonates with one another, we contemplate whether to be proactive or just reactive in formulating choices and decisions or in shaping outside circumstances and consequences.

What are the unique dynamics that influence these four factors in health care? How do we ensure that we are calculating correctly? What are the checks and balances to guarantee that we do not swing too far in one direction or another? How do we in health care appraise whether "what we do" is judicious?

The Essential and the Expendable

Health care occupies the domain of the essential. "Essential" frames how we align our priorities, assess our progress, and plot our game plan. It is essential that the orthopedic surgical suite have the optimum air filtration system, *or else* patients' prostheses will become postoperatively infected. It is essential that lead be removed from the homes of young children, *or else* they risk neurological dysfunction and severe developmental impediments. It is essential that nurse-to-patient ratios be maintained, *or else* patient care will be compromised.

We live in a society that places considerable value on life and the quality of that life: virtue demands that we do what is necessary to enhance survival. We also live in a society with the technical capability to significantly extend and enrich life. Death, in the hands of our machines, has been transformed from a natural event to a conscious and calculated choice. And we live in a society that expects perfection. When that perfection is not achieved, those responsible live in apprehension of the retribution and legal actions likely to follow.

Because of these values, capabilities, and expectations, much of our work in health care is placed in the category of "essential." The risks of overlooking a serious medical condition can be so ominous that we are careful not to be indifferent about anything for which we are responsible. As a dictum of professional and organizational survival, diagnostic tests, medical procedures, safety precautions, and legal protections are transformed into the essential. Given the circumstances, choices, and consequences, prostate cancer screening, tobacco cessation initiatives, cesarian sections, and infection control protocols all arguably are placed in the category of essential. Our decisions are framed foremost by the compulsion to promote and preserve life.

The converse side of essentialness is expendability. If we are not essential to the system, as a provider, administrator, or patient, then we can be expended in the rush to efficiency. The community out-reach program can be closed, because it is expendable. The nurse can be fired, because she is extraneous. The evening clinic can be curtailed, because it is unnecessary. Programs, people, and services can be discarded when they are no longer deemed essential.

There is nothing more professionally disenfranchising than being told you are expendable. The message can come in a number of shapes: the pink slip informing you of your dismissal, the sub-poena alerting you to an impending lawsuit, the announcement advising you and your department that it is being closed. To be informed of your expendability is to be told that you no longer belong and that your services are no longer necessary. Your past training and preparation are meaningless, and your professional future is in doubt.

The very peril of expendability strikes a chord of vulnerability. When *we* are the patient, we fear that those caring for us will ignore our needs because of our insignificance, omit necessary procedures because of their expense, and disregard telling symptoms because of other distractions. For patients, the apprehension of entering the depersonalized expanse of a large institution is the possible loss of individuality and the very identity that makes them essential.

While expendability is, at face value, ominous and offensive, there are times when it can be judicious and humane. Accepting or even asserting expendability at the appropriate time and under the legitimate circumstances is a vital principle of endurance, progress, and purpose.

Certainly, for patients, there is a time to let go—to let nature take its course. For the terminally ill patient whose condition is hopeless, when is it appropriate to shift from the essentialness of survival and care to the expendability of life and treatment? How do we balance appropriate intervention with a fair use of resources? When is it "too soon" to discontinue care, and when has it gone on far "too long?" In spite of our splendid technology and sincere inten-

tions, life itself is a terminal condition. The delusion that our clinical intervention can overcome death itself skews the necessary balance of task and purpose.

Similarly, for those who guide and administer the health system,
there is the balance between life and the quality of life on the one
hand, the "essence" of services and programs, with the bounded
resources society is willing to supply, or to "expend," on the other
hand. We know that to ignore the health needs of a population—
the poor, children, minorities, immigrants—is to render them
expendable. The landscape of human history reveals the many
groups who have been rendered expendable, either by acts of commission or by way of omission. If now, when we have the life-
giving technology and capacity and are unwilling to share it, are we
not doing the same? How do we select among the choices? As
responsible decision makers, we are compelled to reconcile priorities when we cannot do it all.

◆ ◆ ◆ ◆ ◆ ◆ ◆

As do most nurses on the evening shift, Heather Harriford parks
her car in the off-site parking lot and takes the shuttle to the
hospital. She was sitting way back on the left side of the van,
staring vacantly out the window as it slowly made its way about
the lot, picking up employees. From the corner of her eye, she
noticed Gail Godfried make her way up the stairs. She paid no
attention and was content to be alone.

She suddenly felt someone taking the place beside her. She
turned to see Gail, looking timidly in her direction. They hadn't
spoken since Heather left the intensive care unit. There was
none of the small talk that usually opens a conversation: it was
as if Gail were holding something she needed to get off her mind
right away. "I just wanted you to know how much I admire
what you did with Cummings," she said. "There are a lot of
nurses who think your making a stink was a bad idea. It took a
lot of guts. Most people would have just put up with it. You
need to know that I really respect you for what you did."

Gail finished her speech and sat back in the seat. The sentiment weighed heavily upon her, and now that it was out, she relaxed. She had felt guilty in the past about not protesting when the same thing had happened to her. She felt a comforting sense of atonement in lending encouragement to someone who did.

Heather sensed Gail's confusion and wasn't sure how to respond. She retreated to what felt safe. "Thanks a lot." It was a nothing statement. What was Gail trying to express?

Gail felt Heather's discomfort. She wanted to explain. "I know that you and I haven't always seen eye to eye in the past. Sometimes it felt like we came from different planets, you know, very different approaches to what we do and how we go about doing it. I guess I just wrote you off—even worse, became annoyed with you, really. I just thought many times you had too much of, what do they call it, 'chutzpah,' saying what was on your mind and going against the grain.

"And then when this whole affair with Dr. Cummings happened—I mean this whole issue—well, it was that same boldness that let you stand up to him and his kind. Maybe you needed that self-confidence in order to handle it the way you did. I don't know how many times I was in your shoes, with the same thing happening to me. You know, you put up with things. Or you play games to get what you need to get. And then afterwards, even if nothing really terrible happened, you still feel cheapened, like you were used. So to see someone stand up and say 'Hell no,' why that gets a lot of admiration in my book." Gail was smiling a sense of victory. It took guts for her to make even that admission. And she had said it. She felt good about herself.

Heather smiled back. "I really appreciate your saying this. I can't tell you how much self-doubt I've been feeling about this whole thing. I mean, on the one hand, you're right, I did the right thing and I'm glad I did it. Some of the nurses have been great, supporting me and everything. Then, on the other hand, there have been a lot of people who came out against me. I guess it's just human nature that you hear those voices the loudest, because they speak to your own sense of uncertainty. It's scary bucking the system, going against one of those gospels of good nursing behavior." She paused. She hadn't expressed all these feelings to anyone. And now to open up to, of all people, Gail Godfried. Maybe it was fitting, because she had assumed Gail was one of those silent majority types who were gabbing the loudest against her.

Heather continued. "I guess a lot of things flash through your mind when something like this happens. You get really practical. I have rent and my student loans to pay. What if I lose my job? How might this affect my getting into school again? And what would my family think? Courage is a great thing as long as everything works out OK in the end. It just gets rough when there is no guarantee of a happy ending.

"So, I'm glad we were able to settle this thing. My feeling of self-respect and self-confidence is coming back. You're right, it took a lot of guts. Even as I was going through it, it felt like I was watching a movie about somebody else. And I think in the long run that it was even a good thing for Cummings. He wasn't mortally damaged, and actually, he would have gotten hit by this behavior eventually. He's just lucky that it hit him here and now. I realized that. He's a good doctor and he really cares about his patients. He learned his lesson and he'll go on. There was no need to cut off his . . . I mean, you know what I mean." Gail nodded, smiling. "Anyway, I guess it all worked out in the end. I appreciate your saying this to me. The world sends you such mixed signals. It's nice to be reassured sometimes."

Gail realized that her support for Heather was far more important than she had ever imagined. She wanted to make the point very clear. "Heather, you taught me an important lesson about speaking out. If you don't have the backbone to state your mind, then the world does in fact become lopsided." She gestured the movement of a balance up and down with her hands. "That piece of what we have to offer simply is not on the scale if we don't express it. So part of our obligation is speaking out. The question should not be whether we do it. The question is how we do it, and when and to whom. Somehow, Heather, you got it right. I admire you for that."

As it stopped in front of the hospital, the brakes of the van squeaked, punctuating Gail's last comment. The two quietly made their way down the narrow aisle and into the hospital lobby. Before going their separate ways, they hugged each other. Gail whispered to Heather, "You should feel very good about yourself."

Heather whispered back, "Thanks a lot. I needed that."

* * * * * * *

Fluid Purpose

The health care opportunities and constraints we devise translate into services for people and employment for professionals. Priorities are manifest in the buildings we construct, the people we employ, the programs we offer, the machines we buy, the medications we administer, as well as how much we are willing to expend on each. These priorities define the context and circumstances of our work. As they change, so too do our responsibilities, and with them, our choices and decisions.

For those who work in the system, import and opportunity ascend and descend with the shifting tides that define what is considered essential and what is deemed expendable. Specialty care descends as primary care rises, and trailblazing nursing and medical schools change their curriculum to stay ahead of the currents. Hospitalization recedes as outpatient care thrives, and responsive institutions close beds and open ambulatory care clinics with attached home care services. Integrated networks expand as solo practice fades, and providers band together to negotiate a place for themselves in the system. As primary care, deinstitutionalization, and integrated networks become essential, aspects of specialty service, hospital care, and solo practice become expendable. Fewer people are needed, which means that some people are not needed at all.

We each are an extension of the essentialness of what we do and what we offer. Our importance derives from the significance of our tasks, skills, and knowledge. Our worth derives from the value of our contribution, both professionally and personally. At a time when services, priorities, and expenditures are at the center of the health care debate, the question of essentialness then becomes a matter of great personal as well as professional import. Will I have a job in this new system? Are my work and skills recognized and valued? Will my own professional values and personal goals fit the emerging health care contours? How do I measure up among the others who champion their own essentialness? Will the verdict be made simply on the basis of power? Or will purpose and product also be legitimate items on the table?

Expendability and essentialness speak to our most fundamental interests as caregivers. They motivate our career aspirations and form the substance of what we each hope to accomplish with our work. They speak to our membership in a community of caregivers and patients who hopefully will benefit from our endeavors. They are at the heart of much of what we negotiate in our day-to-day endeavors.

How do we craft a workable system to adjust this balance between the essential and the expendable so that the very process does not distort the fundamental question of what we do and why? How can we inspire circumstances, choices, decisions, and consequences that are just, principled, and fair so that the product is worthy of the effort? And how can we be confident that the end results, our accomplishments, reflect well upon our person, our community, and our society?

Recrafting the Puzzle

This paradox between what is essential and what is expendable is the pivotal conflict of health care. At times, it is a source for the creative tension that explores new and innovative ideas, that seeks more effective methodologies and treatments, and that constructs more efficient relationships and systems. Conversely, this paradox can be the crux of spiteful infighting that pits one group against another, that exploits the legitimate interests of patients, and that compromises the basic purposes of health care in the process. It speaks to how much the public and private sectors are willing to invest into basic research versus direct service. It was an unspoken torment of the early debates about response to the AIDS epidemic. It is at the center of deliberation on infant mortality policy, violence prevention efforts, and what to do about the rising cost of health care.

This distinction, between creative tension and bitter infighting, is often reflected in the tone of negotiation. Are the parties flexible, ready to express and recognize the range of legitimate concerns represented at the table? Or are they rigid, distancing themselves from one another in pursuit of narrow objectives? Whole image negotiation or positional confrontation?

Whole image negotiation is more likely to occur when the parties honor each other's essentialness. The operative premise is that my essentialness is not a function of your expendability. The intent of negotiation is not to dominate the pie or merely divide it up. Rather, the purpose is to find a way to understand, reshape, and expand it. Implied in this search for constructive options is respect for the essentialness of both sides. That understanding accepts that we will have our differences. There is only scant concern that those differences will be exploited by one side to destroy the other.

However, if the negotiation becomes a struggle that equates one party's essentialness to the other's expendability, then the interchange is likely to become positional. Each of the participants believes that whoever dominates the process will determine the outcome. The struggle for control assumes the very urgency of survival itself. Groups seek to verify their position by contriving clear measures of their own ascendance and the others' downfall. They each believe their sustainability depends upon the eventual failure or vulnerability of the other.

At a time of significant change in the health system, when the very premises, people, and purpose of our work is open to question, the sensation of vulnerability rises. With the underlying topic of discussion revolving around who and what is essential and who and what is expendable, it is conceivable that everyone will implore his or her own security. Leaping to the assumption of vulnerability, parties presuppose a positional posture, turning the process into a lurid scene of destruction and defeat.

The system becomes mired in confrontation. How can this be turned around?

The key is negotiation purpose. If the parties intend to constructively build and rebuild the puzzle of which they are a part, then the ongoing, productive process facilitates the necessary and constant analysis, adjustment, and reconfiguration. They negotiate the size and shape of the pieces so they better fit and better formulate the image they seek. Rather than a contest, their context is one of collaboration. The focus is not how can I defeat you. Rather the question is how can I balance what I am doing, and what I consider essential, with what you are doing and what you consider essential. Flexibility reigns as the parties focus more on fixing the problem than on fortifying their position.

At times, successfully renegotiating the puzzle means not only reconfiguring the existing pieces, it also requires opening the picture to new players and new ideas. This is a fundamental aspect of rebuilding into a system that is more responsive and more effective. And with these new players at the table, it is vital that their involvement affords them valid participation in the process. It may mean including nurses in medical forums from which they have been excluded, patients in planning processes where they were considered unnecessary, and physicians in administrative sessions in which they were the object of and not a participant in the deliberations. These new players, forums, and ideas embody a new recognition with beneficial returns for those who take part. It is not simply a matter of one side relinquishing and the other intercepting the power: it is not winners and losers. Rather, it is a process of enhancing overall potency for resolving the daily predicaments of health care.

At other times, building new options means closing old ones. The expendability of programs, personnel, or participation must be considerately conceded and honorably conducted. It is not that I won and you lost. Insofar as we are on the same boat, your loss is mine as it is yours. Nonetheless, the consequences I feel, staying here while you leave, cannot be compared to your loss of a job, program, or professional dignity. When this occurs within an organization, it is a painful process. When this pain is fearfully avoided rather than tactfully managed, it can erupt into a tempest of new problems. How so?

Often disregarded is the public nature of expendability. When the reconfigured puzzle requires the retention of some staff and the ouster of others, everybody watches. When one person or program becomes expendable, every person or program becomes vulnerable. They watch how the situation was handled. What led to the action? Were the criteria just? Was the process fair? In order to justify the action, were some people transformed into "the enemy"? A clear message is dispatched. Is it one that eases the process of putting the pieces back together? Or is it one that only heightens uncertainty and turmoil? Is the signal "fight dirty or lose"? Or is it one of fairness and beneficence?

We all pendulate in this precarious balance between essential and expendable. It is the nature of our work in health care. It defines our own job security. From it we derive the satisfaction and hope that we anticipated when we chose our career. Whether it is a constructive and creative process depends on how we play the game.

As we recraft the puzzle, some pieces change shape. New pieces are added. Some are discarded. It is a process that is at once fragile, precarious, and rewarding. How do you structure the process so that what we get on the other side is worthy of the effort?

* * * * * * *

The hallways teemed with their usual midday bustle. When Larry Lumberg and Fred Fisher converged in the crowded first-floor corridor that was the architectural backbone of the hospital, they both instinctively knew where the other was going: lunch.

Fisher's greeting was uncharacteristically enthusiastic. Lumberg responded, "You're looking in a chipper mood today, Dr. Fisher."

"You could say that." Fisher smiled and opened the door to the stairways that led down to the cafeteria and the physicians' dining room.

Lumberg decided to have some fun with his longtime colleague and mentor. "Don't tell me, you won the lottery?" Fisher shook his head and smiled. "I know, your daughter had another baby." Fisher's smile grew, and he again shook his head. They reached the end of the cafeteria line, and Fisher handed Lumberg a tray before taking one for himself.

Finally, Fisher broke his silence. "Two good guesses, Larry, though the second would have required Karen to give birth twice in a five-month period."

Fisher continued. "You know how you can wake up one day and see things slightly differently? Well, this was one of those days. I'm not sure exactly what provoked it. Maybe it was that meeting a few days ago, or this whole thing with the change in reimbursement, or that community health initiative meeting I went to. A few articles I've been reading maybe. I'm not sure exactly." Fisher placed the plate of limp green beans, dreary mashed potatoes, and overcooked chicken on his tray. It's remarkable what gastronomical insults he put up with just for the pleasure of having lunch surrounded by his colleagues.

"You know, Larry, sometimes we get caught up with our own baloney. We create illusions and hide behind them. And then one day, you wake up and realize that they were just illusions.

We're not what we made ourselves out to be. We didn't accomplish all the miracles we claimed to accomplish. And we got taken with ourselves and who we are and what we do."

The small bowl of bright red Jello cubes shook as Lumberg placed them on his tray. He looked over to Fisher. "Fred, what are you talking about?" Lumberg had a hunch. He just couldn't believe these words were coming from a man devoted for so long to just the opposite sentiments.

They waited at the end of the line to pay for their meals. "You know, Larry, we have fashioned such a complicated set of myths to insulate us. We appear to be one thing when we are something very different. We are far more secure in the myths we have created than in the reality of what we do."

They paid for their meals and took their place in the doctors' dining room, at the far end of one of the long tables. They sat across from one another, deep in conversation, emitting an unspoken message that they were not to be disturbed.

Fisher continued, almost excited to get his newfound thoughts out. "I became intrigued with figuring out exactly what we do, stripped of all that myth."

Lumberg prodded Fisher along. "So, what did you come up with?"

Fisher smiled. "You know I was a philosophy minor in college? I'm much better for questions than I am for answers."

Lumberg was quick on the return. "So what are the questions?"

"I think they're about patient care. Not necessarily the care we give patients, rather about the care patients need. They are not always one and the same. And then I think of this complex roller coaster we have placed that simple chariot upon. There is a certain simplicity to keeping people well and healing them in sickness. That is what we are supposed to be about. And yet we have created such a complex maze in which to make that happen, it's as if we forgot what we are doing and where we are going." He paused for a moment to consider the thought. "You know, Larry, trains get someplace. Roller coasters, for all their jiggling around, never get you anywhere: it's a lot of push and pull and up and down. Ultimately, though, you just go around in circles. You think a lot has happened because you are so sick to your stomach. And yet, you haven't made any genuine progress.

"I was reading about this information revolution that we're in the midst of. With just a bit of imagination, tinged with reality, I realized that the impact on medicine could be as significant as the discovery of anesthesia. Machines will soon be able to possess and manage more information more accurately than we physicians could ever hope to. And when those machines are hooked up to robots, their precision in the operating room will so surpass the work of our shaky fingers, that what we are today will soon become as obsolete as the model T.

"So what is left for people like you and me? Yes, we can learn the technicalities of interfacing with all this hardware. In the long run, though, that's a defined set of skills that will fluctuate with the introduction of each new invention. And there will be an army of technicians trained to do just that.

"What about the art of medicine? What will be left of that? There I think of the human dimension, which no computer can replicate. Oddly enough, that is what we have so abandoned in our pursuit of our own myths. We constructed our own pedestal and then reigned upon it. And the machines, and the cost efficiency, and the tough scrutiny of our society are together dismantling that pedestal. So what is left?

"The art of medicine derives from the synthesis of the human dimensions of our work. That synthesis, based on human understanding, relationships, and wisdom, we have turned away from. It's time we get back to those basics, understand them for what they are, and come out from the wizard's room, where we have concocted miracles that were in large part illusion. Do you remember the Wizard of Oz?"

Lumberg nodded as Fisher continued.

"There is something very genuine about the practice of medicine. I've been burning out, like so many of our colleagues, because I lost that core value. It's time we honestly assess what we do, and do it well. If we don't, we will be discovered and judged for what we are. And society won't put up with it."

Larry asked, "So, Fred, what are we, then?"

"It's not what we are, Larry. It's what we are becoming. It is a process of change. And if we manage that process correctly, then we will have a productive and satisfying place in whatever health care is becoming. And if we cannot adapt, then we will be like the dinosaurs. We will become extinct, replaced by technocrats who do not have the understanding or compassion that is at the heart of good medicine. Medicine can thrive alongside all the machines and efficiencies that are emerging. It just has to be a different kind of medicine. And most of the people who talk about it today only see it as a bad thing. It will be bad only if we let it become bad."

"This doesn't sound like the same Fred Fisher who was complaining the other night about becoming an insurance company."

"Oh, it is the same Fred Fisher. The only difference is one of perspective. I responded to the business aspects of the arrangement. Think of the medical aspects. I am being paid to keep people healthy. If I succeed, my patients benefit, I benefit, and the insurance company benefits. Now, I might not like all the business aspects of the arrangement. Yet, the core of my job is keeping people healthy. If the business office can handle the administrative aspects, and if I have the wherewithal to do my job well, then I am willing to give it a try. And if it doesn't work, let's constructively go back to the drawing board. Not to whine. We go back to refine. Big difference of attitude."

The conversation continued through the end of lunch. They talked about the specifics, the politics, and the costs of change. They pondered their own careers and how their difference in age so colored their experiences and expectations. When they finally finished their meal, they picked up their trays and headed for the conveyor belt that would return their dishes to the inner dens of the kitchen.

The stale taste of the hospital carrot cake still lingered in Fisher's mouth. "You know, Larry, it's like this hospital food. It hasn't improved much in the many years I've been here. One day, we have to be wise enough to stand up and say we don't like it. And hospital administration needs to be wise enough to hear us."

Lumberg quipped back. "Or else, we all might realize the gastronomic deception. This has been feed posing as food."

They wished each other a good afternoon and parted ways, each going toward different hallways. As Lumberg left, he realized for the first time that the two were somehow headed in a synchronous direction. He just felt more uncertain than ever before what was their destination.

He also felt a renewed sense of self-confidence.

◆ ◆ ◆ ◆ ◆ ◆ ◆

Adapting Purpose and Process to Product

We strive for fit.

That our purpose fits what our surroundings expect: those expectations as directly expressed to us by patients, staff, or colleagues. Resonance of purpose occurs when our personal direction corresponds with that of our surroundings. *That the choices available to us match those expectations:* so we have the capacity and means to select among feasible options. Legitimate choice occurs when we have the time, resources, and competence to do the job well. *That our decisions reflect our purpose:* our values and capabilities match the task. When the job is well done, the satisfaction is mutual. *That we have made a meaningful contribution for which we are appropriately rewarded:* our work is part of an exchange for which we are fairly compensated.

That the process of creating fit abets our purpose: so that our shared understanding and interpretation of circumstances, choices, decisions, and consequences are symbiotic. We negotiate and resolve our differences in a constructive manner. *That this process helps us better assess our choices and collaboratively reach our decisions:* we invest in the collaboration because our essentialness is recognized and honored. *That good process yields more good process based upon meaningful participation:* success begets more success.

That what we spend returns a positive sum back to society: our efforts are recognized and duly rewarded. *That our priorities are sound and decisions judicious:* there is synchrony of expectation and product. *And that the consequences we reap in turn benefit society and offer us a sense of personal achievement:* our own purpose and product coincide.

"Fit" reflects what we do personally and what we do as a system. You personally reflect that picture when you speak and react to others. When you inform a patient that a procedure is not covered by insurance, when you commend the work of a colleague, when you authorize the purchase of new equipment—for these people, what you say and do formulates their experience with the "system." Each individual is part of a larger whole, affecting that whole and being affected by it.

Just as a picture emerges when the pieces of the puzzle are placed together, our combined work in health care creates a picture. It is the process we use to configure those pieces that will determine what picture will emerge.

Renegotiating the Balance

Compare two premises of negotiation: dichotomous thinking and balanced-integrated thinking.

Using dichotomous thinking, it is either yours *or* mine: the notion of sharing is incompatible with this line of reasoning. Situations are clearly right *or* wrong: the possibility that truth may lie someplace in the middle is logically incongruous. People and services are either essential *or* expendable, and unambiguous lines define the distinction.

By contrast, balanced-integrated thinking affirms that ideas, skills, and expertise are naturally combined and adjusted in order to function: the care of a patient involves clinical as well as contextual and reimbursement matters. In most cases, when a question has become polarized, the answer can be found someplace in between the extremes. And as situations change, what might have been true yesterday is no longer so today.

Because dichotomous thinkers have only two choices, they always advocate that which is in their best interest. Since ownership is "yours or mine," they advocate to control as much as possible. Since there is only a "right and wrong," they always argue the rightness of their position. Because everything they do is essential, their concerns are important while those of others are trivial.

Balanced thinkers pursue shared interests, their own as well as those of others. Since they are part of a larger picture, they are amenable to sharing control with others. And since they grasp that no one person can be the repository of complete knowledge and expertise, they are simultaneously student and teacher, actively learning just as they are informing. They respect the disparities between their view of what is essential and expendable and that of others.

And lest, in the course of making this distinction I make the very same error: yes! There is a time for dichotomous thinking, just as there is a time for balanced thinking.

So what is the point?

Simply that as we renegotiate health care, we change not only what is on the table, we also change how we go about negotiating that substance. Product can only be as good as process.

For years, health care has been dominated by dichotomous thinking. While this line of reasoning has benefitted some, overall it has led us into many of our current health care conundrums. The system is out of balance not because we don't have the knowledge, the expertise, or even the good will to make it work. It is not for lack of money that so many people are without care: we spend enough to be able to take care of everyone in our country. Rather, the system is out of balance because of the premises and processes we have used to construct it.

The current climate of change offers an opportunity to generate a new congruence among the many services, staff, and resources that comprise health care. In order to reliably frame a new arrangement, the method must be compatible with the task.

As a collection of people working in the health care arena, our aspiration is to weave a constructive balance that cultivates health in a socially responsible manner. To do so, we together formulate the picture, the image, that we hope to achieve. It is not your picture; it is not my picture; it is our picture, with mutual investments, pursuits, and rewards. This template for thinking pertains to the particular relationship between a doctor and a patient, just as it does the broader interplay between policymakers and professional groups, administrators and providers, insurers and service systems, and nurses and other nurses. Our inevitable interdependence requires that we move in a congruent direction if we are to get anywhere.

Since we are each one piece of a larger vista, the whole, then it is a matter of fitting the exchange, the give-and-get of our own negotiations, into some larger blueprint. The more trying task in melding together a puzzle is not merely getting all the right pieces on the table. Rather, the primary burden is tailoring those many pieces so that they fit together. And the task is all the more elusive in an emerging health system in which there is no box cover, no existing, exhaustively studied model, to guide our efforts. We are crafting this design as we go. We know that some of our precedents are valuable and should be retained. Likewise, we know that many need alteration. And it is those that need adjustment that are most resistant to finding their new place in this germinating design. That is why this process is so difficult, and why it is so wrought with conflict.

Balanced-integrated thinking is a puzzle-making process. It is not a matter of finding the winner or loser, it is a matter of uncovering the right combination of pieces to make the system work. Changes are deliberated. Ideas and people are reconciled and arranged to mold the best fit between purpose and product. And since changes in circumstance offer different choices that must be accommodated by new decisions, adjusted expectations, and different consequences, the process of balanced thinking becomes simply a means to an ever-fluctuating end.

Balanced-integrated work requires a constant negotiation and a good deal of conflict resolution. It is not the path of least resistance. However, it is the means toward achieving the most profound pay-offs. Clinical understanding combined with administrative know-how enhances effectiveness without compromising efficiency. Nurses are not an appendage to doctors: they are a different set of eyes, understanding, and skills. When combined with those of the physician, they offer a more comprehensive view and more effective treatment for the patient. Similarly, doctors are not an obstacle to good nursing: though not ever-present, the presence, knowledge, and authority of physicians are important pieces of holistic health care. We move beyond dichotomous enemy images of one another to realize complementary purpose and product.

Balanced and integrated thinking not only mixes different professions, organizations and people; very importantly, during a period of change it also combines the old with the new. This is especially important during a time of change. It does not discard the past in its pursuit of fresh ideas and innovations. Tested ways and experiences blended with novel circumstances offer opportunities for trailblazing ingenuity based upon solid reasoning and wise interpretation. Large-scale managed care operations that fuse administrative efficiency with the intimacy of a personal doctor's office will enhance the practice and experience of both patient and physician. Health programs that emphasize prevention and primary care while offering appropriate access to specialty treatment assure the provider, patient, and payor that a fair mix of services are available and accessible. Public health initiatives that address newly recognized "hot" issues, such as smoking cessation and AIDS prevention, while not abandoning past "hot" topics, such as teenage pregnancy and substance abuse, comprehend that many of these problems are intertwined, affecting the same populations and lending themselves to integrated solutions. In our rush to embrace the new, it would be imprudent to abandon what is vital and practical from the past.

To accomplish this balance of pragmatic and pioneering, people and professions, essential and expendable, we negotiate on the basis of our interests. The process requires you to grasp well the frame you bring to the table. Likewise, you are challenged to discern the frames of others. And as you engage in this exercise of informing and understanding, you reach a deeper understanding of your place in the picture, as well as that of others.

To the extent that you can remain flexible, your ability to spawn new and dynamic endeavors is propelled. What is the importance of flexibility?

Just as interests and framing are important, it is the interactive process of reframing that shapes differences and commonalties into new opportunities. These resourceful perspectives spring from the composite frames that emerge from your collaborative efforts: the essence of balanced and integrated thinking. The view you take from the table is changed by the process. The reframe is the output, the product: your combined road map for what it is you want to achieve. And as such, it is in constant flux, adapting with time to the new weights and winds of a changing health care system.

Whole image negotiation fits the challenges of assembling the pieces of a health care system. It is a vehicle for moving us from dichotomous thinking toward balanced, integrated, and collaborative achievement. It is a solution-based method for helping us constructively guide one another in distinguishing what is essential from what is expendable.

Similarly, mediation fits the process for resolving the disputes we encounter along the way. Mediation offers a fulcrum: someplace to articulate our differences and find what lies in between. It is settlement-oriented and helps us move beyond those differences to a balanced closure of our conflicts.

So what is it that we will achieve if we bring our system into better balance?

◆　◆　◆　◆　◆　◆　◆

The hostilities between the health maintenance organizations and the two major hospitals in town reached a deafening roar. The antipathy between the Oppidania Medical Center (OMC)

and the Community Health Plan (CHP) obviated any talks
between them. Likewise, the people at the Urbania Medical
Center (UMC) were riled at CHP for dropping a humiliating
and unwarranted public relations nightmare on their doorstep.
The time-worn rivalry between OMC and UMC was ignited by
the uproar. Urbania was resentful of Oppidania's status and
recognition, and now disdained their foe even more; OMC's
stance of superiority was only bolstered by the negative press
their competitor attracted. Everyone seemed to despise Arena
Health Plan's (AHP) opportunism, as they exploited the disar-
ray and anxiety of the situation to bolster their own market
share.

The predicament, of course, was that no one was in charge
of health care. The federal, state, and municipal agencies that
followed the skirmishes quietly conceded that the standoff presented a political catch-22. In the public's eye, anyone who got
involved would assume responsibility for the issues, though they
wouldn't necessarily have the authority to fix them. The bureau-
crats presumed that the hospital and HMO leaders, with their
greater salaries and perks, always considered themselves superior to the heads of public agencies and therefore would be reticent to heed governmental input on the matter.

Mayor Willie Wynn was aware of the political pitfalls of the
situation. He summoned his public health commissioner, Manuel
Mendez, to assess the situation. Would it be possible to arrange
a private meeting to explore some sort of resolution? If it
worked, only then would the city take the credit. If it failed, the
secrecy of the meeting would guarantee that no one would ever
know Wynn had taken the risk. Mendez commended Wynn for
making an attempt, noting that in the long run, complete inac-
tion on this issue could be a point of political liability in the next
election.

In spite of the potential pitfalls, Mendez was in fact eager to
get involved. He personally invited both Iris Inkwater, the CEO
of Oppidania, and Pete Patterson, the CEO of Urbania, to a private meeting: just the three of them. He explained Wynn's hope
to see these issues resolved. Mendez described the session as

exploratory, and he asked that the meeting be kept strictly confidential. To his relief, both Patterson and Inkwater agreed to
attend.

Though they belong to the same professional associations,
Inkwater never considered Patterson a peer. Pete was old-
school: he grew into his job without the training or background
to lead a top-rate institution. While Iris was aggressively on the
rise, Pete had peaked years before and was probably more concerned about retirement than about going through the turmoil of
running a troubled institution. Similarly, Pete did not much care
for Iris. In his mind, she was a new breed of brash, aggressive
executive, somewhat cold and calculating in her moves, and not
to be trusted. He always felt one-upped by Iris and Oppidania,
and he didn't much care for the association. As the meeting
between Manny, Iris, and Pete opened, the mood was polite
and cool.

Careful not to imply blame, Mendez fairly assessed the problem as belonging to more than just the institutions involved. To
the extent that patients, jobs, and business relationships could be
affected by the standoff, the city had an interest in encouraging
the parties to reach some sort of resolution. He emphasized that
it was not up to the city to solve the problem, though the city
would be prepared to do whatever it could to help the parties
resolve the issues. Inkwater thanked Mendez, as did Patterson.

Mendez asked each to describe the situation from his or her
own perspective. Surprisingly, neither saw the problem as being
with the other. Each felt jostled into this predicament more on
account of the machinations of the health maintenance organizations than on account of any interchanges between themselves.
That revelation turned out to be significant. From that perspective, they each had shared problems and shared interests. They
laughed themselves into commentary on the more bizarre
aspects of the recent round of negotiations, and they noted how
they had been played off each other.

With the mood of the meeting turning, Mendez decided to
pose a delicate question: had the two ever considered some sort
of an alliance? The question was met with dubious silence. Iris

explained that the possibility had not been given any serious consideration at Oppidania. Patterson said the same was true at Urbania. Mendez pursued the question: had either of them specifically *rejected* such an alliance? They agreed that they had not. Mendez then became bolder in his questioning: might it be in the realm of the conceivable? After some discussion, they each agreed that it very well might.

The mood of the meeting once again swerved. Having concurred with something that only moments before had been unthinkable, they retreated from their positions. A heated discussion pursued, during which each explained to Mendez the deeply ingrained and different histories, culture, status, business practices, and positions of the two organizations. Though neither openly stated their reservations, Mendez understood Inkwater to say that she did not want to affiliate with an inferior institution. He discerned Patterson to say that he did not want to get gobbled up by a behemoth.

"So you each have legitimate organizational concerns. Yet, as I have watched you over the years, I see more in common than I see differences. You are both by-products of this city, and you are both very committed to the city. Because of your competitive edge, you each have invested and continue to invest in expensive equipment in order to remain competitive. We have two of too many machines in this town when one could do. Essentially, the competition has become expensive for both of you. Might there be an option?"

Iris felt stunned. There was something so obvious about what Mendez was saying that she was baffled why she had not thought of it herself. Pete felt differently. He wasn't sure where Mendez was going with this line of questioning.

Inkwater turned to Patterson. "You know, Pete, the two of us have acted more like competing high school football rivals than we have two major health care organizations. I think Manny has raised an important question. The fact is, we are both overbedded and overstaffed. We are each trying to be a full-service institution, and that is, as we know, a very expensive proposition. It's been done in other cities between the most unlikely of bedfellows." Inkwater turned to Mendez. "You know, Manny, I feel a little silly for not have raised this question myself."

Patterson appreciated Inkwater's candor. He smiled as if he had just got the punch line of a joke he had heard some time before. "Actually, Iris, there has been talk about discussing some sort of a relationship with Oppidania. It was rejected outright on the assumption that you people wouldn't hear of it. Quite frankly, we didn't want to become your laughingstock. Instead, we decided to put all our marbles in with CHP. Boy, did that ever blow up in our face."

Iris appreciated her counterpart's openness and his sense of humor. "Look, Pete, through the grapevine, you know enough about what's going on in my shop and I know enough about what's going on in yours to figure out that we are both being squeezed hard. On one side it's the insurers and on the other side it's the staff. If by working together we can share some expenses and defer some costs, then it's worth at least exploring the possibility."

Patterson was a bit surprised by her enthusiasm. Is she thinking alliance, he wondered, or takeover? Whichever, Urbania was no longer in the position to enjoy the luxury of full independence. "Iris, I agree with you. It certainly is worth exploring the possibility."

Mendez felt a sense of cautious optimism. He suggested that each give the idea forty-eight hours of considered thought. He recommended that these discussions remain confidential: if word leaked prematurely, it could derail any potential progress. He further offered that if there were continued interest, he would remain available to move the process along.

Two days later, both Inkwater and Patterson called Mendez's office. There indeed was interest. They had each spoken with their board and senior staff, and then spoke again to each other. In that conversation, they agreed to ask Mendez to stay on as intermediary. Mendez arranged a conference call for the three, and he suggested a meeting at a retreat center an hour outside of town. They agreed that such a meeting was a reasonable next step. Mendez offered to make the arrangements and hire a professional facilitator to conduct the session. Each hospital would send a delegation of about ten members. All three underlined the importance of maintaining the secrecy of these discussions. If the meetings were publicized, media sensationalism and staff anxiety would spoil the potential for any progress. .

It was decided to schedule a two-day session and to ask each participant to spend the night at the center. It was felt that the informality and intensity of such a setting would help break the ice and enhance productive discourse. Further, the members of the delegations were to include individuals with decision-making authority: board chairpersons, the CEOs, chief financial officers, chief operating officers, medical directors, nursing vice presidents, two other administrators, and two other board members. The dean of the medical school was also invited. Mendez was there with two members of his staff. The lead facilitator and two associates led the meetings.

In large part because the participants came carefully prepared, the meetings went well, far beyond everyone's expectations. What became clear early on was that each hospital, in fact, was in trouble. There simply were fewer patients and there was less money. By the end of the second day, there was an agreement, in principle, to ally the two hospitals, forming a new corporate entity to oversee the separate though coordinated operations of each. The new entity would bear neither of their names; it would be called the UniCare Corporation. They concluded with a list of questions and issues that would have to be settled as the proposal moved forward, everything from finances to leadership, culture, administration, and clinical issues.

Each side saw a number of benefits to the arrangement. Certainly there would be the economies of scale in purchasing and marketing. Together they would have far more leverage with insurers. More importantly, though, they would be able to reduce unnecessary duplications of services and purchases. In particular, the most expensive, high-tech services could be limited to one facility and accessible to both. It was agreed that Oppidania would have the more acute services: this turned out to be a relief to Urbania, which found over the past few years that they were investing large sums into underutilized and there-fore ultimately unprofitable machinery.

With an understanding in principle, each side agreed to open broader discussions with their leadership. The proposal would be reviewed by both boards as well as the key department heads of each institution. If no major stumbling blocks appeared, the negotiations would be announced simultaneously, first inside each institution through newsletters, and then publicly at a joint press conference. The announcements would be intentionally vague, that the two institutions were "discussing the possibility" of some form of alliance. The press conference announcing these negotiations would involve the board chairs and CEOs of each institution, along with city health commissioner Manual Mendez. It was decided to keep the mayor out of the picture until an actual alliance was formalized.

It took nearly a year of concentrated work. The alliance heartily sprouted at a celebratory news conference attended by the newly aligned leadership, the mayor, and Manny Mendez. After careful deliberation, it was decided to name Iris Inkwater as CEO of the UniCare Corporation, investing in her position general oversight of the overall operation as well as leadership for new ventures by the parent corporation. She outlined her aspiration to create new community outreach programs and ini-tiatives with the community. Pete Patterson continued in his role as CEO of the UMC. Perry Pratt, chief operating officer for Oppidania, was promoted to CEO for OMC. Janice Johnson was asked to work with her counterpart at Urbania to coordi-nate the collaboration of the nursing departments, and Dr. Fred Fisher was asked to do the same for the two medical staffs.

The new alliance was framed as an emerging and flexible relationship that would grow over time, step by step. It was in large measure a learning process, by which the two institutions and their surrounding community gradually could better under-stand and integrate with one another. What was learned would be fed back into the system, serving as the basis for future deci-sions and directions.

The new organization viewed its mission as promoting a

responsive agenda for the health and health care of Oppidania. With the mayor and health commissioner present, this vision was described as an active public-private partnership. They observed that this effort had not been without its bumps, and genuine efforts were being made to hear and respond to the concerns of the many people and constituencies who were being affected by the changes. And they also acknowledged the widespread support expressed by staff, community, and business concerns.

A feeling of professional, personal, and organizational achievement pervaded the room as the plan and vision were outlined. Having persevered to this point, they all proceeded together with the most important asset of all: a sense of confidence and coherence in what they were doing and where they were heading.

♦ ♦ ♦ ♦ ♦ ♦ ♦

Conclusion: Reaching Balanced Health Care

The purpose here is not to prescribe the correct model for health care. There are plenty of treatises available to do just that. Rather, the intention is to offer a constructive means for moving toward that model, and to remind you that once there, it will be time to move on: health care by its nature is always changing. This is a travel guide for a journey that never ends.

Nonetheless, a few cautionary notes are in order to clarify exactly what balance does and does not mean.

Balance is not everyone and everything equal. There is different weight, import, experience, and know-how among the many people, skills, and problems on our ledgers. To equate them would be naive. To calibrate their relative weight as part of negotiating a more balanced health system is what this book is all about.

To do so, incorporate a fair and responsive check and balance system: relevant parties should have voice, and their message should be heard even if the relative influence of some is greater than others. We work, think, and decide in hierarchical terms. Hierarchy in and of itself is not bad: it can be an efficient way to sort innumerable people and tasks. It is only unjust if it is used as a tool to silence some and insulate others.

Giving voice to craft better balance is not just a market survey or a staff-satisfaction questionnaire. It is deeper than that. It goes to a real understanding of what we are doing and what we are trying to accomplish. If the negotiation table provides an opportunity to gain better clarity on that, our chances of developing a worthy health system are greatly improved.

It means that, in the process, we negotiate ends and means; we define and redefine what we are doing; we are open to finding better ways to do it. The outcome is a system that represents the diversity of our work force, population, and health care needs. We promote health; we prevent illness—we heal. We assemble the pieces necessary to accomplish that noble endeavor.

This premise of balance will help us transform into new organizational models, priorities, and opportunities without sacrificing what is already excellent in our health care system.

Is this incrementalist thinking? Yes. Does it mean that change will be a bit more slower, a bit more careful, a bit more reasoned than totally revamping the system? Yes. What is the benefit?

It is better to change at a pace that offers the greatest likelihood of making the right choices than refurbishing the system with no idea whether it will succeed. Insofar as we take seriously what we do, how much do we want to experiment with systems that are untested and that may not work? It means that we fix the big problems first and continue with the same commitment to the remaining problems. It means that society must be clear and reasonable in what it expects from the health system. It means that people must be reasonable in accepting what they get.

Life itself is a delicate balance of chemicals, electricity, liquids, and frames that hold together our bodies. For that system to work, all those reactions and systems must be in synchrony. If they are not we become ill, and life itself is at risk. Similarly, the health system, which intends to nurture our bodies, itself must be in healthy alignment.

14

· ·

Constructing a Resilient Balance

A few thoughts with which to leave you:

On Conflict

Discern apparent from fundamental issues. The rhetoric, accusations, and demands shooting across the tables of conflict depict one representation of the issues. To acquire a deeper understanding of what is really happening and how it might realistically be resolved, hear and understand what lies beneath the spoken assertions: the latent along with the manifest messages. What are the actual agendas for each of the sides? Are there discrepancies between what is said and what is done? How might these underlying issues be configured or reconfigured to encourage settlement? Heed the message as well as the words.

At the heart of much conflict is vulnerability. Beneath the combat, rhetoric, and bravado of conflict, basic emotions and fears motivate and impassion what ostensibly is on the table: the suspicions and insecurities of professional peril, physical risk, and personal uncertainty. At the core of the conflict, then, there is uncertainty, dread of betrayal, and fear of defenseless exposure. For some, vulnerability compels retreat. For others, that inner vulnerability is masked by outward aggression: they attack others to secure themselves. Parties

become locked in escalating defensive and offensive moves motivated and justified by their deep-seated fears. To uncover settlement
options, discern these vulnerabilities and search for ways to miti-
gate, understand, relieve and remove doubts that obscure settlement. This process is at the gist of unearthing interests at a time
when the conflict has intensified into hardened positions.

   Conflict is inevitable. Strive for perfection, and know that in the
long run it is unattainable, humans and natural events being what
they are. Like life itself, the health system cannot be infallible: it
cannot reliably address all the needs of all the people all the time,
though we should never stop trying. Beware the conflicts that arise
from the disappointments of imperfection: given the nature of our
work, the expectation of infallibility is not unreasonable. Anticipate and prepare for the conflicts, knowing that an insurance policy protects you only from the financial and not from the human
rigors of disillusion.

On Framing and Reframing

If it doesn't make sense, you probably don't have all the facts. People are
assumed to operate on the premise of self-interest: usually some
combination of money, advancement, satisfaction, security, and
recognition. It is generally easy to understand motive when the
incentives are relatively straightforward. It becomes confusing, however, when the usual standards of self-interest are of secondary
importance. It is particularly confounding when someone's self-
interest is mingled with destructive purpose, either for themselves
or others. In that case, one person's safety depends on another's
demise. Ironically, in the manner of a self-fulfilling prophecy, when
a destructive impulse becomes an obsession, the outcome itself can
become self-destructive. Likewise, when obsession for a mission
overtakes common sense, the pursuit of the purpose may itself
undermine that purpose. Notwithstanding these many intricacies,

if only you could assemble *all* the explanatory pieces, you would ultimately be able to find a logical explanation for what happened and
why. Negotiation is like good detective work. Careful of decoys distracting you from investigatory pursuit, you look for motive and
means, seeking clues to unravel the mystery.

There are always options: stretch to find them. Modify what you do.
If you cannot change what you do, adjust when you do it. And if
you cannot shift when you do it, reframe how you do it. You are the
mouse in the maze. Sometimes you retrace your steps to inform your
journey. You are not deterred by dead ends. And you are flexible
about how you take to the destination you reach, even if it is not
the piece of cheese you expected. Step back. Take another look.
Turn the puzzle on its side. Try another angle. Seek realistic opportunity. You need not do it alone, and you need not give up the
cause.

Find ways to express differences without provoking contention. There
will always be differences among people: style, attitude, belief,
method, background, and skills. As a species, we tend to the tribal:
we coalesce in order to sustain ourselves. Like small republics con-
gregating with their own to fend off the enemy, we sit in the con-
genial comfort of nurses' lounges, doctors' hideaways, and the inner
dens of our administrative offices. The sense of familiarity in being
with your own—no matter if you define it by profession, gender, age,
ethnic group, race, religion, or alma mater—is not inherently troublesome if its prime purpose is simply to invigorate that relaxing
sensation of the customary. It becomes a problem when this coa-
lescing is the rallying point for portraying outsiders as the enemy: a
place for self-affirming aggrandizement and disparagement of others, building walls and not bridges between people who ultimately
are or could be constructively intertwined. This book challenges
the premise that we must contend within our domain in order to
attain our human potential. It also challenges the premise that we
must conform within our domain in order to attain that potential.

Further, it challenges the premise that these two are incompatible. We can express our differences without denigrating the roots of those dissimilarities. Those differences can be either a strength or a weakness: ultimately, you will be more vital if you shape them into your strength.

Turn jealousy into admiration. We spend boundless time and energy comparing ourselves to one another, measuring whether we are ahead or behind. If your work is merely a race to get somewhere, then this ceaseless comparison is understandable. However, if your intention is to accomplish something of value with others, you will find the constant equating and the jealousy it spawns to be more a hindrance than a boon to your work. When you perceive others' accomplishments as your loss, then you are caught in your own spiral of defeat, since you can never outdo all and everyone you use as your measuring stick. You are jealous of others. They are jealous of you. Conversely, if you can see each other's accomplishments as reflecting well on your common, collaborative efforts, you can turn this negative into a positive.

On Conflict Resolution

Conflicts settle: always in time. Time is that robust dimension of conflict and conflict resolution that often goes undetected for both its problem and its potential. Time offers perspective and a chance to melt that dagger of rage that overwhelms any appetite to settle. When the parties are not simultaneously ripe to resolve, one makes a move for the table of resolution while the other runs, only to return eventually and find the bitterness over the retreat kills any hope for rapprochement. Eventually the conflict fades, settles, or is forgotten: people leave or die; the original issues are seen for their fruitlessness; new opportunities cloud the sources of discord; the parties tire of the fight and relent. And so, someone reflects on the time and energy devoted to the battle and wonders what could have been accomplished if those same resources had been devoted to the good that motivated each of the sides. In those hopeless moments of battle, it is wise to remember that life itself is short and fleeting, and that in the long run, we each possess little more on the planet than time itself. How best to use it?

Truth is found usually in the middle, not at the extremes. Truth is that rendition of reality so easily manipulated and crafted to reflect what we want to believe. Different parties to a dispute perceive it differently. No one owns it: there are fewer absolutes than we might desire. Keep your mind open, and cultivate the possibility that your version of the truth may deviate from that of others. Do not abandon your convictions; at the same time, do not allow them to blind you. Permit ideas and possibilities to commingle: multiple perspectives are more likely to reveal a perspective that meets the measure of many people's truths. Wisdom is tolerating that your version of the truth may be different than mine, and that for all practical purposes, they could both be true. And it is recognizing that everything is relative: what may have been extreme yesterday is mainstream today.

Mediation is like baking bread: you have to trust the process even though you can't see it. (Barry C. Dorn, M.D., deserves credit for this insight.) Take simple ingredients: facts, circumstances, people, choices, emotions, consequences. Blend them in a perceptive manner and allow them to conceive something better than their individual parts.

On Change

There is little that is permanent: change is a given. The curve on the pace of change is climbing. Consider the past two hundred years and the quickening pace of change in the most recent fifty. And consider the past fifty years in health care and the quickening pace of just the past five. With sensational new technologies and expectations already in sight, we can be confident that the rate of transformation is likely to continue its ascent. Amid this change, flexibility is the key to enduring achievement. On the interpersonal level of work relationships, flexibility is manifest through negotiation. Differences on the direction and pace of change are manifested as conflict. And conflict resolution seeks to convey flexibility into the process. What works today may not work tomorrow. For those who hate change and crave stability, this prospect offers little comfort. Let go. Your security rests more with your ability to be agile than with your instinct to remain stationary. Further, your long-term achievement will soar highest from your ability to be ahead of the flow, or even more so, in your charting its destination.

Individuals are defined by their context, and individuals define their context. People often discount their influence upon others and the influence of others upon them. On the personal level, in every conversation you reflect to someone something about themselves: from the appropriateness of their dress to the depth of their professional acumen or the place they hold in the pertinent social order. Likewise, your self-perceptions are often molded by what others resonate to you, whether it be overt, through direct comments, or oblique, through innuendo or body language. On the societal level, people are influenced and characterized by their culture of origin or the period in which they grew up: the imprint of "the sixties" is an example. This web of subtle-yet-ever-present influence molds our negotiations. The negotiation expectations of others are shaped by the cues we give them, just as ours are shaped by those we get from them: the "give-and-get" of the process. This interplay excels when it is active and balanced, not dominated or controlled. While the equation need not be even, when one person eclipses or disenfranchises the other, constructive feedback does not work: the overbearing boss is not told bad news, or learns it too late. An animated dynamic of exchange works best: up-down, down-up, and across. Fine-tuned organizations and individuals are so because they encourage conduits of influence to keep them responsive and vital, because they have the wisdom to know the bounds, and because, when it is legitimate to do so, they have the courage to draw the line and hold it.

Distinguish the leader with vision from visionary leadership. (Thanks to Robert Taylor, Dean of the School of Business, University of Kentucky, for sharing these thoughts, 1988.) The "leader with vision" has a specific objective, in pursuit of which he or she takes followers. That objective is molded and sanctioned by the leader. Followers, neatly lined up behind the leader, are uniformly directed. Anyone questioning purpose or method is a dissenter to be silenced or cut down: there is no negotiation. The aspiration of the followers is to reach the vision of the leader: they passively have only marginal influence over either means or ends. "Visionary leadership," on the other hand, is an interactive process by which leaders bring together the contributions of many people, and in the process enrich both the objective as well as the realization of purpose. The objective itself is furthered because more people have contributed and are invested in it, and so it is broader in scope and relevance. The means are enhanced because the scope of creative talent is broadened. The role of leadership is to facilitate this process, diplomatically orchestrating efforts toward synthesized purpose. It is a modus operandi that requires constant negotiation and conflict resolution. Unanimity itself takes time to nurture, and at times it is elusive: visionary leadership too has its challenges and pitfalls. Nonetheless, with the combined expanse of professions, knowledge, expertise, and interests, visionary leadership is an approach congruent with the purposes and processes of health care (see Bennis and Nanus, 1986).

On Health Care Systems

Build process to refine balance. The complex, high-consequence enterprise of health care requires fine-tuned checks and balances to ensure the proficiency of its work: what are *you* doing? what are *they* doing? how might you *all* do it better? The "quality improvement" movement has contributed substantive mechanisms to enhance this process: peer review procedures, data gathering and communication techniques, and analytic models and management methods to transform both attitudes and practice. To be effective, these procedures must work both on the systems level as well as on the interpersonal level. This is where your negotiation skills come into play: systems are no better than what you are able to do with them. And since these checks and balances naturally bring conflict to the fore, quality improvement in reality also requires a good deal of conflict resolution. For a system of checks and balances to realize its objectives, one person must be sanctioned to check what the other does, and the process must be affirmed so that the message is in fact accepted. There is neither beginning nor end to this cycle: you negotiate, raise differences, resolve differences, negotiate, and start all over again. It keeps us proficient and in tune.

Strive for congruency of purpose and method. Good health care benefits from healthy organizations and healthy negotiations. If the manner for conducting our business is not consonant with its intention—health—then we eventually are trapped in the very contradictions we create. Negotiation that is genuine, honest, just, legitimate, moral, respectful, and mutually beneficial is congruent with our purpose. Our work is information-intensive, and the authenticity of that information must be indisputable. We balance a multitude of criteria in our decision making, so our standards must be fair. The very essence of our work—life, death, and the quality of life—requires us to uphold moral principles and then guide our practice by them. Our endeavors are about healthy people and ailing patients, so fostering the interests and concerns of well-being is part of our obligation. And finally, our agreements must meet the measure of integrity if they are to endure, because in the long run, endurance amid the brevity of life is the nature of our work.

The bottom line of our work is healthy people. There are many bottom lines in the negotiation of health care: professional reputation, political influence, personal vulnerability, and a balanced budget, to name a few. There is one bottom line we share, and that bottom line justifies the recognition, power, prestige, and expense we claim at the negotiation table. That bottom line is the best interests of the patient. While we can legitimately place our own agenda on the back of that common standard, asserting that what we offer is in fact in the best interests of the patient, it is incumbent upon us to see our own agenda and that of others in their proper perspective. The common frame we seek revolves about healthy people. The decisive question is how to achieve that end, for each individual patient and for society, insofar as we are part of a connected system of people and expertise. It is all too easy to mask our own animosities, aspirations, or discords behind a deceptive altruistic concern for the patient's best interest. As a community of professionals devoted to health and health care, elevating our common bond is a personal, professional, organizational, and societal responsibility.

So . . . negotiation and renegotiation is a constant. Like breathing, negotiation is something you do all the time. As a negotiator, you are constantly learning and adjusting your strategy, methods, and moves. You know that what worked wonderfully yesterday could flop today. You understand that you have your own filters on reality, and that while you might not always be able to control them, you can at least account for how they might skew your assessment of facts and options. You have a good sense of your own priorities and are willing to accept that others order their list differently. You know that health care systems, the political animals that they are, engage in moral conduct because people with a moral and ethical agenda place their perspectives persuasively on the table. You appreciate that the system will not be created and recreated in one day and that you and others are on board for the long haul, a perspective that requires constant personal, professional, and systemic flexibility. And finally, you grasp that you are part of a bigger picture; that the quality of that picture depends on a joint capacity to assemble the pieces, and that sometimes you have to hold on and sometimes you just have to let go.

◆　◆　◆　◆　◆　◆　◆

It was 11:00 P.M. The lingering smell of a day of hard work was still in the air as Ken Kavanaugh and Dave Donley entered the deserted locker room to change out of their hospital greens.

They made their way to the small cove at the far end of the cramped room. Donley took a seat in front of his open locker at one end of the bench. Kavanaugh preferred to stand, hanging onto the squeaking open door that dangled back and forth as he took off his shoes. They both were exhausted, drudging through the routine of transforming back into their civilian lives.

Donley suddenly lit up impulsively. "You know, Ken, I've been working on a whole new theory of the universe."

Kavanaugh barely had the energy to listen. Before he had even finished the thought, Donley was blurting ahead.

"You know how in those science fiction movies the alien creatures all look about our size and shape?" Donley paused a moment to get Kavanaugh's assent. "I think they have it all wrong. I think even aiming telescopes into the sky may be inane."

"Tell me, why is it inane?" Kavanaugh tried to convey his growing disinterest through the tone of his voice.

Donley plunged on, oblivious to Kavanaugh's indifference. "Have you ever looked at a picture of the universe. We look like an atom, with the sun as a nucleus and the planets like little protons spinning around the middle." Donley was gesturing in the air as he pulled his shirt over his head. His animated voice continued as he became absorbed in his own speculation. "And then when you look at the whole Milky Way, it looks like a set of atoms assembled together to make up a molecule."

"Yeah, so what?" Kavanaugh grumbled.

"Well, have you ever considered that the universe as we know it may be a small piece of matter in a much larger particle? Say all these atoms and molecules together are just a piece in some colossal being's thumbnail."

Kavanaugh finally looked up. He was incredulous. "Donley, you think we are an atom in somebody's thumbnail?"

"Well, perhaps." Donley hesitated. "And it gets more intriguing." His enthusiasm grew. He was convinced that he had captured Kavanaugh's interest.

"If *we* are a particle in someone's thumbnail, just as likely there could be whole universes in our own thumbnail." Donley now looked like he had persuaded himself. "There could be suns and planets, malls, gyms—the whole bit—right inside here." He gestured toward his hand.

Though Kavanaugh was beginning to find the prospect amusing, he feigned annoyance. "Donley, where do you come up with these crazy ideas?"

Donley continued unabated. "And then dimensions of time differ." Donley's arms began gesturing theatrically into the air. "For the larger being, the billions of years of our planet's existence are only a millisecond. And for the beings in our thumbnail, why, whole civilizations could have come and gone in the course of this conversation, and we wouldn't know it." Donley stared at his thumb, hoping for a shred of tangible evidence.

The two picked up their limp hospital-issued attire and tossed the clothes into the laundry hamper as they paced out the room. They stepped along like two programmed robots who had done this very routine many times before, heading into the brightly lit hallway leading toward the parking lot and home.

Kavanaugh decided to challenge Donley's absurd line of thinking. "OK, Donley, that would be fine. So, what does it have to do with anything?"

"I was just thinking." His eyes squinted as he became more absorbed in what he was saying. "A little five-year-old-girl came in through emergency today—motor vehicle, hit by a car, pretty bad trauma. I was in and out with her since this morning." Kavanaugh paid closer attention.

"When I was a kid, I got hit by a car too. That's how I got into medicine—I really admired everything they did for people. They ended up saving my life . . . as you can see." Donley gestured to himself as proof. "I was in some hospital for ten days, and by the time they released me, I had convinced myself that one day I would be a doc too."

"So what does that have to do with planets in your thumbnail?"

"I was ten years old when it happened, and for some reason, it came back to me today. I dreamed up that wild idea right after the accident. Someone had brought me a book about the planets and the universe. All I could do was look at the pictures and think. I saw the sun and nine planets looking like an atom that's part of a larger molecule and all that."

Kavanaugh realized that something had struck a deep chord for Donley. Donley continued.

"Anyway, as I was taking care of this little girl today, that image came back up on my screen. And then, while I was filling out some stupid insurance forms, it somehow brought up all my feelings about this whole health care cosmos we are a part of. You know, sometimes when I'm in the hospital, it feels like we are some tiny outpost in all those larger games played out about the health care system. A small little particle in some larger picture that at times I can barely fathom."

They had reached the end of the hallway and were about to make their way into the cold night air.

"And then I look at this little girl, scared and afraid, with all that swirl going around her in emergency. For her, this is a whole incomprehensible world. Today was a lifetime for her. She'll never forget what happened. She'll relive it over and over again—it will be with her forever. For us, it was just a few hours. When it's all over, we pack up and call it another day at work."

"So she's that world in your thumbnail?" Kavanaugh was beginning to see the point.

"That's right, Ken. She is that world in my thumbnail. It just brought it home how we always see things from our own perspective. We expect the universe to somehow be in our own scale, on our time line and along our own dimension. It's very hard to step back and take another slant on what it is we are seeing. We are locked into our own biases of what makes the world go around. It happens all the time here in the hospital. Everyone talks one line, but when push comes to shove, we all see things through that limited viewfinder of our own looking glass."

Kavanaugh turned to Donley, now fascinated. Donley had somehow captured Kavanaugh's own feeling of fantasy and frustration. "I'm not sure I buy the thumbnail theory, though I'll grant you that we do get stuck on our own way of thinking. I had exactly that problem in the ICU today. Everybody was mired in their own mud and we weren't getting anywhere."

Donley was lost in thought. Kavanaugh continued. "You know, I'm going to think about this whim of yours. It's lunacy, though I find it intriguing." Kavanaugh decided to have some fun with Donley. "And by the way, tell me: in that mall in your fingernail, is there a multiplex?"

Donley looked down at his thumb to check. "Several," he said and peered up.

Kavanaugh grinned. "Do me a favor." He paused. "If they're showing any good movies this weekend, do give me a call. I'm bored with what's out here."

As Donley was unlocking his car door, he shouted out to his friend, "Ken, my friend, you've got a deal." And now, satisfied that he had convinced Kavanaugh of his theory, he shouted out, "And I supply the popcorn!"

◆ ◆ ◆ ◆ ◆ ◆

Strength to you for all your journeys.

List of Characters

• •

Listed in alphabetical order

Arlan Abbington   Chairman of the board of trustees at OMC

Anna Ashwood   Artie Ashwood's mother

Artie Ashwood   Patient admitted to Oppidania Medical Center (OMC) with an enlarged heart

Bob Bennett   Mediator with an agency that has a contract with the state board of medical registration to conduct mediation of medical practice disputes

Benjamin Bennington   Retired physician and OMC board member

Beatrice Benson   Attending physician in the emergency department

Betty Brown   Patient of Dr. Tuckerman who died of lung cancer

Carrie Carrington   Artie Ashwood's girlfriend

Catherine Cartwright   Oppidania board member

Charlotte Channing   Triage nurse in the emergency department

Cliff Clemens   A second-year resident

Charlie Collins   A resident

Cathy Crow   Nurse on Six West

Chuck Cummings   Resident on Six West

Diane Darling   Operating room nurse responsible for room scheduling

David Dickenson   Vice president for Human Resources at OMC

Dave Donley   Resident in the emergency department

Debby Donnelly   Nurse on Six West

Evelyn Edelman   Director of OMC's dietary department

Eli Ewing   Chief resident in the cardiac intensive care unit

Fred Fisher   Medical director for the Oppidania Medical Center

Gail Godfried   Nurse in the cardiac intensive care unit

Gloria Green   President of the internal medicine group

Heather Harriford   Nurse in the cardiac intensive care unit, later transferred to the general medical floor

Mrs. Hayward   A seventy-eight-year-old woman on Six West, suffering from colon cancer

Iris Inkwater   Chief executive officer of the Oppidania Medical Center

Janice Johnson   Vice president for nursing at the Oppidania Medical Center

Judy Johnson   Nurse on Six West

Ken Kavanaugh   Chief of the intensive care unit

Katherine Knight   Nurse manager in the intensive care unit

Lauren Lieber   Chief resident for orthopedics at OMC

Larry Levine   Ted Tuckerman's medical malpractice attorney

Leslie Long   Betty Brown's daughter

Larry Lumberg   Medical director of the emergency department

Melinda Martin   Director of the Harborside Youth Action League

Melanie Melancourt   Chief of the surgical intensive care unit

Manuel Mendez   City health commissioner for Oppidania

Nathaniel Norquist   Chief financial officer of the Community Health Plan health maintenance organization

Nick Norton   Chief of orthopedics at Oppidania

Oscar O'Neill   Primary nurse on Six West

Pauline Patrick   Nurse on Six West

Pete Patterson   Chief executive officer of the Urbania Medical Center

Patty Pinkerton   A colleague of Janice Johnson and a leader in the regional nurse executive association

Perry Pratt   Chief operating officer for OMC

Ralph Richman   Chief financial officer for OMC

Ralph Rollins   A senior physician at OMC and a close friend of Dr. Fred Fisher

Steve Schilling   A second-year resident

Stuart Schilling   Bioethicist at OMC

Sylvia Sheffield   Nurse on Six West

Sarah Smith   Lieutenant governor for the state, with responsibility for health reform

Tanya Tarrington   Head nurse on Nine West

Tim Thatcher   Administrator for the OMC internal medicine group

Ted Tuckerman   An internist

Mr. Ulrich   Terminally ill patient about whom a do-not-resuscitate order was in question

Victor Vining   A cardiologist

Will Wainwright   A primary care physician

Will Walter   An anesthesiologist

Wendell White   An internist

Mayor Willie Wynn   Mayor of Oppidania

Ziva Zartman   A social worker

Negotiation Handles

. . . .

Use these terms as quick reference reminders for the concepts and methods discussed in the book.

Negotiation Profiles

Negotiation Process to determine the exchange of tangibles and intangibles.

Complex Negotiation Interlocking exchanges among disconnected intermediaries: the more intermediaries, the more complex.

Simple Negotiation Negotiation that *only* involves those right at the table and nobody else.

Representational Negotiation Negotiation on behalf of or affecting people not at the table.

Home Team Those people not at the table on whose behalf you negotiate (and they won't let you forget it).

Negotiation Map The web of connections and relations among people who influence or must approve a negotiated decision.

Symbolic Negotiation Negotiating with a category of people or characteristics: What do *they* signify for you? What do *you* signify for them?

Negotiation Buttons Those values, behaviors, or appearances that evoke emotional reactions, reducing your negotiation effectiveness.

Interest-Based Negotiation Appreciating differences and finding common purpose based on shared needs, concerns, and objectives.

Integrative Negotiation Combining ideas, resources, and investments to find fair and mutually satisfying solutions.

Positional Negotiation Draw a line in the sand and stand firm: go for the win to avoid the loss. A dangerous strategy in health care, given the close work and need for cooperation.

Distributional Negotiation With a fixed sum to divide, the more you get, the less I get. I want more.

Whole Image Negotiation Inventive, integrative exchange based on overlapping and mutual interests. Particularly appropriate to health care negotiations.

Whole Synthesizing separate interests to pursue common interests for mutual gain: the process creates a sum that is larger than its parts. "We are one."

Image The generative quality of combined vision: what is discovered from the blended efforts of the parts.

Relationship Building Early phase negotiation, when the parties assess one another and plan their strategy. Its growth during negotiation facilitates further progress.

Negotiation Dancing Mid-phase negotiation, as parties shift from early assessment and prepare for deal making.

Bargaining Late phase negotiation: takes place close to when parties are ready to finalize the decision or action.

Conflict Profiles

Conflict An expressed difference, disagreement, or dispute among two or more people.

Not a Conflict When the person toward whom you are frustrated, disappointed, or angry does not know your feelings: the sentiments are not expressed and are not known.

Start a Conflict Step one in conflict resolution: the other side needs to know there is a problem. How it is started, from contentious to collaborative, will greatly determine its potential and means for resolution.

Inner Conflict Private ambivalence, accentuated when a decision or action must be taken. Often unknown to the other side.

Shadow Effect The movement of conflict through an organization or over time, propelled by contradicting policies or interpersonal animosities.

Enemy Image A conviction that the other side is out to destroy you. You are obsessed to get them before they get you!

Polarization The parties move to opposite sides in an adversarial stand-off or disagreement.

Conflict Escalation The growth and persistence of conflict: costs, stakes, and damage increase as the parties become increasingly obsessed with defeating the opposition.

Conflict Interruption A plateau that momentarily halts the escalation. It could go anywhere from here: heat up or cool down.

Conflict Deescalation Humanize, gain perspective, save face, share savings, apologize: animosities abate.

Conflict Creators

Blame, Finger-Pointing I'm right, you're wrong. The sparks for positional confrontation.

Arms Race Continued investment in an escalating dispute, beyond the real value of the matter at hand.

Cause (in conflict escalation) To rationalize investment that exceeds the real value of that matter, parties ascribe a higher purpose and meaning to it.

Costs of Conflict Investments made in waging the dispute: often outweighs the real benefits.

Thrill of Conflict The spectacular game of survival: overcoming the odds and reaching victory. The enticement of positional negotiation. The exhilaration of victory; the agony of defeat.

Purpose of Conflict Range of rationalizations to keep it going.

Feuding Good guys and bad guys: we're the good guys.

Simplification Good versus bad; black versus white; right versus wrong. In a polarized conflict, the complexities of the gray zone (and the possibility that I may not be right) are ignored.

History The collective memory of past association. Could be good; could be bad.

Baggage Unforgotten stories, incidents, and concerns that incite continued disputing. Baggage accumulates with time.

Getting Even The wild west school of conflict resolution.

Gotchya Contenders search and wait for the other's mistakes or vulnerabilities: when one is found, it is used to promote one's rightness and the other's evil.

Crowding/Capacity Too many people in too small a space, or too few people in too big a space. Typical of overcapacity in health care services—too many beds amidst diminishing resources and demand too small.

Scarcity Limited resources provokes competition for what little exists.

Threat Self-protective response to danger: that response can further provoke the threat.

Ambiguity Amid uncertainty, different parties come to different conclusions to which they adhere: a starting point for conflict.

Complexity The more interlocking people involved in a decision, the greater the likelihood of conflict.

Competition A premise for win-lose negotiation: conflict over the criteria for who wins inflames the dispute.

Evaluation What are the criteria for assessment? Success for one person is considered failure by another—a source of bitter conflict.

Stress and Pressure When work is fast and without time for careful deliberation, inflammatory words and actions can foster conflict.

Change Conflict emerges between (1) the change promoters, reforming an existing and deficient system, and (2) the change resisters, content with current conditions and their influence therein.

Emotion The passions that fuel disputing.

Obsession to Win The instinctual compulsion to score a victory: that impulse becomes irrational, as investments in winning far exceed the rewards or value of victory.

Humiliation The fear of losing face: a high-stakes loss among professionals.

Fears Anxieties promote self-protection and little mutual recognition.

Vulnerabilities Painful matters that raise fears of doom. These matters are closely defended by one party and may be the point of attack for the other.

Anger The impetus for instinctual attack. Never negotiate when you have it. Beware its presence in others.

Situational Anger Rage about circumstances not caused by anyone in particular: nonetheless, the rage is directed at anyone in the room.

Anger at Someone Else You did not provoke the anger. Since the person who did is not present, you are the surrogate and get the rage.

Legitimate Anger You did it, and now they are angry, justifiably, at you.

Negotiation Essentials

Trust The glue of negotiation.

Relationship The ingredients for the glue.

Imagination The recipe for the glue (especially when there's been conflict).

Negotiation Methods

Framing Interpretations, perceptions, objectives, and assorted baggage that you bring to the negotiation process.

Reframing Finding a frame for the parties to share: new light that helps them reach resolution.

Flexible Frames Negotiation chameleon adjusts frames based on experience, learning, and information gained in the negotiation process.

Negotiation Chameleon Change of style and strategy based on circumstances: fit the environment to change it.

Negotiation Handle Learn it, and when you are least able to think clearly, grab and use it.

Collaborative Problem Solving First, gain mutual understanding of what is the problem(s). Next, agree on the process. Finally, seek solutions.

Negotiation Style The persona you bring to negotiation.

Template Your overarching and deeply rooted beliefs, values, and convictions that mold the frames of specific negotiations.

Collaborative Combined resources that form a new common identity to foster shared and enhanced process and outcome.

Cooperative Coordinated efforts that maintain the participants' distinct identities and that also achieve shared objectives.

Competitive A contest in which superiority of process leads to supremacy of gains: win–lose.

Contentious–Adversarial Antagonistic battle in which the objective is to defeat: win–destroy.

Frame Elements

The Problem/Purpose The reason parties are at the table. Settlement is easiest when these are similar; when they differ or contradict, reaching settlement is more difficult.

Priorities The fundamentals on your list of importance: the essentials for negotiation satisfaction.

Relative Importance Not every issue is a priority: distinguish which are not to initiate trading of benefits and concessions.

People Who is and who is not at the negotiation table.

Primary Players Those at the table with an active role.

Secondary Players Those just outside the room, with an immediate interest, though no direct participation in the deliberations: presumably represented by the primary players.

Tertiary Players The public interest on whose behalf the primary players speak, such as "the patients" or "the community": these constituents are not directly involved or aware of the deliberations.

Negotiation Technique

Expand the Pie Through constructive negotiation, discover, create, or enlarge resources so that when they are divided, each of the parties is better satisfied.

Gain Perspective/Step to the Other Side See the same problem from the eyes of other parties.

Go to the Balcony Watch the fray from a distance, as if in a theater, to see yourself as well as others on stage: in the process, you gain insights into downsides and potential upsides.

Timing The pace of negotiations. It differs for each of the parties involved.

Ripeness Simultaneous readiness to settle by all parties.

Too Soon One party is ready to talk while others feel it premature.

Too Late Negotiation delays have rendered an unwillingness to settle for some parties.

Imagination A most important quality of the very best negotiators: the ability to find and see options not readily apparent.

Objective Criteria Agreement on the facts upon which negotiation and settlement can proceed.

Generating Options Finding potential solutions from which the parties may select: settlement comes when each of the parties can accept the same or compatible options.

Inventing Options Creating new solutions from the combined resources and insights of the parties: the valued-added quality of the negotiation process.

The Art of Negotiation The intuition, experience, and insight to guide what to do when.

The Skill of Negotiation The learned use of methods and techniques.

Negotiation Process Timing, order, and tenor of events, actions, and decisions.

Negotiation Substance The agreement, exchange, or outcome of the process.

Mutual Gain Each of the parties acquires, attains, or achieves something they value, in sufficient quantity to bring them to settlement.

Dispute Conduct Conflict behavior, from controlled and calculating to defiant and erratic.

Reorder the Issues Based on new perspectives gained in negotiation, a combined list of priorities that integrates the essential concerns of each party.

Active Listening Attend, understand, synthesize, and respond: working with what the other person says.

Negotiation Jujitsu Absorb and reframe: useful to control your own defensive or emotional response and to avoid conflict escalation.

Acknowledgment Expressing your recognition of the problem (though not responsibility).

Apology Expressing your responsibility for the problem.

Agreement Often happens in stages: don't expect it all at once.

Restate You can't agree, acknowledge, or apologize to the other person, yet you want them to know you are actively listening. Be accurate. Avoid patronizing.

Substance Tangibles and intangibles that will be given, exchanged, and received in the negotiation process.

Interests The concerns, motivations, and objectives that underlie each person's negotiation. Revealed and integrated in interest-based negotiation.

Reactions Expressed and latent assessments of what occurs during negotiation: attend to other's reactions to evaluate what is acceptable to them; plan your strategy accordingly.

Building Motive Creating the desire and momentum to settle: incentives fuel the process.

Decision-Making Authority Negotiate with the person who has it.

"But" Less; "And" More Take *but* out of your vocabulary and replace it with *and*: congruity in thinking, speaking, and interaction.

Humor Negotiation lubrication.

Negotiation Styles

Negotiation Claimers Those who negotiate for the maximum grab. Fear provokes claimer.

Negotiation Creators Those who negotiate to combine interests and resources for maximum gain. Hope inspires creator.

Conflict Commander A judge, or judge-type person who resolves conflict by edict, excluding the parties from deciding the outcome.

Conflict Conquistador Someone who seeks resolution by out-powering or outmaneuvering the other side in a win-lose match, creating resentment in the process.

Conflict-Phobe Based on fear of dissonance, someone afraid to raise concerns, thereby generating resentment and causing the original problem to grow.

Avoider Someone with low assertiveness and low need for social acceptance: "It's OK, I'll sit alone in the dark."

Accommodator Someone with low assertiveness yet high need for social acceptance: "Let's all sit in the dark together."

Collaborator Someone with high assertiveness and high need for social acceptance: "Let's change the light bulb together."

Competer Someone with high assertiveness and low need for social acceptance: "My room is better lit than yours."

Compromiser Combines qualities of the above: "Today we'll sit in the dark; tomorrow we'll sit in the light."

Positional Negotiation

Leverage Power to influence that which others care about: used to change thinking and action. Use with caution.

Diversionary Tactics Grandstand what you don't care about and give loudly: be quiet and hold on to what's really important.

Adversarial Dispute Resolution Use of confrontational techniques to win the contest.

High Your opening demand in a positional negotiation: make it high enough to come down, yet not so high that you appear unreasonable.

Target The range where you would like to conclude your negotiations: your preferred conclusion.

BATNA Best Alternative To a Negotiated Agreement: the point when you walk from the negotiation table, either to pursue more adversarial methods or to abandon the cause. Have your better alternative planned and ready.

Learn Other's Strategy Wouldn't it be nice to know their high, target, and BATNA points?

Secretive In a positional negotiation, never lie and never tell the whole truth.

Bluff Create impressions to influence the negotiation.

Threat Your "or-else" statement: be certain you are ready for the "or" and have the "else."

Create Consequences Know what your opponents value, and show your ability to strike where it counts.

Cooptation A diversionary tactic. Get your opponent to go along with you by satisfying matters of secondary importance and holding on to matters of greater importance.

Negotiation Strategy

Mixed Models of Negotiation Strategically combine positional and interest-based approaches, based on experience gained with other parties and one's own negotiation objectives.

Negotiation Stages Each round of negotiation differs from that which preceded and that which follows. Adjust your strategy to those changes.

Good Options/Bad Options Place them all on the table so that parties are aware of the range of choices and consequences.

Test the Limits How far is the other side willing to go? How far are you willing to go?

Linked Destiny Motive for interest-based negotiation: if you fail, I fail, so I have a stake in your success.

Negotiation Problems

Complete Control No need to negotiate: the decision is yours. Problems occur when others think it theirs.

No Control You have no say in the decision. Problems occur when you think you should.

Negotiable Decision When you expect a give-and-take in reaching a decision. Problems occur when they order and don't negotiate.

Exclusion You have been kept out of the negotiation process and you resent it.

Hierarchical Relation The ups and downs of negotiation. Problems occur when the ladder itself hinders good decision making.

Imbalance Disproportionate attention to certain people, issues, or problems that preclude wise decision making.

Uneven Table People with legitimate and valuable contributions are ignored.

People

Negotiation Coach Gives perspective: trusted personal-professional confidant with whom you discuss your negotiation reactions and strategy. Don't leave home without one.

Evolving Health Practitioner One who negotiates (not orders) to enhance the collaborative aspects of health care work.

Professional Language The different vocabulary, experiences, priorities, expertise, and attitudes of health care professionals: as in, nurses speak "nurse," doctors speak "doctor," managers speak "manager," and so on.

Negotiation Expectations

Process Preferences Not what was decided; rather how it was decided. The "who, what, when, where, how, and if" of negotiation.

Psychological Needs Motives, incentives, concerns, and history that speak to the inner desires of the parties.

Substantive Desires The desired outcome, defined by tangibles and intangibles exchanged.

Interest Intent Personal significance of the issues. The intensity of desire, demand, or necessity.

Preferences Interests that are easiest to meet or concede. Desires and hopes not fundamental to your persona.

Values Interests that reflect fundamental purpose and integrity: issues to which you hold fast as a matter of principle, with little room for compromise.

Survival Interests you hold instinctively: concede only when survival is assured.

High Level of Benefit One's interpretation defines how one plays the game.

Accomplish Contentious negotiators disregard the overlapping in objectives; collaborative negotiators link common purpose to common endeavors.

Assumptions Unsubstantiated beliefs based on limited information and impression: rectifying misperceptions is a step toward settlement.

Expectations What you hope to achieve through negotiation.

In-Bounds What is reasonable to expect.

Out-of-Bounds What is unreasonable to expect.

Negotiable Bounds What is possible though not certain.

Mutual Expectations What parties equitably expect of one another.

Negotiation Outcomes

Conflict Investment/Loss/Gain Conflict costs! What you stand to lose and gain from the process, and what it will cost you to achieve it.

Claimer–Claimer Negotiation Grab + Grab = Small gains.

Creator–Creator Negotiation Negotiation results that exceed the expected.

Zero Sum Negotiation Nothing new created in the negotiation process: split what we've got.

Positive Sum Negotiation 1 + 1 = 3. The added value of process and outcome.

Negative Sum Negotiation Ending the negotiation with less than you started.

Win-Win Negotiation Magnificent goal and often a fantasy: it would take a lot to make everyone a true winner.

Win-Lose Negotiation The anticipated outcome of a positional negotiation: winner beware the revenge of the next round.

Gain-Gain Negotiation Realistic outcome of a negotiation process: everyone gets something; no one gets it all.

Principled Settlement Settlement based on adherence to principle, law, or ethical tenets.

Resolution Bring to rest both the interpersonal disputes and the intrapersonal dilemmas.

Punishment Inflicting pain that has meaning. Could be measured in terms of money, time, or professional humiliation.

Revenge Instinctual desire to get even.

Balance Moving beyond the dichotomy of right-wrong, yours-mine, to judicious reckoning of blame and equity.

Give Accepted offerings to the other side for the sake of resolution.

Get Acceptance of what the other side offers you for the sake of resolution.

Take Against the will of one side, what the other appropriates.

Hold An issue, principle, or matter that you are unwilling to concede.

Validation Substantiation that you are right: gratifying.

Invalidation Negation of one's position or interests: humiliating.

Discovery New and useful information unearthed in the negotiation process.

Learning An essential for effective negotiation: about the people, issues, and potential solutions. A by-product of recurring negotiation.

Stakes The tangible outcomes facing the parties: what you hope to gain; what you fear to lose.

Good Stakes The bounty you could reap from the deal.

Bad Stakes The adversities that could befall you on account of the deal.

Opportunity Stakes The possibilities, gained or lost, that could result from the deal.

Good Opportunities The chance to create success.

Bad Opportunities The possibility to decline into failure.

Forward Motion Negotiation progress: without it, deliberations could break off.

Negotiation Decision Point Where the rubber meets the road: now is the time to go one way or the other.

Synergy of Ideas, Solutions, and Benefits The prize of productive negotiation.

Mutually Acceptable Outcomes It works for everyone.

Loops of Information Learn from your successes and your failures to foster fruitful change.

Common Ground Matters of agreement.

Conflict Resolution Methods

ADR Alternative Dispute Resolution: formal and informal processes, such as mediation or arbitration, to resolve differences without resorting to the courts, power plays, or other shows of force.

Mediation The use of an impartial neutral to facilitate negotiation between disputing parties.

Arbitration The use of an impartial neutral to determine the settlement between the disputing parties.

Informal Mediation When the facilitator or go-between is not recognized as a formal mediator, though methods of mediation are used to bring parties to resolution.

Conflict Manager Someone within an organization who observes, analyzes, and helps resolve conflict.

Dispute System Design Easily accessible, low-cost, and nonadversarial resolution mechanisms incorporated into organizational routine: reduce factors known to cause conflict.

Third Party Impartial neutral: the mediator, arbitrator, or facilitator.

Facilitator An outsider to the dispute or negotiation who structures and eases discussion.

Common Interests Issues, concerns, and objectives that the parties share: they may discover this concurrence during negotiation.

Interest-Based Negotiation Parties interact based on interests they share: least adversarial and most collaborative.

Rights-Based negotiation Parties advocate their cause using laws and regulations, for example, through use of the courts or grievance process: mid-level adversarial and most legalistic.

Power-Based Negotiation Parties battle their cause, with the most forceful winning: the method most adversarial and confrontational.

Continuum of Dispute Resolution Dispute resolution begins with interest-based negotiation on one end, to prevent contention and promote collaboration, and proceeds to organizational change and alternative dispute resolution on the other: real dispute resolution is limited not only to high end conflict.

Anticipate Conflict In the course of human events, conflict is certain to occur: reduce causal factors and when it does occur, resolve it using prearranged, nonadversarial methods.

Grievance System Formal system of redress to resolve internal organizational disputes.

Beginning–Middle–End Dispute resolution, such as mediation, has each, though not necessarily in that order. Example: resolution occurs when fundamental issues are placed on the table late in the process.

Training Encourage early resolution of organizational disputes by fostering interest-based negotiation.

Culture Change A shift in organizational norms.

Mediation Techniques

Investigation Mediator detective work.

Empathy Acknowledgment and understanding for the feelings and circumstances of the parties. Empathy is an essential ingredient of a trusting relationship.

Neutrality Nonpartisan and unbiased. How the mediator is perceived.

Impartiality Not favoring one side or the other: as such, the mediator symbolizes the possibility that truth lies in neither of their dogmas. How the mediator speaks and behaves.

Manage the Interaction The mediator establishes order, monitoring the timing and sequence of discussion between the parties: the mediator as rule keeper.

Inventiveness Amid conflict, generating an innovative compatibility of ideas, proposals, and people.

Inventive Options Settlement proposals, sparked by the mediation process, that hadn't been found by the disputants on their own.

Persuasion Change in beliefs, attitudes, and decisions based on what occurs during mediation: the mediator persuades by questioning, so the parties reach their own conclusions.

Safe Environment Mediator creates conditions in which parties can reveal their interests, objectives, and vulnerabilities, confident that these will not be used against them.

Table Metaphor for the meeting point of the parties, where they engage in negotiation.

Return to the Table Disputants usually have been in productive negotiation on their own at an earlier time: mediation brings them back together with the structure and protection of an impartial facilitator.

Motivators Desires and interests that influence thinking and action: keys to building resolution.

Incentives Tangible and intangible inducements that can alter behavior and decisions.

Diagnosis Understanding the sources of conflict: useful in planning a strategy for resolution.

What's the Problem? Early question of the mediator. If the disputants are, in fact, trying to resolve different issues or problems, the mediator seeks to reduce their dissonance of purpose.

Caucus–Private Sessions Meeting between the mediator and one of the disputants, or a subgroup of the disputants, so that information can be shared with the mediator that would not be revealed to the others.

Shuttle Diplomacy The neutral moves between the separated disputants, delivering messages and options for building a workable agreement.

Confidential Disputants know they can reveal their interests with confidence: with this information, the mediator is able to find otherwise unknown points of agreement.

Voluntary Disputants participate in mediation of their own volition.

Conflict Resolution Techniques

Choices Good ones, bad ones: make them clear to the parties.

Consequences Link choices to consequences. Often, parties fantasize only the consequences of their win: review the range of real consequences, including the lousy ones, to offer new incentives to resolve.

Humanize See the other not as the enemy, that simplified persona of evil, rather as someone who shares similar fears, concerns, and objectives.

Share Savings Motive to settle: conflict is expensive, and its potential resolution can reveal rewards to entice settlement.

Brainstorm Consider all the possible choices, the good, the bad, and the wild. To encourage openness and creativity, do not even consider obstacles to making them happen.

Laundry List Take the ideas from the brainstorm and place them in useful categories: feasible, infeasible, feasible under certain conditions, or whatever category works.

Face Saving A way out of humiliation. Place initial dogmatic statement in a box: what you said made sense in the prior context. Demonstrate the changed current context as a way to allow a change in stance—with dignity.

Negotiation Movement The pace of progress: if it slows, stops, or slides back, finding resolution is more difficult.

Recognize Predicament See the writing on the wall: the cruel face of reality. A mediator may help parties recognize their predicament to move them toward considering real settlement options.

Workable Solutions Real options for resolution.

Truce Cease-fire in hostilities: parties agree to desist from shooting antagonistic words and actions at one another.

Dividing Line As part of a settlement, an agreement to maintain distance between the parties. Sometimes the line can be narrow, sometimes wide, and sometimes as big as a desert.

Spur to Settlement Comment, information, event, or insight that can be an effective catalyst.

Crafting Fit: Moving from Congruity to Incongruity Parties in conflict experience incongruity in their expectations. In moving toward resolution, they reshape pieces of the puzzle so they become more compatible.

Joint Discovery The shared satisfaction of finding solutions.

Options for Settlement What works for all sides.

Hope Necessary ingredient of resolution.

Common Purpose Overlapping agendas that combine for collaborative effort.

Message Not what is said, rather what is meant. What one person hopes the other will understand. The mediator facilitates this transmission.

Leadership Handles

Leader with Vision The leader sets the goals and arranges for everyone to follow behind. Other options and ideas are unwelcomed dissonance.

Visionary Leadership Encouraging a variety of ideas to invigorate the movement toward shifting goals.

Risk Taking Willingness to try untested yet promising ideas and proposals: an essential for leadership.

Paradigm Shift Adoption of new premises and assumptions that foster options for mutual gain.

The Problem of Power

Those With It Afraid to lose it: maintaining and enhancing power takes precedence over fair decision making and negotiation.

Those Without It Trying to get it: "When we're in power, everything will be better." Empowerment takes precedence over solving real problems.

Wrest Control Those with power and those trying to get it are in the same game: trying to keep it from each other. This game gets in the way of health care decision making.

Balanced Model Decision making less focused on who has the power and more attentive to effective decision making.

Silence The frustration of those who have no voice in the negotiation. Often, the plight of tertiary players whose concerns are used to advance the positions of others who presume to represent them.

Give Voice Creating a more even table: attending to the real concerns of those often excluded from the table.

References

Bacharach, S., and Lawler, E. *Bargaining: Power, Tactics, and Outcomes*. San Francisco: Jossey-Bass, 1981.

Bazerman, M., and Lewicki, R. (eds.). *Negotiating in Organizations*. Newbury Park, Calif.: Sage Publications, 1983.

Bazerman, M., and Neale, M. *Negotiating Rationally*. New York: The Free Press, 1992.

Bennis, W., and Nanus, B. *Leaders: The Strategies for Taking Charge*. New York: Harper and Row, 1985.

Blake, R., and Mouton, J. *Solving Costly Organizational Conflicts: Achieving Intergroup Trust, Cooperation, and Teamwork*. San Francisco: Jossey-Bass, 1984.

Brams, S. *Negotiation Games: Applying Game Theory to Bargaining and Arbitration*. London: Routledge, Chapman and Hall, 1990.

Carpenter, S., and Kennedy, W. J. D. *Managing Public Disputes: A Practical Guide to Handling Conflict and Reaching Agreements*. San Francisco: Jossey-Bass, 1988.

Charns, M., and Tewksbury, L. *Collaborative Management in Health Care: Implementing the Integrative Organization*. San Francisco: Jossey-Bass, 1993.

Crowley, T. *Settle It Out of Court: How to Resolve Business and Personal Disputes Using Mediation, Arbitration, and Negotiation*. New York: John Wiley and Sons, 1994.

Dauer, E. *Health Industry Dispute Resolution: Strategies and Tools for Cost-Effective Dispute Management*. New York: Center for Public Resources, Health Disputes Project, 1993.

Dubler, N. N., and Marcus, L. J. *Mediating Bioethical Disputes: A Practical Guide*. New York: United Hospital Fund, 1994.

Dubler, N. N., and Nimmons, D. *Ethics on Call: A Medical Ethicist Shows How to Take Charge of Life-and-Death Choices*. New York: Harmony Books, 1992.

Fisher, R., and Brown, S. *Getting Together: Building Relationships as We Negotiate*. New York: Penguin Books, 1988.

Fisher, R., Kopelman, E., and Schneider, A. *Beyond Machiavelli: Tools for Coping with Conflict*. Cambridge, Mass.: Harvard University Press, 1994.

Fisher, R., Ury, W., and Patton, B. *Getting to Yes: Negotiating Agreement Without Giving In*. New York: Penguin Books, 1991.

Folberg, J., and Taylor, A. *Mediation: A Comprehensive Guide to Resolving Conflicts Without Litigation*. San Francisco: Jossey-Bass, 1984.

Folger, J., and Bush, R. B. "Ideology, Orientations Conflict and Mediation Discourse." In J. Folger and T. Jones (eds.), *New Directions in Mediation: Communication, Research and Perspectives*. Newbury Park, Calif.: Sage, 1994.

Folger, J., and Jones, T. (eds.). *New Directions in Mediation: Communication, Research, and Perspectives*. Newbury Park, Calif.: Sage Publications, 1994.

Goldberg, S., Green. E., and Sander, F. *Dispute Resolution*. Boston: Little Brown, 1985.

Goldberg, S., Green, E., and Sander, F. *Dispute Resolution: 1987 Supplement with Exercises in Negotiation, Mediation, and Mini-Trials*. Boston: Little Brown, 1987.

Gray, B. *Collaborating: Finding Common Ground for Multiparty Problems*. San Francisco: Jossey-Bass, 1989.

Hall, L. *Negotiation: Strategies for Mutual Gain*. Newbury Park, Calif.: Sage Publications, 1993.

Honeyman, C. "On Evaluating Mediators." *Negotiation Journal*, 1990, 6(1), 23–36.

Honoroff, B., Matz, D., and O'Connor, D. "Putting Mediation Skills to the Test." *Negotiation Journal*, 1990, 6(1), 37–46.

Karrass, C. *The Negotiating Game*. New York: World Publishing, 1970.

Kelman, H. "Contributions of an Unofficial Conflict Resolution Effort to the Israeli-Palestinian Breakthrough." *Negotiation Journal*, 1995, 11(1), 19–28.

Kemper, R., and Kemper, D. *Negotiation Literature: A Bibliographic Essay, Citations and Sources*. Metuchen, N.J.: Scarecrow Press, 1994.

Kolb, D., and Bartunek, J. (eds.). *Hidden Conflict in Organizations: Uncovering Behind-the-Scenes Disputes*. Newbury Park, Calif.: Sage Publications, 1992.

Kressel, K., Pruitt, D., and Associates. *Mediation Research: The Process and Effectiveness of Third-Party Intervention*. San Francisco: Jossey-Bass, 1989.

Kritek, P. B. *Negotiating at an Uneven Table: Developing Moral Courage in Resolving Our Conflicts*. San Francisco: Jossey-Bass, 1994.

Laue, J. "The Emergence and Institutionalization of Third Party Roles in Conflict." In D. Sandole and I. Sandole-Starost (eds.), *Conflict Management and Problem Solving: Interpersonal to International Applications*. New York: New York University Press, 1987.

Laue, J., and Cormick, G. "The Ethics of Intervention in Community Disputes." In G. Bermant, H. Kelman, and D. Warwick (eds.), *The Ethics of Social Intervention* (pp. 205–232). Washington, D.C.: Halsted Press, 1978.

Lax, D., and Sebenius, J. *The Manager as Negotiator: Bargaining for Cooperative and Competitive Gain*. New York: The Free Press, 1986.

Likert, R., and Likert, J. *New Ways of Managing Conflict*. New York: McGraw-Hill, 1976.

Luce, R. D., and Raiffa, H. *Games and Decisions*. New York: Wiley, 1957.

Maslow, A. *Motivation and Personality*. New York: Harper and Row, 1970.

Moore, C. *The Mediation Process: Practical Strategies for Resolving Conflict*. San Francisco: Jossey-Bass, 1986.

Potapchuk, W., and Carlson, C. "Using Conflict Analysis to Determine Intervention Techniques." *Mediation Quarterly*, 1987, *16*, 31–43.

Pruitt, D. *Negotiation Behavior*. New York: Academic Press, 1981.

Rahim, M. *Managing Conflict in Organizations* (2nd ed.). Westport, Conn.: Praeger, 1992.

Raiffa, H. *The Art and Science of Negotiation: How to Resolve Conflicts and Get the Best Out of Bargaining*. Cambridge, Mass.: Harvard University Press, 1982.

Schelling, T. *The Strategy of Conflict*. London: Oxford University Press, 1960.

Singer, L. *Settling Disputes: Conflict Resolution in Business, Families, and the Legal System* (2nd ed.). Boulder, Colo.: Westview, 1994.

Slaikeu, K. "Designing Dispute Resolution Systems in the Health Care Industry." *Negotiation Journal*, 1989, *5*(4), 395–400.

Strauss, A. *Negotiations: Varieties, Contexts, Processes, and Social Order*. San Francisco: Jossey-Bass, 1994.

Stulberg, J. *Taking Charge/Managing Conflict*. Lexington, Mass.: Lexington Books, 1987.

Susskind, L., and Cruikshank, J. *Breaking the Impasse: Consensual Approaches to Resolving Public Disputes*. New York: Basic Books, 1987.

Tannen, D. *You Just Don't Understand: Women and Men in Conversation*. New York: Ballantine, 1990.

Thorne, S. *Negotiating Health Care: The Social Context of Chronic Illness*. Newbury Park, Calif.: Sage Publications, 1993.

Ury, W. *Getting Past No: Negotiating with Difficult People*. New York: Bantam Books, 1991.

Ury, W., Brett, J., and Goldberg, S. *Getting Disputes Resolved: Designing Systems to Cut the Costs of Conflict*. San Francisco: Jossey-Bass, 1988.

U.S. Department of State, Foreign Service Institute, Center for the Study of Foreign Affairs. J. McDonald, Jr., and D. Bendahmane (eds.). *Conflict Resolution: Track Two Diplomacy.* Washington, DC: Government Printing Office, 1987.

Index

Those names appearing in italic typeface indicate characters from the novel portion of this book.

Values, defined, 430
Vining, Victor, 115–119
Visionary leadership: defined, 439;
    versus leader with vision, 405
Voluntary, defined, 437
Vulnerabilities, defined, 422

W

Wainwright, Will, 259–260
Walter, Will, 243–244
What's the problem, defined, 436
White, Wendell, 115–118
Whole image negotiation, 43, 53–56,
    176–177, 418

Win-lose negotiation, 68, 111, 112,
    432. *See also* Distributive negotia-
    tion
Win-win negotiation, defined, 431
Winning obsession, 24
Workable solutions, 438
Workplace grievance procedures,
    324
Wrest control, 43
Wynn, Willie, 391

Z

Zartman, Ziva, 115–118
Zero sum negotiation, 111, 112, 431